HEALTH
POLICYMAKING
in the UNITED STATES

HEALTH
POLICYMAKING
in the UNITED STATES

Beaufort B. Longest, Jr.

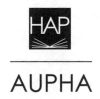

AUPHA

Health Administration Press, Chicago, Illinois

Association of University Programs in Health Administration, Arlington, Virginia

20 19 18 17 16   5 4 3 2 1

Library of Congress Cataloging-in-Publication Data
Longest, Beaufort B., Jr., author.
  Health policymaking in the united states / Beaufort B. Longest, Jr. — Sixth edition.
    p. ; cm.
  Includes bibliographical references and index.
  ISBN 978-1-56793-719-0 (alk. paper)
  I. Association of University Programs in Health Administration, issuing body. II. Title.
  [DNLM: 1. Health Policy—United States. 2. Health Planning—legislation & jurisprudence—United States. 3. Policy Making—United States. WA 540 AA1]
  RA395.A3
  362.10973—dc23
                        2015004331

The paper used in this publication meets the minimum requirements of American National Standard for Information Sciences—Permanence of Paper for Printed Library Materials, ANSI Z39.48-1984. ∞™

Acquisitions editor: Janet Davis; Project manager: Andrew Baumann; Manuscript editor: Rachel Hinton; Cover designer: James Slate; Layout: PerfecType

Found an error or a typo? We want to know! Please e-mail it to hapbooks@ache.org, and put "Book Error" in the subject line.

For photocopying and copyright information, please contact Copyright Clearance Center at www.copyright.com or at (978) 750-8400.

Health Administration Press
A division of the Foundation of the American
   College of Healthcare Executives
One North Franklin Street, Suite 1700
Chicago, IL 60606-3529
(312) 424-2800

Association of University Programs
   in Health Administration
2000 North 14th Street
Suite 780
Arlington, VA 22201
(703) 894-0940

For Carolyn

Always

BRIEF CONTENTS

DETAILED CONTENTS

ACRONYMS AND ABBREVIATIONS

AAFP	American Academy of Family Physicians
AAHSA	American Association of Homes and Services for the Aging; now known as LeadingAge
AAMC	Association of American Medical Colleges
AAP	American Academy of Pediatrics
AARP	American Association of Retired Persons
ACA	Affordable Care Act of 2010; also known as Patient Protection and Affordable Care Act
ACHE	American College of Healthcare Executives
ACO	Accountable Care Organization
ACP	American College of Physicians
ACR	adjusted community rate
ACS	American Cancer Society
	American College of Surgeons
ADA	American Dental Association
	Americans with Disabilities Act
AFDC	Aid to Families with Dependent Children
AHA	American Heart Association
	American Hospital Association
AHCA	American Health Care Association
AHCPR	Agency for Healthcare Policy and Research; now the Agency for Healthcare Research and Quality
AHERA	Asbestos Hazard Emergency Response Act
AHIP	America's Health Insurance Plans
AHRQ	Agency for Healthcare Research and Quality
AIAMC	Alliance of Independent Academic Medical Centers
AIDS	acquired immunodeficiency syndrome
ALJ	administrative law judge
AMA	American Medical Association
AMWA	American Medical Women's Association
ANA	American Nurses Association
ANRC	American National Red Cross
AoA	Administration on Aging
APA	Administrative Procedure Act
AUPHA	Association of University Programs in Health Administration

BBA	Balanced Budget Act
BBRA	Medicare, Medicaid, and SCHIP Balanced Budget Refinement Act
BCBSA	Blue Cross and Blue Shield Associations
BIO	Biotechnology Industry Organization
BIPA	Medicare, Medicaid, and SCHIP Benefits Improvement and Protection Act
CAA	Clean Air Act
Cal/OSHA	California Occupational Safety and Health program
CARE	Ryan White Comprehensive AIDS Resources Emergency Act
CBA	cost–benefit analysis
CBO	Congressional Budget Office
CDC	Centers for Disease Control and Prevention
CDER	Center for Drug Evaluation and Research
CEA	cost-effectiveness analysis
CERCLA	Comprehensive Environmental Response, Compensation and Liability Act
CERT	Comprehensive Error Rate Testing
CFR	*Code of Federal Regulations*
CHAMPUS	Civilian Health and Medical Program of the Uniformed Services
CHIP	Children's Health Insurance Program
CLIA	Clinical Laboratory and Improvement Amendments
CMI	Center for Medicare and Medicaid Innovation
CMS	Centers for Medicare & Medicaid Services
COBRA	Consolidated Omnibus Budget Reconciliation Act
COGR	Council on Governmental Relations
CON	certificate of need
COTH	Council of Teaching Hospitals and Health Systems
CPSC	Consumer Product Safety Commission
CR	Continuing Resolution
CRS	Congressional Research Service
CWA	Clean Water Act
DHEW	Department of Health, Education, and Welfare
DHHS	Department of Health and Human Services; usually referred to as HHS
DOJ	Department of Justice
DOSH	Division of Occupational Safety and Health
DRA	Deficit Reduction Act
DRG	diagnosis-related group
DSH	disproportionate share hospital

EAB	Environmental Appeals Board
EDC	Enterprise Data Center
EMTALA	Emergency Medical Treatment and Labor Act
EPA	Environmental Protection Agency
EPCRA	Emergency Planning and Community Right-to-Know Act
EPL	effective patient life
EPSDT	early and periodic screening, diagnostic, and treatment
ERISA	Employee Retirement Income Security Act
ESRD	end-stage renal disease
FAH	Federation of American Hospitals
FCLAA	Federal Cigarette Labeling and Advertising Act
FDA	Food and Drug Administration
FDCA	Food, Drug, and Cosmetic Act
FEC	Federal Election Commission
FECA	Federal Election Campaign Act
FFM	Federally Facilitated Marketplace
FHSA	Federal Hazardous Substances Act
FIFRA	Federal Insecticide, Fungicide, and Rodenticide Act
FMAP	Federal Medical Assistance Percentage
FPL	federal poverty level
FQHC	federally qualified health center
FR	*Federal Register*
FSA	Federal Security Agency
FY	fiscal year
GAO	Government Accountability Office
GDP	gross domestic product
GME	graduate medical education
GPO	Government Printing Office
HCBS	home and community-based services
HCERA	Health Care and Education Reconciliation Act of 2010
HCFA	Health Care Financing Administration; now Centers for Medicare & Medicaid Services
HELP	Health, Education, Labor, and Pensions Committee of the US Senate
HHA	home health agency
HHS	Health and Human Services
HIPAA	Health Insurance Portability and Accountability Act
HIRIF	Health Insurance Reform Implementation Fund
HIV	human immunodeficiency virus
HMO	health maintenance organization

HOLC	House Office of the Legislative Counsel
HPNEC	Health Professions and Nursing Education Coalition
HRSA	Health Resources and Services Administration
IHS	Indian Health Service
IOM	Institute of Medicine
IPAB	Independent Payment Advisory Board
IPPS	inpatient prospective payment system
IRS	Internal Revenue Service
MA	Medicare Advantage (plan)
MAACS	maximum allowable actual charges
MAC	Medicare Administrative Contractor
MAPD	Medicare Advantage prescription drug (plan)
MedPAC	Medicare Payment Advisory Commission
MEI	Medicare Economic Index
MIP	Medicare Integrity Program
MIPPA	Medicare Improvement for Patients and Providers Act
MMA	Medicare Prescription Drug, Improvement, and Modernization Act
MN	medically needy
MPRSA	Marine Protection, Research, and Sanctuaries Act
MSA	Medical Savings Account
MS-DRGs	Medicare severity diagnosis-related groups
NAACP	National Association for the Advancement of Colored People
NACHRI	National Association of Children's Hospitals and Related Institutions
NACOSH	National Advisory Committee on Occupational Safety and Health
NCHWA	National Center for Health Workforce Analysis
NCOA	National Council on Aging
NCQA	National Committee for Quality Assurance
NFIB	National Federation of Independent Businesses
NHCWC	National Health Care Workforce Commission
NHSC	National Health Service Corps
NIBIB	National Institute of Biomedical Imaging and Bioengineering
NIH	National Institutes of Health
NMA	National Medical Association
NOW	National Organization for Women
OAA	Older Americans Act
OALJ	Office of Administrative Law Judges

OASI	Old Age and Survivors Insurance
OBRA	Omnibus Budget Reconciliation Act
ODA	Orphan Drug Act
OECD	Organisation for Economic Co-operation and Development
OIG	Office of the Inspector General
OMB	Office of Management and Budget
OSHA	Occupational Safety and Health Administration
PAC	political action committee
PACE	Programs of All-Inclusive Care for the Elderly
PARDOC	Participating Physician/Supplier Program
PCORI	Patient-Centered Outcomes Research Institute
PDP	prescription drug plan
PHP	prepaid health plan
PhRMA	Pharmaceutical Research and Manufacturers of America
PHSA	Public Health Service Act
PPC	Provider Contract Center
PPO	preferred provider organization
PPS	prospective payment system
PRO	peer review organization
ProPAC	Prospective Payment Assessment Commission
PSO	patient safety organization
	provider-sponsored organization
PSRO	professional standards review organization
QDWI	Qualified Disabled and Working Individual
QI	Qualifying Individuals (program)
QMB	Qualified Medicare Beneficiary
RBRVS	resource-based relative value scale
RCRA	Solid Waste Disposal Act, as amended by the Resource Conservation and Recovery Act
RO	regional office
ROE	return on equity
RVS	relative value scale
RWCA	Ryan White Care Act
SCHIP	State Children's Health Insurance Program
SDWA	Safe Drinking Water Act
SERC	state emergency response commission
SGR	sustainable growth rate
SHCC	state health coordinating council
SMI	Supplementary Medical Insurance

SNF	skilled nursing facility
SPAP	state pharmaceutical assistance program
SSA	Social Security Administration
SSI	Supplemental Security Income
TANF	Temporary Assistance for Needy Families
TEFRA	Tax Equity and Fiscal Responsibility Act
TSCA	Toxic Substances Control Act
UPMC	University of Pittsburgh Medical Center
USPHS	United States Public Health Service
VA	Veterans Affairs
VHA	Veterans Health Administration
WHO	World Health Organization
WTC Program	World Trade Center Program

PREFACE

Personal health is an important goal of most people, and the pursuit of health is of growing significance to the US economy and the nation's system of social justice. Thus, health policy has long received attention from government. In the past two decades, the nation experienced a uniquely active period in health policy. The aftermath of this unprecedented era of health reform continues as health policy is enacted, implemented, and modified.

This textbook is written for those interested in health policy, especially the complicated process by which public policy pertaining to health is made. I define *health policy* as authoritative decisions regarding health or the pursuit of health made in the legislative, executive, or judicial branches of government that are intended to direct or influence the actions, behaviors, or decisions of others. The phrase *authoritative decisions* refers to decisions that are made anywhere within the three branches of government—at any level of government—and are within the legitimate purview (which means within the official roles, responsibilities, and authorities) of those making the decisions.

Through a long history of incremental and modest steps, an extensive array of authoritative decisions that make up health policy has evolved in the United States. Although dramatic developments in health policy, especially the emergence of Medicare and Medicaid in 1965 and, more recently, the enactment of the Patient Protection and Affordable Care Act (ACA) in 2010, have occasionally accelerated this history, health policymaking largely takes the form of slow but persistent evolution and modification. Health policy's role in the pursuit of health is played out in many arenas, because health is determined by many variables: the physical environment in which people live and work, individuals' biology and behavior, social factors, and access to health services. The effects of health policies can be seen in each of these determinants.

At the federal, state, and local levels, governments formulate, implement, and continually modify health policies in an intricately choreographed policymaking process. The purpose of this book is to provide a comprehensive overview of this process. An understanding of it is essential to policy competence. For typical health professionals, this topic is at most a secondary interest. However, a sufficient understanding of policymaking will permit people to effectively analyze the public policy environment that affects them and their work and to exert some influence in that environment. This understanding is an increasingly important attribute for those whose professional lives are devoted to the pursuit of better health for society and its individual members.

I first developed the model of the health policymaking process presented in this book for the benefit of my students, and I have continued to refine it. The usefulness of the model as a framework for students' understanding of the extraordinarily complicated process of health policymaking stimulated me to present it to a broader audience. The result was the first edition of this book. Now in its sixth edition, the book has been and will continue to be used in health policy courses to provide students with an overview of the policymaking process. The model puts the various aspects of policymaking in perspective and serves as a foundation on which students can build a more detailed understanding of the process and how it is related to decisions that affect them and their patients, clients, and customers.

The structure of this textbook largely reflects the model of the policymaking process. Chapter 1 defines health and health policy and considers their connection. Chapter 2 lays out the context in which policymaking occurs. I call this the policy market. Chapter 3 presents the model of the policymaking process that is the heart of this book. Recognizing their increasing importance in the process, Chapter 4, written by Mary Crossley, discusses the role of the courts in health policy. Chapters 5 through 9 describe in detail specific components of the policymaking process. Chapters 5 and 6 cover agenda setting and development of legislation, which comprise policy formulation. Chapter 7 includes a general discussion of policy implementation and the organizations responsible for implementation. Chapter 8 is devoted to the implementation activities of designing, rulemaking, operating, and evaluating. Chapter 9 addresses policy modification, reflecting the fact that all policies are subject to modification. Chapter 10 is devoted to the development of a degree of competence in policymaking for health professionals. This competence is needed by those who wish to have a say in the nation's health policy.

The book includes 30 appendixes, which are intended to enrich the reader's learning experience. Appendix 1 provides an overview of the Affordable Care Act, and Appendixes 2 and 3 provide overviews of Medicare and Medicaid, reflecting the importance of these health policies. Appendix 4 lists chronologically the United States' most important federal laws pertaining to health. In addition to providing synopses of these laws, the chronology illustrates several important characteristics of the nation's health policy. The list clearly shows, for example, that the vast majority of health policies are but modifications of or amendments to previously enacted laws; incrementalism has indeed been a feature of the development of American health policy. The list of policies in Appendix 4 also shows that health policy mirrors the determinants of health. There are policies that address the environments in which people live, their lifestyles, and their genetics, and there are policies related to the provision of and payment for health services. The remaining appendixes, referred to throughout the book, present excerpts from congressional testimony, examples of rules or proposed rules issued by implementing agencies, and reprints of illustrative letters, executive orders, and other documents that show important aspects of the policymaking process. The intent is to enliven the text and to provide useful and illustrative examples.

Instructor's Resources

Instructor's resources that include a test bank, answers to the chapter-end discussion questions, and slides of the book's exhibits are available to instructors who adopt this book. These resources can be obtained through the Health Administration Press website. For access information, please e-mail hapbooks@ache.org.

ACKNOWLEDGMENTS

I wish to acknowledge the contributions of several people to this sixth edition and to thank them. Mark Nordenberg, Patrick Gallagher, Arthur Levine, Donald Burke, and Mark Roberts provided a professional environment conducive to scholarship. I have enjoyed a professional home at the University of Pittsburgh for more than 35 years.

In preparing this sixth edition, I decided it was time to add a chapter about the increasingly important role played by courts in health policy. In considering experts who could address the topic, I had to look no further than my own university's School of Law. There was no better choice than Mary Crossley, JD, former dean and now a professor in Pitt's School of Law. I thank Professor Crossley for contributing Chapter 4 to this book. She exceeded my high expectations.

I thank Emily Friedman for permitting me to use her excellent essay, "U.S. Hospitals and the Civil Rights Act of 1964," as a case study at the end of Chapter 1.

I thank Janet Davis, Andrew Baumann, Rachel Hinton, Sharon O'Donnell, and the rest of the team at Health Administration Press for their professionalism in bringing this book to fruition.

Most of all, however, I want to thank Carolyn Longest. Sharing life with her continues to make many things possible for me and to make doing them worthwhile.

Beaufort B. Longest, Jr.
Pittsburgh, Pennsylvania

HEALTH AND HEALTH POLICY

After reading this chapter, you should be able to

- define health and describe health determinants,
- define public policy and health policy,
- begin to appreciate the important historical roles of Medicare and Medicaid in healthcare in the United States,
- begin to appreciate the important role of the Patient Protection and Affordable Care Act (ACA) of 2010 in healthcare in the United States,
- identify some of the important challenges for health policy,
- understand the four forms of health policies,
- distinguish between allocative and regulatory categories of health policies, and
- understand the impact of health policy on health determinants and health.

Health and its pursuit have long been woven tightly into the social and economic fabric of nations. Health is essential not only to the physical and mental well-being of people but also to nations' economies. The United States will spend about $3.2 trillion in pursuit of health in 2015, representing about 17.6 percent of the nation's gross domestic product (GDP), and may spend more than $5 trillion annually, or almost 20 percent of GDP, by 2023. About half of this spending will be from federal, state, and local governments (Sisko et al. 2014). Thus, it is not surprising that government at all levels is keenly interested in health and how it is pursued. As will be discussed throughout this book, government's interest is expressed largely through public policy.

Despite government's substantive role through policy, most of the resources used in the pursuit of health in the United States are controlled by the private sector. This rather unique public–private endeavor means that when government is involved in the pursuit of health for the citizenry, it often seeks broader access to health services that are provided predominantly through the private sector.

The long-established Medicare (providing healthcare for many of the nation's elderly and people with disabilities) and Medicaid (providing healthcare for some of the nation's poorer people) programs provide clear examples of this public–private approach, which is continued in the more recent expansion of insurance coverage in the Patient Protection and Affordable Care Act (P.L. 111-148) of 2010. The ACA, as it is known, will continue the pattern of using public dollars to purchase services in the private sector for beneficiaries, as is done under Medicare and Medicaid. (Appendixes 1, 2, and 3, respectively, provide overviews of the ACA, Medicare, and Medicaid. These policies are so important to understanding health policy and its effect on health in the United States that you may wish to read the overviews soon; the information provided will be helpful throughout the book.)

This book explores the intricate public policymaking process through which government influences the pursuit of health in the United States. The primary focus is on policymaking at the federal level, although much of the information also applies to state and local levels of government. This chapter discusses the basic definitions of health, health determinants, and health policy and their relationships to one another. Chapter 2 describes the context within which policymaking takes place. Chapter 3 presents a model of the public policymaking process and specifically applies this model to health policymaking. Chapter 4 describes the increasingly important roles played by the courts in health policymaking. Building on the foundational material presented in the first four chapters, subsequent chapters cover in more detail the various interconnected components of the policymaking process. Chapter 10 concludes the book with attention to how health professionals, whether managers or clinicians, can build a more useful level of policy competence. In this book, policy competence simply means that health professionals understand the policymaking process to the point that they can exert some influence on the process to achieve higher levels of human health. The path toward policy competence begins with some key definitions—of health, health determinants, public policy, and health policy.

Health Defined

A careful definition of health is important because it gives purpose to any consideration of health policy. Being precise about what causes or determines health is similarly important. As will be discussed more fully later, policy affects health through its impact on the determinants of health.

The World Health Organization (WHO; www.who.int) defines *health* as the "state of complete physical, mental, and social well-being and not merely the absence of disease or infirmity," a definition first appearing in the organization's constitution in 1946 and continuing unchanged through today (WHO 1946). Other definitions have embellished the original, including one that says health is "a dynamic state of well-being characterized by a physical and mental potential, which satisfies the demands of life commensurate with age, culture, and personal responsibility" (Bircher 2005). Another variation on the definition views health as a "state in which the biological and clinical indicators of organ function are maximized and in which physical, mental, and role functioning in everyday life are also maximized" (Brook and McGlynn 1991). Yet another definition adds the concept of health as a human right by saying health is "a condition of well-being, free of disease or infirmity, and a basic and universal human right" (Saracci 1997). The former European commissioner for health and consumer protection provides a definition with an important expansion by considering good health as "a state of physical and mental well-being necessary to live a meaningful, pleasant, and productive life" and further noting that "good health is also an integral part of thriving modern societies, a cornerstone of well performing economies, and a shared principle of . . . democracies" (Byrne 2004).

The WHO definition, especially as embellished with considerations of health as a right, a cornerstone of thriving economies, and a key principle of democracies, not only permits consideration of the well-being of individuals and the health of the larger societies they form but also facilitates assessments of the performance of governments in promoting health (Shi 2014). Throughout this book, health is defined as WHO defined it long ago.

Health is important in all nations, although the resources available for its pursuit vary widely. Current international health expenditure comparisons for the member countries of the Organisation for Economic Co-operation and Development (OECD), all of which share a commitment to democratic government and market economies, reflect some of this variation and are available online at www.oecd.org.

The value leaders and citizens of nations place on the health of their populations is partially reflected in the proportions of available resources devoted to the pursuit of health. Exhibit 1.1 shows per capita health spending and percentage of GDP devoted to health in selected countries. As reflected in the high expenditure levels in the United States and the large expenditures by other countries as shown in the OECD data, many nations make significant efforts to help their citizens attain good health.

Important to appreciating the role health policy plays in the pursuit of health is the fact that health is a function of several variables, or as they are often called, health determinants. The existence of multiple determinants provides governments with a large set of ways to intervene in any society's pursuit of health.

Health Determinants

Health determinants can be defined simply as factors that affect health or more formally as a "range of personal, social, economic, and environmental factors that influence health" both at the individual and population levels (US Department of Health and Human Services [HHS] 2014a). The question of what determines health in humans has been of interest for a long time.

EXHIBIT 1.1
Health Spending in Selected OECD Countries, 2012

Country	Total Health Spending	
	Per Capita	**Percent of GDP**
Australia	$3,997	9.1%
Canada	$4,602	10.9%
Czech Republic	$2,077	7.5%
Denmark	$4,698	11.0%
France	$4,288	11.6%
Germany	$4,811	11.3%
Israel	$2,304	7.3%
Japan	$3,649	10.3%
Netherlands	$5,099	11.8%
New Zealand	$3,172	10.0%
Norway	$6,140	9.3%
Poland	$1,540	6.8%
Spain	$2,998	9.4%
Sweden	$4,106	9.6%
Switzerland	$6,080	11.4%
United Kingdom	$3,289	9.3%
United States	$8,745	16.9%
OECD median	$3,484	9.3%

Source: Data from OECD (2014).

An important early theory about the determinants of health was the Force Field paradigm (Blum 1974). In this theory, four major influences, or force fields, determine health: environment, lifestyle, heredity, and medical care. In another conceptualization the determinants are divided into two categories (Dahlgren and Whitehead 2006). One category, named *fixed factors*, is unchangeable and includes such variables as age and gender. A second category, named *modifiable factors*, includes lifestyles, social networks, community conditions, environments, and access to products and services such as education, healthcare, and nutritious food.

The research on determinants of health, which is now extensive, has led to a holistic approach to health determinants. For individuals and populations, health determinants include the physical environments in which people live and work; people's behaviors; their biology (genetic makeup, family history, and acquired physical and mental health problems); social factors (including economic circumstances, socioeconomic position, and income distribution; discrimination based on such factors as race/ethnicity, gender, and sexual orientation; and the availability of social networks or social support); and their access to health services.

This inclusive perspective on what factors determine health in humans is clearly reflected in *Healthy People 2020* (www.healthypeople.gov), a comprehensive national agenda for improving health. The following list of health determinants is adapted from its identification and definition of determinants (HHS 2014a):

- *Biology* refers to the individual's genetic makeup (those factors with which he is born), family history (which may suggest risk for disease), and physical and mental health problems acquired during life. Aging, diet, physical activity, smoking, stress, alcohol or illicit drug abuse, injury or violence, or an infectious or toxic agent may result in illness or disability and can produce a "new" biology for the individual.

- *Behaviors* are individual responses or reactions to internal stimuli and external conditions. Behaviors can have a reciprocal relationship with biology; in other words, each can affect the other. For example, smoking (behavior) can alter the cells in the lung and result in shortness of breath, emphysema, or cancer (biology), which then may lead an individual to stop smoking (behavior). Similarly, a family history that includes heart disease (biology) may motivate an individual to develop good eating habits, avoid tobacco, and maintain an active lifestyle (behaviors), which may prevent his or her own development of heart disease (biology).

  An individual's choices and social and physical environments can shape her behaviors. The social and physical environments include all factors that affect the individual's life—positively or negatively—many of which may be out of her immediate or direct control.

- *Social environment* includes interactions with family, friends, coworkers, and others in the community. It encompasses social institutions, such as law enforcement, the workplace, places of worship, and schools. Housing, public transportation, and the presence or absence of violence in the community are components of the social environment. The social environment has a profound effect on individual and community health and is unique for each individual because of cultural customs, language, and personal, religious, or spiritual beliefs. At the same time, individuals and their behaviors contribute to the quality of the social environment.

- *Physical environment* can be thought of as that which can be seen, touched, heard, smelled, and tasted. However, it also contains less tangible elements, such as radiation and ozone. The physical environment can harm individual and community health, especially through exposure to toxic substances, irritants, infectious agents, and physical hazards in homes, schools, and work sites. The physical environment can also promote good health—for example, by providing clean and safe places for people to work, exercise, and play.

- *Public- and private-sector programs and interventions* can have a powerful and positive effect on individual and community health. Examples include health promotion campaigns to prevent smoking; public laws or regulations mandating child restraints and safety belt use in automobiles; disease prevention services such as immunization of children, adolescents, and adults; and clinical services such as enhanced mental health care. Programs and interventions that promote individual and community health may be implemented by public agencies, such as those that oversee transportation, education, energy, housing, labor, and justice, or through such private-sector endeavors as places of worship, community-based organizations, civic groups, and businesses.

- *Quality health services* can be vital to the health of individuals and communities. Expanding access to services could eliminate health disparities and increase the quality of life and life expectancy of all people living in the United States. Health services in the broadest sense include not only those received from health services providers but also health information and services received from other venues in the community.

Nations differ in the relative importance they assign to addressing the various determinants of health. For example, among the OECD nations, the United States ranks first in health expenditures but twenty-fifth in spending on social services. This expenditure pattern reflects a particular prioritization among determinants and is not the most effective pattern. It has been shown, for example, that the 1.5 million people in the United States who experience homelessness in any given year make disproportionately high use of costly acute care services (Doran, Misa, and Shah 2013).

Not only do nations prioritize health determinants differently, but people, as individuals and populations, vary in their health and health-related needs. The citizenry of the United States is remarkably diverse in age, gender, race/ethnicity, income, and other factors. Current census data put the US population at approximately 314 million people; 13.7 percent of them are older than 65. By 2020, about 55 million will be older than 65 and about 23 million will be older than 75. Persons of Hispanic or Latino origin make up about 16.9 percent of the population, and African Americans constitute approximately 13.1 percent of the population (US Census Bureau 2014). These demographics are important when considering health and its pursuit.

Older people consume relatively more health services, and their health-related needs differ from those of younger people. Older people are more likely to consume long-term care services and community-based services intended to help them cope with various limitations in the activities of daily living.

African Americans and people of Hispanic or Latino origin are disproportionately underserved for health services and underrepresented in all health professions. They experience discrimination that affects their health and continuing disparities in the burden of illness and death (James et al. 2007). "Healthcare disparities" and "health disparities," although related, are not the same. Healthcare disparities refer to differences in such variables as access, insurance coverage, and quality of services received. Health disparities occur when one population group experiences higher burdens of illness, injury, death, or disability than another group.

In recent years, policymakers have paid greater attention to racial/ethnic disparities in care, with notable, although unfinished, progress. Congress legislatively mandated the Institute of Medicine (IOM; www.iom.edu) to study healthcare disparities and established the National Center on Minority Health and Health Disparities at the National Institutes of Health. Congress also required the Department of Health and Human Services (HHS; www.hhs.gov) to report annually on the nation's progress in reducing healthcare and health disparities (HHS 2014b). These steps have established the foundation for better addressing disparities in health and healthcare (James et al. 2007).

The IOM (2002) report, *Unequal Treatment: Confronting Racial and Ethnic Disparities in Health Care*, called for a multilevel strategy to address potential causes of racial/ethnic healthcare disparities, including

- raising public and provider awareness of racial/ethnic disparities in healthcare,
- expanding health insurance coverage,
- improving the capacity and quantity of providers in underserved communities, and
- increasing understanding of the causes of and interventions to reduce disparities.

Progress in pursuing this multifaceted strategy continues, and it received a substantial boost from the passage of the ACA. Among the ACA's numerous goals, two of the most important are to reduce the number of uninsured people and to improve access to healthcare services for all citizens (Garfield and Damico 2012; Williams 2011).

In recent years, the impact of income and of wide disparities in levels of income on health has been increasingly understood. Wealthier Americans tend to be in better health than their poorer counterparts primarily because of differences in education, behavior, and environment. Higher incomes permit people to buy healthier food; live in safer, cleaner neighborhoods; and exercise regularly (Luhby 2013). However, low income does not necessarily mean poorer health. In part, the impact of income depends on what government does about supporting people with low incomes. A national survey has shown that the income variable interacts importantly with the extant health policy in the various states (Schoen et al. 2013). Using 30 indicators of access, outcomes, prevention, and quality, the survey documents sharp healthcare disparities among states, revealing up to a fourfold disparity in performance for low-income populations. The most important conclusion of this survey is that "if all states could reach the benchmarks set by leading states, an estimated 86,000 fewer people would die prematurely and tens of millions more adults and children would receive timely preventive care" (Schoen et al. 2013).

Although its population is diverse, several widely shared, although not universally shared, values directly affect the approach to healthcare in the United States. For example, many Americans place a high value on individual autonomy, self-determination, and personal privacy and maintain a widespread, although not universal, commitment to justice. Other societal characteristics that have influenced the pursuit of health in the United States include a common deep-seated belief in the potential of technological rescue and an obsession with prolonging life regardless of the costs (although this attitude is changing). These values shape the private and public sectors' efforts related to health, including the elaboration of public policies germane to health and its pursuit. They also influence the prioritization of attention to the various determinants of health.

Defining Health Policy

A suitable context is necessary to fully understand what health policy is. First, it is important to realize that policy is made in both the private sector and the public, or governmental, sector. Policy is made in all sorts of organizations, including corporations such as Google, institutions such as the Mayo Clinic, and governments at federal, state, and local levels. In all settings, *policies* are officially or authoritatively made decisions for guiding actions, decisions, and behaviors of others (Longest and Darr 2014). The decisions are official or authoritative because they are made by people who are entitled to make them based on their positions in their entities. Executives and other managers of corporations and institutions are entitled to establish policies for their entities because they occupy certain positions. Similarly, in the public sector, certain people are positionally entitled to make policies. For example, members of Congress are entitled to make certain decisions, as are executives in government or members of the judiciary.

Policies made in the private sector can certainly affect health. Examples include authoritative decisions made in the private sector by executives of healthcare organizations about such issues as their product lines, pricing, and marketing strategies. Official or authoritative decisions made by such organizations as The Joint Commission (www.jointcommission.org), a private accrediting body for health-related organizations, and the National Committee for Quality Assurance (www.ncqa.org), a private organization that assesses and reports on the quality of managed care plans, are also private-sector health policies. This book focuses on the public policymaking process and the public-sector health policies that result from this process. Private-sector health policies, however, also play vital roles in the ways societies pursue health.

Public Policy

There are many definitions of public policy but no universal agreement on which is best. For example, Peters (2013, 4) defines public policy as the "sum of government activities, whether acting directly or through agents, as those activities have an influence on the lives of citizens." Birkland (2001) defines it as "a statement by government of what it intends to do or not to do, such as a law, regulation, ruling, decision, or order, or a combination of these." Cochran and Malone (1999) propose yet another definition: "political decisions for implementing programs to achieve societal goals." Drawing on these and many other definitions, we define *public policy* in this book as authoritative decisions made in the legislative, executive, or judicial branches of government that are intended to direct or influence the actions, behaviors, or decisions of others.

The phrase *authoritative decisions* is crucial in this definition. It specifies decisions made anywhere within the three branches of government—and at any level of government—that are within the legitimate purview (i.e., within the official roles, responsibilities, and authorities) of those making the decisions. The decision makers can be legislators, executives of government (presidents, governors, cabinet officers, heads of agencies), or judges. Part of these roles is the legitimate right—indeed, the responsibility—to make certain decisions. Legislators are entitled (and expected) to decide on laws, executives to decide on rules to implement laws, and judges to review and interpret decisions made by others. Exhibit 1.2 illustrates these relationships.

In the United States, public policies—whether they pertain to health or to defense, education, transportation, or commerce—are made through a dynamic public policymaking process. This process, which is discussed in Chapter 3, involves interaction among many participants in three interconnected phases: formulation, implementation, and modification.

EXHIBIT 1.2
Roles of Three
Branches of
Government in
Making Policies

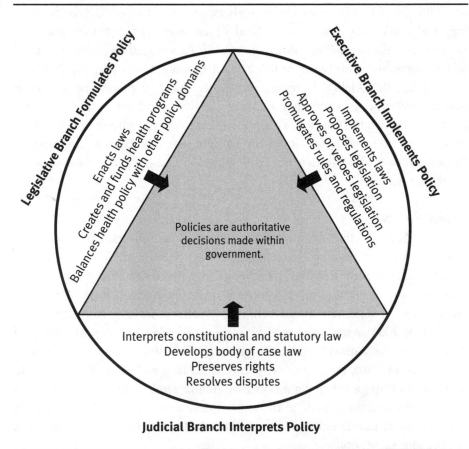

Health Policy

Health policy is but a particular version of public policy. Public policies that pertain to health or influence the pursuit of health are health policies. Thus, we can define public-sector *health policy* as authoritative decisions regarding health or the pursuit of health made in the legislative, executive, or judicial branches of government that are intended to direct or influence the actions, behaviors, or decisions of others.

Health policies are established at federal, state, and local levels of government, although usually for different purposes. Generally, a health policy affects or influences a group or class of individuals (e.g., physicians, the poor, the elderly, children), or a type or category of organization (e.g., medical schools, health plans, integrated delivery and financing healthcare systems, pharmaceutical manufacturers, employers).

At any given time, the entire set of health-related policies made at any level of government constitutes that level's health policy. Thus, a government's health policy is a large set of authoritative decisions made through the public policymaking process. Throughout this book, we will say much more about health policy and about the context in which and the process through which these decisions are made. Much of what can be said about health policy in the United States is positive. People are healthier because of the impact of many health policies. However, the United States faces significant challenges in its efforts to improve the health of the citizenry. Although many health policies have had enormous benefit (e.g., Medicare for the elderly and those with disabilities, advances in science and technology fostered by public funding), many challenges remain. Policies, which are decisions made by humans, can be good (with positive consequences) or misguided (with negative or unintended consequences).

Challenges for Health Policy

There is no shortage of thoughtful assessments of what health policy should achieve. One of the best recent determinations of what policy should achieve in the area of healthcare delivery and financing is one made by the Partnership for Sustainable Health Care (2013), a diverse group of healthcare stakeholders including the hospital, business, consumer, and insurance sectors. Brought together under the auspices of the Robert Wood Johnson Foundation (www.rwjf.org), this group envisions "a high-performing, accountable, coordinated health care system where patient experience and population health are improved, and where per-capita health care spending is reduced." The specific elements of their vision for healthcare in the United States are as follows:

- Health care that is affordable and financially sustainable for consumers, purchasers, and taxpayers

- Patients who are informed, empowered, and engaged in their care
- Patient care that is evidence based and safe
- A delivery system that is accountable for health outcomes and resource use
- An environment that fosters a culture of continuous improvement and learning
- Innovations that are evaluated for effectiveness before being widely and rapidly adopted
- Reliable information that can be used to monitor quality, cost, and population health

To date, these are neither widespread nor entrenched characteristics of the American healthcare system. For example, to focus on one of the elements—evidence-based and safe patient care—systematic and sustained improvement in patient care has been sought over the past 50 years, but only limited success has been achieved (Chassin and Loeb 2011; Smith et al. 2012).

The ACA holds promise for achieving, at least in part, these and other goals through improved policy. However, implementation of many aspects of the ACA is proving difficult (Jost 2014; Thompson 2013). Furthermore, not only is it challenging to establish the appropriate policies and implement them successfully, but some policies worsen the problems they are intended to address or foster other problems. For example, one of the important provisions of the ACA was significant expansion of the population covered by Medicaid. One of the expected results of this expansion was a reduction in use of expensive emergency department visits as more people acquired health insurance coverage for routine medical care in physicians' offices. A study of the effects of expanded Medicaid coverage in Oregon, however, found just the opposite: Emergency department use increased by about 40 percent with Medicaid coverage (Taubman et al. 2014).

Evidence-based learning can improve policies and minimize such problems as unintended consequences, "but learning in complex systems is often weak and slow. Complexity hinders our ability to discover the delayed and distal impacts of interventions, generating unintended 'side effects'" (Sterman 2006, 505). The healthcare system may well be the most complex system in the United States (Smith et al. 2012).

Some countries, most notably Canada and Great Britain, have developed expansive, well-integrated policies to fundamentally shape their societies' pursuit of health (Ogden 2012). The United States has begun to take this approach only recently, with the enactment of the ACA in 2010. Instead, the traditional approach in the United States has been to have a few large health-related policies, including Medicare and the regulation of pharmaceuticals, but to take a more incremental or piecemeal approach to health policy in general. The net result is a large number of policies, few of which have dealt with the pursuit of health in a broad, comprehensive, or integrated way until the ACA. The current efforts to fully implement the ACA are facing serious difficulties, and as Gawande (2009) has observed, health reform has not occurred in one dramatic step in any Western democracy.

With the enactment of the ACA, the United States has entered a period of major national health reform. The healthcare system has accurately been described as "unsustainable" and "flawed" and is characterized by uncontrolled costs, variable quality, and millions of uninsured and under-insured people. We may reasonably view the ACA as a grand experiment in the large-scale, comprehensive reforms that would systematically address the cost, quality, and access problems that now characterize the nation's health-care system. We will have to wait a few years to see if this approach works.

Forms of Health Policies

Health policies, which we defined earlier as authoritative decisions, take several basic forms (see Exhibit 1.3). Some policies are decisions made by legislators that are codified in the statutory language of specific pieces of enacted legislation—in other words, laws. Federal public laws are given a number that designates the enacting Congress and the sequence in which the law was enacted. P.L. 89-97, for example, means that this law was enacted by the Eighty-Ninth Congress and was the ninety-seventh law passed by that Congress. A briefly annotated chronological list of important federal laws pertaining to health can be found in Appendix 4.

Stemming from laws are rules or regulations established to implement the laws. Whereas laws are policies made in the legislative branch, rules or regulations are policies made in the executive branch. Both are important forms of policies. A third form of public policies includes numerous decisions

| Laws |
| Rules or Regulations |
| Other Implementation Decisions |
| Judicial Decisions |

EXHIBIT 1.3
Forms of Health Policies

made authoritatively by government officials, organizations, and agencies as they implement laws and operate government and its programs. Policies in the form of implementation decisions are in addition to formal rules or regulations and are typically made by the same executive branch members who establish rules or regulations. Still other policies are the judicial branch's decisions.

Selective examples of health policies include

- the 2010 federal public law P.L. 111-148, the Patient Protection and Affordable Care Act;
- an executive order regarding operation of federally funded health centers;
- a federal court's ruling that an integrated delivery system's acquisition of yet another hospital violates federal antitrust laws;
- a state government's procedures for licensing physicians;
- a county health department's procedures for inspecting restaurants; and
- a city government's ordinance banning smoking in public places within its borders.

Laws

Laws enacted at any level of government are policies. One example of a federal law is the Food and Drug Administration Amendments Act of 2007 (P.L. 110-85), which amended the federal Food, Drug, and Cosmetic Act to revise and extend the user-fee programs for prescription drugs and medical devices. Another example is the Breast and Cervical Cancer Prevention and Treatment Act of 2000 (P.L. 106-354), which created an optional Medicaid category for low-income women diagnosed with cancer through the Centers for Disease Control and Prevention's (www.cdc.gov) breast and cervical cancer early-detection screening program. State examples include laws that govern the licensure of health-related practitioners and institutions. When laws trigger elaborate efforts and activities aimed at implementing the law, the whole endeavor is called a program. The Medicare program is a federal-level example. Many laws, most of which are amendments to prior laws, govern this vast program.

Appendix 5 provides an example of a complete federal law, the National Institute of Biomedical Imaging and Bioengineering Establishment Act of 2000. This law established the National Institute of Biomedical Imaging and Bioengineering (www.nibib.nih.gov) to accelerate the development and application of biomedical technologies. Electronic versions of this and other federal laws dating back to 1973, the ninety-third Congress, can be found at www.congress.gov, a website maintained by the Library of Congress that provides access to official federal legislative information.

Rules or Regulations

Another form policies can take is that of rules or regulations (the terms are used interchangeably in the policy context) established by administrative agencies responsible for implementing laws. Administrative agencies, whether created by the federal Constitution, Congress, or a state legislature, are official governmental bodies authorized and empowered to implement laws. These governmental bodies come in many forms, including agencies, departments, divisions, commissions, corporations, and boards. In this book, we will refer to them most often simply as *implementing organizations and agencies.* In Chapter 4, which discusses the role of courts in policymaking, these bodies are referred to primarily as administrative agencies because that is the term for them preferred by the legal profession. More information about implementing organizations and agencies is provided in Chapter 7, and more information about rules and rulemaking is provided in Chapter 8.

The Administrative Procedure Act of 1946 defined *rule* as "the whole or part of an agency statement of general or particular applicability and future effect designed to implement, interpret, or prescribe law," a definition that still stands. Because such rules are authoritative decisions made in the executive branch of government by the organizations and agencies responsible for implementing laws, they fit the definition of public policies. The rules associated with the implementation of complex laws routinely fill hundreds and sometimes thousands of pages. Rulemaking, the processes through which executive branch agencies write the rules to guide law implementation, is an important activity in policymaking and is discussed in detail in Chapter 8.

Rules, in proposed form (for review and comment by those who will be affected by them) and in final form, are published in the *Federal Register* (*FR;* www.federalregister.gov), the official daily publication for proposed and final rules, notices of federal agencies, and executive orders and other presidential documents. The *FR* is published by the Office of the Federal Register, National Archives and Records Administration. Appendix 6 contains the summaries of a proposed rule that would revise parts of the Medicare hospital inpatient prospective payment system and a final rule that modifies and updates certain elements of the Health Insurance Portability and Accountability Act of 1996 (HIPAA). The entire proposed rule and the final rule are available online at the *FR* website.

Implementation Decisions

When organizations or agencies in the executive branch of any level of government implement laws, they must make numerous implementation decisions in addition to establishing rules or regulations needed to implement laws. These decisions, authoritatively made in the implementing organizations and agencies although different from the formal rules that influence implementation, are policies as well. For example, effectively managing Medicare requires the federal government to undertake a complex and diverse set of management tasks, including the following:

- Implementing and evaluating Medicare policies and operations
- Identifying and proposing modifications to Medicare policies
- Managing and overseeing Medicare Advantage and prescription drug plans, Medicare fee-for-service providers, and contractors
- Collaborating with key stakeholders in Medicare (i.e., plans, providers, other government entities, advocacy groups, consortia)
- Developing and implementing a comprehensive strategic plan to carry out Medicare's mission and objectives
- Identifying program vulnerabilities and implementing strategies to eliminate fraud, waste, and abuse in Medicare

In carrying out these tasks, the Centers for Medicare & Medicaid Services (CMS; www.cms.gov), the agency responsible for implementing the Medicare and Medicaid programs as well as many aspects of the ACA, makes myriad decisions about implementation. Again, because they are authoritative, these decisions are policies.

Examples of implementation decisions can be found in all implementing agencies. For example, the several federal agencies with implementation responsibilities for the Water Quality Improvement Act (P.L. 91-224) establish operational protocols and procedures for dealing with those affected by the provisions of this law. These protocols and procedures are a form of policy because they are authoritative decisions. Appendix 7 provides another example by illustrating an implementation decision made within the federal Food and Drug Administration (FDA; www.fda.gov)—in this instance, a decision to permit the marketing of a medical device to prevent migraine headaches.

Judicial Decisions

Judicial decisions are another form of policy. An example in the health domain is the US Supreme Court's (www.supremecourt.gov) 2005 decision not to hear an appeal filed by six health insurers in a bid to stop a class-action lawsuit brought by more than 600,000 doctors who claimed the companies underpaid them for treating patients. This decision allowed a lower court's ruling to stand, meaning that a class-action suit could proceed in federal court. Another example is the Supreme Court's 2008 *MetLife v. Glenn* decision regarding how federal courts reviewing claims denials by plan administrators under the Employee Retirement Income Security Act "should take into account the fact that plan administrators (insurers and self-insured plans) face a conflict of interest because they pay claims out of their own pockets and arguably stand to profit by denying claims" (Jost 2008, w430). These decisions are policies because they are authoritative and direct or influence the actions, behaviors, or decisions of others.

Although the judicial branch of government has played an important role in health policy for decades, its role is increasingly relevant. For example, the US Supreme Court ruled in 2012 that the ACA was indeed constitutional. This ruling was a crucial milestone for the law, permitting it to proceed (Liptak 2012). Chapter 4 is devoted to the vital role played by the judiciary in health policy.

Categories of Health Policies

All policies, whether law, rule or regulation, implementation decision, or judicial decision, can be categorized in various ways. One approach divides policies into distributive, redistributive, and regulatory categories (Birkland 2001). Sometimes the distributive and redistributive categories are combined into an allocative category; sometimes the regulatory category is subdivided into competitive regulatory and protective regulatory categories. For our purposes, all of the various forms of health policies fit into two basic categories—allocative or regulatory.

In market economies, such as that of the United States, the presumption is that private markets best determine the production and consumption of goods and services, including health services. Of course, when markets fail, as the financial markets in the United States and worldwide began to do in 2008, government intervention becomes essential. In market economies, government generally intrudes with policies only when private markets fail to achieve desired public objectives. The most credible arguments for policy intervention in the nation's domestic activities begin with the identification of situations in which markets are not functioning properly.

The health sector is especially prone to situations in which markets function poorly. Theoretically perfect (i.e., freely competitive) markets, which do not exist in reality but provide a standard against which real markets can be assessed, require that

- buyers and sellers have sufficient information to make informed decisions,
- a large number of buyers and sellers participate,
- additional sellers can easily enter the market,
- each seller's products or services are satisfactory substitutes for those of its competitors, and

- the quantity of products or services available in the market does not swing the balance of power toward either buyers or sellers.

The markets for health services in the United States violate these requirements in several ways. The complexity of health services reduces consumers' ability to make informed decisions without guidance from the sellers or other advisers. Entry of sellers into the markets for health services is heavily regulated, and widespread insurance coverage affects the decisions of buyers and sellers. These and other factors mean that markets for health services frequently do not function competitively, thus inviting policy intervention.

Furthermore, the potential for private markets on their own to fail to meet public objectives is not limited to production and consumption. For example, markets on their own might not stimulate sufficient socially desirable medical research or the education of enough physicians or nurses without policies that subsidize certain costs associated with these ends. These and similar situations provide the philosophical basis for the establishment of public policies to correct market-related problems or shortcomings.

The nature of the market problems or shortcomings directly shapes the health policies intended to overcome or ameliorate them. Based on their primary purposes, health policies fit broadly into allocative or regulatory categories, although the potential for overlap between the two categories is considerable.

Allocative Policies

Allocative policies provide net benefits to some distinct group or class of individuals or organizations at the expense of others to meet public objectives. Such policies are, in essence, subsidies through which policymakers seek to alter demand for or supply of particular products and services or to guarantee certain people access to them. For example, government has heavily subsidized the medical education system on the basis that without subsidies to medical schools, markets would undersupply physicians. Similarly, for many years government subsidized the construction of hospitals on the basis that markets would undersupply hospitals in sparsely populated or low-income areas.

Other subsidies have been used to ensure that certain people have access to health services. A key feature of the ACA is its subsidization of health insurance coverage for millions of people. Preceding the ACA and continuing into the future, however, the Medicare and Medicaid programs have been massive allocative policies. Medicare expenditures will be more than $1 trillion in 2023, and Medicaid expenditures could surpass $918 billion by then (Sisko et al. 2014).

Federal funding to support access to health services for Native Americans, veterans, and migrant farmworkers and state funding for mental institutions are other examples of allocative policies that are intended to help individuals gain access to needed services. Although some subsidies are reserved for the people who are most impoverished, subsidies such as those that support medical education, the Medicare program (the benefits of which are not based primarily on financial need), the expansive subsidies in the ACA, and the exclusion of employer-provided health insurance benefits from taxable income illustrate that poverty is not necessarily a requirement.

Some of the provisions of the American Recovery and Reinvestment Act of 2009 (P.L. 111-5) provide examples of allocative policy. This law, enacted in response to the global financial crisis that emerged in 2008, contains many health-related subsidies. Exhibit 1.4 lists some examples.

Regulatory Policies

Policies designed to influence the actions, behaviors, and decisions of others by directive are regulatory policies. All levels of government establish regulatory policies. As with allocative policies, government establishes such policies to ensure that public objectives are met. The five basic categories of regulatory health policies are

1. market-entry restrictions,
2. rate- or price-setting controls on health services providers,
3. quality controls on the provision of health services,
4. market-preserving controls, and
5. social regulation.

The first four categories are variations of economic regulation; the fifth seeks to achieve such socially desired ends as safe workplaces, nondiscriminatory provision of health services, and reduction in the negative externalities (side effects) associated with the production or consumption of products and services.

Market entry–restricting regulations include licensing of health-related practitioners and organizations. Planning programs, through which preapproval for new capital projects by health services providers must be obtained, are also market entry–restricting regulations.

Although price-setting regulation is generally out of favor, some aspects of the pursuit of health are subject to price regulations. The federal government's control of the rates at which it reimburses hospitals for care provided to Medicare patients and its establishment of a fee schedule for reimbursing physicians who care for Medicare patients are examples.

Program or Investment Area	Amount and Purpose of Funding
Continuation of health insurance coverage for unemployed workers	$24.7 billion to provide a 65% federal subsidy for up to 9 months of premiums under the Consolidated Omnibus Budget Reconciliation Act. The subsidy will help workers who lose their jobs to continue coverage for themselves and their families.
Health Resources and Services Administration	$2.5 billion, including $1.5 billion for construction, equipment, and health information technology at community health centers; $500 million for services at these centers; $300 million for the National Health Service Corps (NHSC); and $200 million for other health professions training programs.
Medicare	$338 million for payments to teaching hospitals, hospice programs, and long-term care hospitals.
Medicaid and other state health programs	$87 billion for additional federal matching payments for state Medicaid programs for a 27-month period that began October 1, 2008, and $3.2 billion for additional state fiscal relief related to Medicaid and other health programs.
Prevention and wellness	$1 billion, including $650 million for clinical and community-based prevention activities that will address rates of chronic diseases, as determined by the secretary of health and human services; $300 million to the Centers for Disease Control and Prevention for immunizations for low-income children and adults; and $50 million to states to reduce health care–associated infections.

Source: Steinbrook, R. 2009. "Health Care and the American Recovery and Reinvestment Act." *New England Journal of Medicine* 360 (11): 1057–60. Copyright © 2009 Massachusetts Medical Society. All rights reserved. Used with permission.

Quality-control regulations are those intended to ensure that health services providers adhere to acceptable levels of quality in the services they provide and that producers of health-related products, such as imaging equipment and pharmaceuticals, meet safety and efficacy standards. For example, the FDA is charged with ensuring that new pharmaceuticals meet these standards. In addition, the Medical Devices Amendments (P.L. 94-295) to the Food, Drug, and Cosmetic Act (P.L. 75-717) placed all medical devices under a comprehensive regulatory framework administered by the FDA.

Because the markets for health services do not behave in truly competitive ways, government establishes and enforces rules of conduct for participants. These rules serve as market-preserving controls. Antitrust laws such as the Sherman Antitrust Act, the Clayton Act, and the Robinson-Patman Act—which are intended to maintain conditions that permit markets to work well and fairly—are good examples of this type of regulation.

These four classes of regulations are all variations of economic regulation. The primary purpose of social regulation, the fifth class, is to achieve such socially desirable outcomes as workplace safety and fair employment practices and to reduce such socially undesirable outcomes as environmental pollution and the spread of sexually transmitted diseases. Social regulation usually has an economic effect, but this is not the primary purpose. Federal and state laws pertaining to environmental protection, disposal of medical wastes, childhood immunization, and the mandatory reporting of communicable diseases are examples of social regulations at work in the pursuit of health.

The Impact of Health Policy on Health Determinants and Health

From government's perspective, the central purpose of health policy is to enhance health or facilitate its pursuit. Of course, other purposes may be served through specific health policies, including economic advantages for certain individuals and organizations. But the defining purpose of health policy, as far as government is concerned, is to support the people in their quest for health.

Health policies affect health through an intervening set of variables called health determinants (see Exhibit 1.5). Health determinants, in turn, directly affect health. Consider the role of health policy in the following health determinants and, ultimately, its impact on health through them:

- Physical environments in which people live and work
- Behavioral choices and biology
- Social factors, including economic circumstances; socioeconomic position; income distribution within the society; discrimination based on factors such as race/ethnicity, gender, or sexual orientation; and the availability of social networks or social support
- Availability of and access to health services

Health Policies and Physical Environments
When people are exposed to harmful agents, such as asbestos, dioxin, excessive noise, ionizing radiation, or toxic chemical and biological substances,

EXHIBIT 1.5
The Impact of Policy on Health Determinants and Health

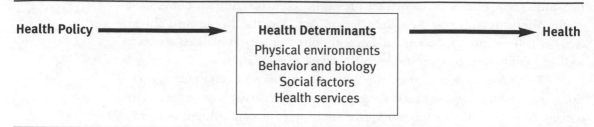

their health is directly affected. Exposure risks pervade the physical environments of many people. Some of the exposure is through such agents as synthetic compounds that are by-products of technological growth and development. Some exposure is through wastes that result from the manufacture, use, and disposal of a vast range of products. And some of the exposure is through naturally occurring agents, such as carcinogenic ultraviolet radiation from the sun or naturally occurring radon gas in the soil.

The hazardous effects of naturally occurring agents are often exacerbated by combination with agents introduced by human activities. For example, before its ban, the widespread use of Freon in air-conditioning systems reduced the protective ozone layer in the earth's upper atmosphere. As a result, an increased level of ultraviolet radiation from the sun penetrated to the earth's surface. Similarly, exposure to naturally occurring radon appears to act synergistically with cigarette smoke as a carcinogen.

The health effects of exposure to hazardous agents, whether natural or human made, are well understood. Air, polluted by certain agents, has a direct, measurable effect on such diseases as asthma, emphysema, and lung cancer and aggravates cardiovascular disease. Asbestos, which can still be found in buildings constructed before it was banned, causes pulmonary disease. Lead-based paint, when ingested, causes permanent neurological damage in infants and young children. This paint is still found in older buildings and is especially concentrated in poorer urban communities.

Over many decades, government has made efforts to exorcise environmental health hazards through public policies. Examples of federal policies include the Clean Air Act (P.L. 88-206), the Flammable Fabrics Act (P.L. 90-189), the Occupational Safety and Health Act (P.L. 91-596), the Consumer Product Safety Act (P.L. 92-573), the Noise Control Act (P.L. 92-574), and the Safe Drinking Water Act (P.L. 93-523).

Health policies that mitigate environmental hazards or take advantage of positive environmental conditions are important aspects of any society's ability to help its members achieve better health. Other determinants provide additional avenues to improved health.

Health Policies and Human Behavior and Biology

As Rene Dubos (1959, 110) observed more than a half century ago, "To ward off disease or recover health, men [as well as women and children] as a rule find it easier to depend on the healers than to attempt the more difficult task of living wisely." The price of this attitude is partially reflected in the major causes of death in the United States. Ranked from highest to lowest by the CDC (2014), the leading causes are heart disease, cancer, chronic lower respiratory diseases, stroke, accidents, Alzheimer's disease, diabetes, nephritis/nephritic syndrome/nephrosis, influenza/pneumonia, and suicide.

Behaviors—including choices about the use of tobacco and alcohol, diet and exercise, illicit drug use, sexual behavior, and violence—and genetic predispositions influence many of these causes of death and help explain the pattern. Furthermore, underlying the behavioral factors are such root factors as stress, depression, and feelings of anger, hopelessness, and emptiness, which are exacerbated by economic and social conditions. In short, behaviors are heavily reflected in the diseases that kill and debilitate Americans.

Changes in behaviors can change the pattern of causes of death. The death rate from heart disease, for example, has declined dramatically in recent decades. Although aggressive early treatment has played a role in reducing this rate, better control of several behavioral risk factors—including cigarette smoking, elevated blood pressure, elevated levels of cholesterol, poor diet, lack of exercise, and elevated stress—explains much of the decline. Even with this impressive improvement, however, heart disease remains the most common cause of death and will continue to be a significant cause. Cancer death rates continue to be problematic, with much of the problem attributable to lung cancer, which is strongly correlated with behavior. Appendix 8 describes the extent of state, commonwealth, territory, and municipality laws intended to restrict where smoking is allowed.

Health Policies and Social Factors

A number of social factors can affect health. Chronic unemployment, the absence of a supportive family structure, poverty, homelessness, and discrimination, among other social factors, affect people's health as surely—and often as dramatically—as harmful viruses or carcinogens.

People who live in poverty experience measurably worse health status, meaning more frequent and more severe health problems, than those who are more affluent (Do and Finch 2008). African Americans, Hispanics, and Native Americans, who are disproportionately represented below the poverty line, experience worse health than the white majority (National Center for Health Statistics 2013).

The poor also typically obtain their health services in a different manner. Instead of receiving care that is coordinated, continuing, and comprehensive, the poor are far more likely to receive a patchwork of services, often provided by public hospitals, clinics, and local health departments. In addition, poor people are more often treated episodically, with one provider intervening in one episode of illness and another provider handling the next episode.

The effect of economic conditions on the health of children is especially dramatic. Impoverished children, on average, have lower birth weights and more conditions that limit school activity compared with other children. These children are more likely to become ill and to have more serious illnesses than other children because of increased exposure to harmful environments, inadequate preventive services, and limited access to health services.

Economic circumstances are part of a larger set of social factors that unequally affect people in their quest for health. Living in an inner-city or rural setting often increases the challenge of finding health services because many such locations have too few providers. Lack of adequate information about health and health services is a significant disadvantage, one compounded by language barriers, functional illiteracy, or marginal mental retardation. Cultural backgrounds and ties, especially among many Native Americans, Latinos, and Asian immigrants, for all the support they can provide, can also create a formidable barrier between people and the mainline healthcare system.

An example of health policy intended to address social factors is the Balanced Budget Act of 1997 (P.L. 105-33). This policy provided for expanded health insurance coverage of children by establishing the State Children's Health Insurance Program. In 2009, President Obama signed a renewal of this program into law as the Children's Health Insurance Program (CHIP) Reauthorization Act of 2009 (P.L. 111-3). The CHIP reauthorization significantly expanded coverage to include an additional 4 million children and, for the first time, allowed the spending of federal money to cover children and pregnant women who are legal immigrants. The ACA extended CHIP through 2015. This policy, with many others, has addressed some of the social factors that affect health. However, a great deal remains to be done.

Health Policies and Health Services

As shown in Exhibit 1.5, another important determinant of health is availability of and access to health services, which are any of a host of "specific activities undertaken to maintain or improve health or to prevent decrements of health" (Longest and Darr 2014, 253). Health services can be preventive (e.g., blood pressure screening, mammography), acute (e.g., surgical procedures, antibiotics to fight an infection), chronic (e.g., control of diabetes or hypertension), restorative (e.g., physical rehabilitation of a stroke or trauma patient), or palliative (e.g., pain relief or comfort in terminal stages of disease).

The production and distribution of health services require a vast set of resources, including money, workforce, and technology, all of which are heavily influenced by health policies. The organizations and networks that transform these resources into health services and distribute them to consumers is collectively known as the *health system*. The system itself is also influenced by health policies. Health policies determine the nature of health services through their effect on the resources required to produce the services and on the health system through which the services are organized, delivered, and paid for. Policies' effects on the resources used to provide health services and on the health system are examined in the next sections.

Money

As Exhibit 1.6 shows, the United States allocates enormous sums of money to health, and growth of these national health expenditures is expected to continue. As noted earlier, these expenditures may exceed $5 trillion by 2023, at which time the nation will be spending about 20 percent of its GDP on health. About half of these expenditures will be by governments, directed by their policy decisions.

The United States spends more on health than does any other country (OECD 2014). Other countries have been far more likely to adopt policies such as global budgets for their healthcare systems or to impose restrictive limitations on the supplies of health services (Squires 2011).

Current health expenditures and projected future increases have significant implications. The increasing expenditures, in part, reflect higher prices. Higher prices reduce access to health services by making it more difficult for many people to purchase the services or the insurance needed to

	2008	2012	2019[a]	2023[a]
NHE (billions)	$2,412	$2,793	$4,043	$5,159
NHE personal healthcare (billions)	2,017	2,360	3,413	4,360
Government public health activities (billions)	71.5	75.0	102.1	123.9
NHE per capita	7,936	8,915	12,131	14,944
NHE as percentage of GDP	16.4%	17.2%	18.1%	19.3%

EXHIBIT 1.6 National Health Expenditures (NHE), Aggregate and per Capita Amounts, and Share of Gross Domestic Product (GDP) for Selected Calendar Years

Source: Data abstracted from Sisko et al. (2014).
[a]Projected.

cover those services. As the nation works its way through the aftermath of the worst economic downturn since the Great Depression, reduced employment is dramatically affecting the number of uninsured. Implementation of the ACA will help address this problem for millions of people, but expenditure levels will remain problematic. They negatively affect the nation's competitiveness in the global economy (Vietor and Weinzierl 2012), and health expenditures have absorbed much of the growth of many workers' real compensation, meaning that as employers spend more to provide health insurance benefits, wages decrease.

Growing health expenditures are a continuing source of budgetary pressure for the federal and state governments. As health expenditures consume a growing portion of government resources, it is becoming more difficult for government to support other priorities, such as education or homeland security.

Workforce

The talents and abilities of a large and diverse workforce make up another basic resource used to provide health services. The healthcare workforce is directly affected by health policies, whether through public funding of educational programs or licensing of health professionals. There are about 19 million healthcare workers in the United States, representing more than 13 percent of the nation's workforce. Despite the recent economic downturn, which saw jobs decline throughout the economy, jobs in the health sector grew by more than 25 percent and are expected to grow by another 30 percent between 2010 and 2020 (Center for Health Workforce Studies 2012).

The nation's rapidly aging population, coupled with the large increase in insured people triggered by the ACA, will "strain a healthcare delivery system already struggling under the weight of its current load" (Association of Academic Health Centers 2013, 1). These pressures will require a new approach to national health workforce policy. The traditional approach focused on numbers of workers, producing health workforce policy that featured responses to projected shortages in the workforce, especially among physicians and nurses. For example, the number of physicians doubled from the mid-1960s to the mid-1990s, an accomplishment driven by federal policies intended to increase their supply, including the Health Professions Educational Assistance Act of 1963 (P.L. 88-129) and its amendments of 1965, 1968, and 1971. Similarly, the main federal response to a projected nurse shortage was the Nurse Reinvestment Act of 2002 (P.L. 107-205), which authorized the following provisions:

- Loan repayment programs and scholarships for nursing students
- Public service announcements to encourage more people to enter the nursing profession

- Career ladder programs for those who wish to advance in the profession
- Best-practice grants for nursing administration
- Long-term care training grants to develop and incorporate gerontology curriculum into nursing programs
- A fast-track faculty loan repayment program for nursing students who agree to teach at a school of nursing

Going forward, a comprehensive and integrated national health workforce policy will be needed. A good prescription for such a policy for the nation is the following (Association of Academic Health Centers 2013, 2–3):

- Create and fund a national health workforce planning body that engages diverse federal, state, public, and private stakeholders.
- Promote harmonization in public and private standards, requirements, and prevailing practices across jurisdictions.
- Invest in a comprehensive health workforce research component that will
  - address development and dissemination of consensus definitions and terminology;
  - monitor developing technological breakthroughs that require changes in provider numbers, types, and expertise;
  - identify gaps in data collection and current modeling strategies for supply and demand; and
  - promote consistent approaches to research across all health professions.

Provisions in the ACA that created the National Health Care Workforce Commission and the National Center for Health Workforce Analysis hold promise for producing a more comprehensive and integrated workforce policy, but the work of these entities in the future will depend on as-yet-unrealized adequate funding.

Technology

A third type of resource that health policies significantly affect is health-related technology. Broadly defined, *technology* is the application of science to the pursuit of health. Technological advances result in better pharmaceuticals, devices, and procedures. A major influence on the pursuit of health in the United States, technology has helped eradicate some diseases and has greatly improved diagnoses and treatment for others. Diseases that once were not even diagnosed are now routinely and effectively treated. Advancing technology has brought medical science to the early stages of understanding disease at the molecular level and intervening to treat diseases at the genetic level.

The United States produces and consumes more health-related technology than does any other nation, and it spends far more on it. It has provided technology with a uniquely favorable economic and political environment. As a result, health-related technology is widely available in the United States.

Health policy provides funding for much of the research and development (R&D) that leads to new technology, although the private sector also pays for a great deal of R&D. The United States has a long history of support for the development of health-related technology through policies that support biomedical research and encourage private investment in such research. The National Institutes of Health (NIH; www.nih.gov) invests more than $30 billion annually in medical research. About 80 percent of the NIH's funding is awarded through almost 50,000 competitive grants to more than 300,000 researchers at more than 2,500 universities, medical schools, and other research institutions in every state and around the world. About 10 percent of the NIH's budget supports projects conducted by nearly 6,000 scientists in its own laboratories, most of which are on the NIH campus in Bethesda, Maryland (NIH 2014).

Encouraged by policies that permit firms to recoup their investments, private industry also spends heavily on biomedical R&D. In fact, the Pharmaceutical Research and Manufacturers of America (PhRMA; www.phrma.org), which represents the nation's leading biopharmaceutical research companies, reports that industry-wide research investment was $48.5 billion in 2012 (PhRMA 2014).

Health policy also affects technology through the application of regulatory policies, such as those promulgated by the FDA to ensure technology's safety and efficacy. The FDA is responsible for protecting the public health by ensuring the safety, efficacy, and security of human and veterinary drugs, biological products, medical devices, the food supply, cosmetics, and products that emit radiation. The FDA also has responsibility for regulating the manufacture, marketing, and distribution of tobacco products to protect the public health and to reduce tobacco use by minors. Finally, the FDA plays a significant role in the nation's counterterrorism capability by ensuring the security of the food supply and by fostering the development of medical products to respond to deliberate and naturally emerging public health threats (FDA 2014).

The following are laws the FDA is responsible (or partially responsible) for implementing, including writing rules for implementation:

- Food, Drug, and Cosmetic Act of 1938 (P.L. 75-717)
- Infant Formula Act of 1980 (P.L. 96-359)
- Orphan Drug Act of 1983 (P.L. 97-414)

- Federal Anti-Tampering Act of 1983 (P.L. 98-127)
- Drug Price Competition and Patent Term Restoration Act of 1984 (P.L. 98-417)
- Prescription Drug Marketing Act of 1987 (P.L. 100-293)
- Generic Animal Drug and Patent Term Restoration Act of 1988 (P.L. 100-670)
- Sanitary Food Transportation Act of 1990 (P.L. 101-500)
- Nutrition Labeling and Education Act of 1990 (P.L. 101-535)
- Safe Medical Devices Act of 1990 (P.L. 101-629)
- Medical Device Amendments of 1992 (P.L. 102-300)
- Prescription Drug Amendments of 1992 (P.L. 102-353)
- Mammography Quality Standards Act (MQSA) of 1992 (P.L. 102-539)
- Prescription Drug User Fee Act (PDUFA) of 1992 (P.L. 102-571)
- Animal Medicinal Drug Use Clarification Act (AMDUCA) of 1994 (P.L. 103-396)
- Dietary Supplement Health and Education Act of 1994 (P.L. 103-417)
- FDA Export Reform and Enhancement Act of 1996 (P.L. 104-134)
- Food Quality Protection Act of 1996 (P.L. 104-170)
- Animal Drug Availability Act of 1996 (P.L. 104-250)
- Food and Drug Administration Modernization Act (FDAMA) of 1997 (P.L. 105-115)
- Best Pharmaceuticals for Children Act of 2002 (P.L. 107-109)
- Public Health Security and Bioterrorism Preparedness and Response Act of 2002 (P.L. 107-188)
- Medical Device User Fee and Modernization Act (MDUFMA) of 2002 (P.L. 107-250)
- Animal Drug User Fee Act of 2003 (P.L. 108-130)
- Pediatric Research Equity Act of 2003 (P.L. 108-155)
- Project BioShield Act of 2004 (P.L. 108-276)
- Food Allergen Labeling and Consumer Protection Act of 2004 (P.L. 108-282)
- Minor Use and Minor Species Animal Health Act of 2004 (P.L. 108-282)
- Dietary Supplement and Nonprescription Drug Consumer Protection Act of 2006 (P.L. 109-462)
- FDA Amendments Act of 2007 (P.L. 110-85)
- Family Smoking Prevention and Tobacco Control Act of 2009 (P.L. 111-31)
- FDA Food Safety Modernization Act of 2011 (P.L. 111-353)

Advances in technology drive up the costs of health services as the new technology is used and paid for. One paradox of advancing health-related technology is that as people live longer because of these advances, they then may need additional health services. The net effect drives up health expenditures for the new technology and for other services consumed over a longer life span. The costs associated with the use of technology generate policy issues of their own. For example, Medicare policies guide the determination of whether it will pay for new services, treatments, and technologies. Using an evidence-based process, with opportunities for public participation, CMS makes a national coverage determination based on whether an item or service is reasonable and necessary for the diagnosis or treatment of an illness or injury. This complex process can be reviewed at the CMS website (www .cms.gov/Medicare/Coverage/DeterminationProcess/). A specific example of this decision making is CMS's decision to cover implantable cardioverter defibrillators (Hlatky, Sanders, and Owens 2005).

Health System

The health system in any country can be defined as the total national effort undertaken in the private and public sectors that is focused on pursuing health. In the United States, the health system is distinctly divided into public health and healthcare delivery and financing components. The distinctions between these two components are beginning to blur, but major differences remain. Each component is heavily influenced by policies.

The public health component of the health system produces services on a community-wide or population-wide basis, such as health promotion and prevention, communicable disease control, sanitation, food and water safety, the collection and analysis of health statistics, and air pollution control. The healthcare delivery and financing component of the health system provides services primarily to individuals, including diagnosis, treatment, and rehabilitation.

Structurally, the public health component of the health system includes the following (Congressional Research Service 2005):

- About 3,000 county and city health departments and local boards of health
- Fifty-nine state, territorial, and island nation health departments
- Various US Public Health Service agencies in HHS
- Tribal health agencies, coordinated at HHS by the Indian Health Service
- More than 160,000 public and private laboratories

In addition to these public health infrastructure components, some accounts include volunteer organizations such as the American Red Cross,

American Diabetes Association, and American Cancer Society as part of the public health component. Reflecting the blurring of the lines between public health and healthcare components, some accounts also include hospitals and other providers of healthcare services. Structurally, however, the healthcare delivery and financing component of the health system in the United States remains largely distinct from the public health component. The healthcare component is also much larger and more elaborate. One way to envision the variety and diversity of healthcare delivery organizations is to consider a continuum of health services that people might use over the course of their lives and to think of the organizational settings that provide them (Longest and Darr 2014).

The continuum could begin before birth with organizations that minimize negative environmental impact on human fetuses or that provide genetic counseling, family planning services, prenatal counseling, prenatal ambulatory care services, and birthing services. This stage would be followed early in life by pediatric ambulatory services; pediatric inpatient hospital services, including neonatal and pediatric intensive care units (ICUs); and ambulatory and inpatient psychiatric services for children.

Healthcare delivery organizations for adults include those providing adult ambulatory services, such as ambulatory surgery centers and emergency and trauma services; adult inpatient hospital services, including routine medical, surgical, and obstetrical services as well as specialized cardiac care units, medical ICUs, surgical ICUs, and monitored units; stand-alone cancer units with radiotherapy capability and short-stay recovery beds; ambulatory and inpatient rehabilitation services, including specific subprograms for orthopedic, neurological, cardiac, arthritis, speech, otologic, and other services; ambulatory and inpatient psychiatric services, including specific subprograms for psychotics, day programs, counseling services, and detoxification; and home health care services.

In their later years, people might add to the list of relevant healthcare delivery organizations those providing skilled and intermediate nursing services; adult day-care services; respite services for caregivers of homebound patients, including services such as providing meals, visiting nurse and home health aides, electronic emergency call capability, cleaning, and simple home maintenance; and hospice care, palliative care, and associated family services, including bereavement, legal, and financial counseling.

Healthcare delivery traditionally took place in autonomous organizations with little attention paid to coordination of the continuum of services. In recent decades, however, most healthcare delivery organizations have significantly changed how they relate to one another. Mergers, consolidations, acquisitions, and affiliations are now commonplace. This activity has led to vertical integration, in which multiple organizations unify in organizational arrangements or systems. Vertically integrated systems capable of providing a largely seamless continuum of health services—including primary, acute, rehabilitation, long-term, and hospice care—increasingly characterize healthcare in the United States. At the extreme end of this integrative activity are large integrated systems and networks in which providers, spanning the full continuum of health services, are integrated with financing mechanisms such as health plans or insurers (Longest and Darr 2014).

Each component of the health system is heavily influenced by policy. Public health policy concerns the government's power to protect and preserve the health of the citizenry while recognizing individual rights to autonomy, privacy, and other legally protected interests. Policy for healthcare delivery and financing includes licensing of institutions, regulation of health plans, reimbursement arrangements for services, and many other activities. Among its many provisions, the ACA includes some that clearly support the public health component of the health system (e.g., establishing the National Prevention, Health Promotion, and Public Health Council to coordinate federal prevention, wellness, and public health activities) and other provisions that support the healthcare delivery and financing component (e.g., improvements and expansion of the Medicare and Medicaid programs, fostering accountable care organizations).

In terms of government's support, as expressed through policy, for the two components of the health system, it is fair to say that support for public health is inadequate and support for healthcare has historically been generous but is now tightening under pressure for government at all levels to operate under budgetary constraints. Evidence of government's support for healthcare includes enactment in 1946 of the Hospital Survey and Construction Act (P.L. 79-725), a policy that placed Congress squarely in support of expanded availability of health services and improved facilities. Called the Hill-Burton Act after its authors, this legislation provided funds for hospital construction and marked the beginning of a decades-long program of extensive federal developmental subsidies aimed at increasing the availability of health services.

Public policy has also supported and facilitated the expansion of health insurance coverage. During World War II, when wages were frozen for many workers, health insurance and other benefits in lieu of wages became attractive features of the American workplace. Encouraged by policies that excluded these fringe benefits from income taxes and by a US Supreme Court ruling that employee benefits, including health insurance, could be legitimately included in the collective bargaining process, employer-provided health insurance benefits grew rapidly in the mid-twentieth century (Murray 2007).

Medicare and Medicaid are policies providing greater access to mainstream health services through publicly subsidized health insurance for aged individuals and many poor. With enactment of these programs, 85 percent of the American population had some form of health insurance. Fuller implementation of the ACA will extend health insurance coverage still further.

Summary

WHO (1946) defines health as the "state of complete physical, mental, and social well-being and not merely the absence of disease or infirmity," a definition first appearing in the organization's constitution in 1946 and continuing unchanged to today. Health is a function of many health determinants: the physical environments in which people live and work; their behaviors and genetics; social factors (including economic circumstances, socioeconomic position, and income distribution); discrimination based on factors such as race/ethnicity, gender, or sexual orientation; and the availability of social networks or social support and the type, quality, and timing of health services that people receive. Examples of how health policy affects the various determinants of health are provided in the chapter.

A distinction is made between public- and private-sector policy. Public-sector health policy is defined as authoritative decisions regarding health or the pursuit of health made in the legislative, executive, or judicial branches of government that are intended to direct or influence the actions, behaviors, or decisions of others. In this definition, the phrase "authoritative decisions" is crucial. It specifies decisions made anywhere in the three branches of government—and at any level of government—that are within the legitimate purview (i.e., the official roles, responsibilities, and authorities) of those making the decisions.

Public-sector health policies are the principal means through which governments help shape the pursuit of health. In the United States, policies can take the form of laws, rules or regulations, implementation decisions, and judicial decisions. Health policies, like other public policies, can fit into broad allocative or regulatory categories.

As this chapter concludes, it will be useful to revisit Exhibit 1.5 briefly. With the information provided in this chapter, the reader should be able to define health, health determinants, and health policy and understand the important interrelationships among them. Most important, health policy affects health by affecting one or more of the health determinants listed in Exhibit 1.5.

Review Questions

1. Define health. What are the determinants of health in humans?
2. Define public policies and health policies.
3. What forms do health policies take? Give an example of each.
4. Compare and contrast the two basic categories of health policies.
5. Discuss the connections among health policies, health determinants, and health.

Case Study: U.S. Hospitals and the Civil Rights Act of 1964

The Civil Rights Act of 1964 (P.L. 88-352) is a landmark civil rights policy in the United States. It is also an important health policy because it addresses an important determinant of health: discrimination. This case study of the act's emergence and subsequent impact provides vivid examples of many of the concepts and features of health policy-making presented in this book. For example, the case illustrates the formulation, implementation, and modification phases of policymaking. It illustrates both public- and private-sector policy. And it illustrates the various forms that public policy takes: laws, rules and regulations, implementation decisions, and judicial decisions. The case includes examples of health policy emerging from the work of legislative bodies, executive branch employees, and the courts. It shows how policy is influenced by and, in turn, influences the larger environment in which policymaking occurs. Most important, the case illustrates the extraordinary role that policy can play in human health as well as the sometimes equally extraordinary difficulties policies face in achieving their intended impact. Written in the summer of 2014, this case looks back 50 years and more.

Next month, the Civil Rights Act of 1964 will celebrate its 50th birthday. It was the product of more than 150 years of advocacy, violence, court fights and public demonstrations during which many people were imprisoned, injured and even killed as they endeavored to force the United States, to use the words of the great Princeton economist Uwe Reinhardt, "to live up to its own Constitution."

(continued)

The act had an impact on virtually every aspect of American life, and nowhere did it change things more than in many U.S. hospitals.

A Common Misperception

There has long been a misperception about the act's role in the racial desegregation of American health care. The widespread belief is that passage of the Social Security Amendments of 1965 (Public Law 89-97, which created Medicare and Medicaid) was the determining factor. That was not the case; by the time it was passed, many hospitals that had practiced racial segregation already had abandoned it. Medicare was more of a clean-up operation with recalcitrant facilities. The Civil Rights Act, specifically Title VI, was the key to racial equality in the health care setting.

Uncomfortable as it is to remember less enlightened times, racial segregation was commonplace in U.S. hospitals well into the 20th century. It took several forms. One was simply that, particularly in the South, there were hospitals for white people and hospitals for African-Americans, the latter often founded by African-American physicians who could not obtain admitting privileges at white hospitals. Care at the black hospitals tended to be of lower quality, usually due to lack of resources. Some hospitals admitted both groups, but the African-American patients were segregated, often in subpar attic or basement wards.

In the case of Grady Memorial Hospital in Atlanta, a wall was constructed between the "black" and "white" sides of the hospital, leading many people to refer to the facility as "the Gradies." Segregation in health care took other forms. In some hospitals, white and black patients could not share the same room. African-American physicians could not get privileges except in black hospitals. African-American nurses, no matter how senior, were not allowed to supervise white nurses. Transfusion of blood donated by a member of one racial group to a patient belonging to a different group often was prohibited, regardless of the clinical quality of the match. Even newborns often were segregated in different nurseries.

A Widespread Practice

How widespread was all this? According to Professor P. Preston Reynolds, M.D., Ph.D., of the University of Virginia School of Medicine, who has chronicled the history of hospital desegregation in a series of instructive articles, and on whose work I am drawing heavily for

(continued)

this story, it wasn't rare. She reports that in 1959, pioneering African-American physician Paul Cornely, M.D., conducted a survey of racial segregation in health care. He found that 83 percent of Northern hospitals were integrated in terms of patient admissions, but only 6 percent of Southern hospitals were. Of the other 94 percent of facilities in the South, 33 percent admitted no African-Americans, 50 percent admitted them to segregated wards, and segregation was present in some form in the others.

It wasn't much better for African-American physicians. Only 10 percent of Northern hospitals accepted African-American interns or residents; only 20 percent had them on staff. Only 6 percent of Southern hospitals accepted them as interns or residents, and only 25 percent granted them staff privileges.

However, by the late 1950s, 42 percent of medical schools in the South were admitting African-Americans, and 53 percent of Southern medical societies accepted them. Some change was in the wind. But for the most part, it was business as usual.

Segregation had clinical consequences. It is widely believed that the great blues singer Bessie Smith, critically injured in an auto accident, died as a result of being refused admission to a white hospital; the physician who treated her on the scene said that was not the case and that she died of non-survivable injuries. There is also a myth that Charles R. Drew, M.D., another pioneering African-American physician whose work greatly improved blood storage and blood bank efficiency, thus saving thousands of lives, bled to death because he was refused "white" blood. This is also untrue.

But Reynolds reports that prominent African-Americans did die as a result of hospital segregation. One was Juliette Derricotte, dean of women at Fisk University, who died following an auto accident because she was refused care at a hospital that did not accept African-Americans. Another was the father-in-law of Walter White, executive director of the National Association for the Advancement of Colored People, who, after being hit by a car, died after being transferred during a rainstorm from Grady's "white" side to its "black" side. There were undoubtedly many others.

Pressure for Change
Change finally came as the result of years of work by African-American physicians, the NAACP and the courts.

(continued)

It should have come earlier than it did, because the Hill-Burton Act of 1946, which provided funds for construction and improvement of hospitals all over the United States, had a provision requiring equal treatment of all patients. However, it also had a "separate but equal" provision, allowing segregated hospitals to receive Hill-Burton funds as long as the quality of care was the same. It wasn't, and neither was the distribution of Hill-Burton funds, which grossly favored white hospitals.

Interpretation of the Hill-Burton requirements sometimes defied logic. The general counsel of the Department of Health, Education, and Welfare decided that Hill-Burton hospitals could not deny admission to any person *to the part of the hospital that used federal funds* (it must have been fun figuring that out), but patients could be denied access to other areas.

Also, even if a Hill-Burton hospital accepted African-American patients, often their black physicians could not continue to treat them once they were admitted, because they did not have privileges and could not get them.

In 1956 (two years after *Brown vs. Board of Education* ended separate-but-equal practices in education), the NAACP decided it was time to challenge the separate-but-equal provision of the Hill-Burton Act. The first lawsuit was *Eaton vs. Board of Managers of the James Walker Memorial Hospital*, filed by a trio of African-American physicians who had been denied privileges. They argued that because the hospital received federal funds, discriminating against them violated the Fourteenth Amendment. They lost at the district and appeals level, and the Supreme Court declined to review the case. However, three justices dissented.

Buoyed by the possibility of future success at the Supreme Court, the NAACP pushed forward, and soon the ideal case emerged. George Simkins, D.D.S., a North Carolina African-American dentist, had been denied privileges at Moses H. Cone Memorial Hospital, which admitted black patients and received Hill-Burton funds. Working with the NAACP, and with support from the Department of Justice, Simkins recruited African-American patients and other practitioners to join a suit, and on February 12, 1962, *Simkins vs. Moses H. Cone Memorial Hospital* was filed in district court. The plaintiffs asked that the separate-but-equal provision of the Hill-Burton Act be struck down, that discrimination in admitting and treatment privileges be ended, and that refusal to admit African-American patients be banned.

(continued)

The district court found for the defendants, but the plaintiffs appealed and won at the Fourth Circuit Court of Appeals. The case was appealed to the Supreme Court. At that point, HEW [now HHS] Assistant Secretary James Quigley offered support to the NAACP effort and, as all the stakeholders awaited a decision from the Supreme Court, Quigley stopped Hill-Burton payments to eight hospitals being constructed under the separate-but-equal provision.

On March 2, 1964, the Supreme Court declined to review the case, and the appeals court verdict stood. Separate-but-equal under Hill-Burton was dead. Hospitals receiving funds from the program would have to desegregate.

HEW officials were quick to enforce the decision, although there was little they could do to desegregate hospitals that no longer received Hill-Burton funds or those that never had. That would have to be voluntary on the part of the hospitals.

The Last Nail in the Coffin

But four months later, President Lyndon B. Johnson signed the Civil Rights Act, which was pretty much the last nail in segregation's coffin. The key provision of Title VI read: "No person in the United States shall, on the ground of race, color, or national origin, be excluded from participation in, be denied the benefits of, or be subjected to discrimination under any program or activity receiving federal financial assistance."

Passage of a law is one thing; enforcement [and its overall implementation] is quite another. The Eisenhower administration had been lackadaisical in its enforcement of the *Brown vs. Board of Education* decision; the Johnson administration was ready for a full-court press to use Title VI to end, in the words of African-American physician W. Montague Cobb, "the greatest of all discriminatory evils, differential treatment toward African-Americans with respect to hospital facilities."

Less than a month after passage of the Civil Rights Act, Surgeon General Luther Terry, M.D. (back then, the surgeon general was much more than a figurehead), who was one of the federal health officials charged with seeking hospital compliance with the act, wrote an article in *Hospitals* in which he urged American Hospital Association members to comply. He pointed out that Title VI applied to hospitals receiving federal funds of any type.

(continued)

He also noted that before the act was even passed, the AHA "had gone on record as favoring the adoption by hospitals of nondiscrimination policies in the admission and care of patients and the granting of staff privileges." He urged health care associations to "create a favorable climate of opinion" to ensure that all hospitals were in compliance with the act. The AHA subsequently took that request seriously.

Federal reviewers fanned out across the country, seeking to document compliance. They encountered a mixed bag, ranging from hospitals that had long since desegregated (or had always been integrated) to those that were trying to comply (hospital administrators would tell the feds that they wanted to end racist policies, but that their boards would not let them) to those that had no interest in complying and were determined to hold out.

On September 1, 1965, HEW Assistant Secretary Quigley spoke at the AHA annual meeting in San Francisco and related some tales of recalcitrance. Some hospitals said there were no African-American newborns in the nurseries because all of their mothers wanted to nurse them, so they were kept in their mothers' rooms. A few administrators said that they did not segregate African-American patients, but rather "reserved" a section of the hospital for them. Other administrators claimed that African-Americans preferred to use entrances that had only recently been marked "Colored." One hospital executive said he could not convince his staff to write "Mr.," "Mrs." or "Miss" in front of an African-American patient's name on the chart. Someone else told reviewers that there were no African-Americans on the hospital board because black people were not public-spirited enough to volunteer. A few administrators said that African-American patients did not want to share rooms with white patients.

One hospital, in Quigley's words, "removed 'Colored' and 'White' signs from their rest rooms and installed locks on the doors—then issued keys only to the white staff." But in what Quigley described as "the ultimate step in our education to date," a hospital placed African-American and white patients in the same rooms, closed the segregated dining room for African-Americans and integrated the nursery—then changed everything back to segregated circumstances once the review team had left town.

(continued)

Quigley ended his remarks by asking AHA's members, "You have been unsparing in the past—will you join us now in this biggest job of all?"

And Then Came Medicare

Many hospitals did—but not all. And that posed a problem when Medicare and Medicaid were passed a year later; President Johnson signed the Social Security Amendments of 1965 on July 30. Medicare funds were federal funds; if a hospital received them, it had to be in compliance with Title VI of the Civil Rights Act.

Although federal representatives directed by Sherry Arnstein, HEW's new director of hospital civil rights compliance, had successfully desegregated 21 Southern hospitals, by April 1966—shortly before Medicare and Medicaid were to take effect—only 49 percent of American hospitals were in full compliance with Title VI. In seven Southern states, only 15 percent were.

Federal authorities did everything they could to change the situation, because, very simply, reimbursement for care of Medicare and Medicaid patients would not be forthcoming if a hospital remained segregated. President Johnson had been worried ever since the passage of Medicare that there would not be enough physicians to treat newly enfranchised patients (the AMA had fiercely opposed the legislation); now there might not be enough hospitals willing to accept those patients.

Deputy Surgeon General Leo Gehrig, M.D. (who later served for 10 years as director of the AHA's Washington, D.C., office) approached Edwin Crosby, M.D., president of the AHA, and asked for help. Crosby said he would do anything he could. He arranged many meetings between federal compliance staff and hospital leaders. The AHA also produced a short film and a pamphlet for Southern state hospital associations to help them educate their members about what had to be done.

Federal authorities also made the point that segregation was expensive for hospitals, given the cost of duplicating so many services. And the idea of not being eligible for Medicare and Medicaid reimbursement was also a powerful incentive, once it was obvious that the feds meant business and would not pay noncompliant facilities.

The pressure started to pay off. Even conservative Southern politicians conceded that the fight was over. As Reynolds writes, by June 1965, "The word was out. [The Department of Health, Education, and Welfare] would not cave in."

(continued)

By that same month, 85 percent of hospitals were in compliance with Title VI, and Crosby continued to facilitate meetings between federal representatives and officials of hospitals that were still holding out.

Blue Cross and Blue Shield plans, which at the time had an extremely close relationship with the AHA (ah, the good old days!), joined the effort and informed noncompliant hospitals that they would not pay them for patients older than 65 because they would be eligible for Medicare. And if the hospitals wanted Medicare reimbursement for those patients, they would have to comply with Title VI. Sometimes a Catch-22 makes sense.

On June 30—the day before Medicare became effective—federal officials produced the latest numbers. In 14 states and three territories, 100 percent of hospitals were in compliance. In all but five Southern states, 80 percent of hospital beds would be available for Medicare patients. President Johnson told a television audience that night, "Medicare will succeed if hospitals accept their responsibility under the law not to discriminate against any patient because of race." And with the help of their national and state associations, they did just that.

There were many unsung heroes in this effort: the NAACP legal team, which included Thurgood Marshall (later the first African-American Supreme Court Justice), Jack Greenberg and Michael Meltsner (of the hundreds of Hill-Burton complaints sent to the Justice Department, Meltsner wrote most of them); Surgeon General Luther Terry, M.D. (who in 1964 also issued the landmark federal report on the dangers of smoking) and his deputy, Leo Gehrig, M.D.; a host of HEW officials, including James Quigley, Sherry Arnstein and Peter Libassi, who was appointed special assistant to HEW Secretary John Gardner for civil rights; HEW secretaries Anthony Celebrezze and John Gardner; the African-American physicians, dentists and patients who would no longer tolerate being treated as second-class health care citizens; and the American Hospital Association and Edwin Crosby, M.D., who risked his job to do the right thing.

And just for the record, in our current partisan and sometimes hateful times, a lot of these folks were white.

An Unfinished Crusade

So is racism in health care history? Not unless you just took a header off the turnip truck. A 2013 study by the Institute for Diversity in Health Management and the Health Research & Educational Trust found

(continued)

that "although minorities represent a reported 31 percent of patients nationally, they comprise only 14 percent of board members, an average of 12 percent of executive leadership positions, and 17 percent of first- and midlevel management positions." Whites continued to be overrepresented on boards, whereas African-Americans and Latinos were grossly underrepresented. Although 58 percent of chief diversity officers were members of minority groups (surprise), only 17 percent of chief medical officers, 13 percent of COOs, 11 percent of chief nursing officers, 9 percent of CEOs and 6 percent of CFOs were.

Racial and ethnic disparities in access to care, insurance and outcomes are still with us, and although progress has been made, some of them seem intractable. And as recently as 2010, there was still racial friction on health care's front lines. That year, Brenda Chaney, a certified nursing assistant in a long-term care facility, sued her employers when they sought to honor a white patient's request to have only white caregivers. The courts found the nursing home in violation of Title VI.

There were casualties of Title VI as well, notably the historically African-American hospitals, of which there were once as many as 500, which in the years after passage of the Civil Rights Act were closed or merged with other facilities. They represented a significant part of health care history, and they are gone. Nathaniel Wesley Jr., however, has chronicled their story, so it has not been lost (see below).

But there has been progress as well. The AHA has had three African-American chairs (the late Carolyn Boone Lewis, Kevin Lofton and John Bluford) and the American Medical Association an African-American president, Lonnie Bristow, M.D. African-Americans have served as both surgeons general and as secretary of HEW (now HHS).

A Cultural Shift

More importantly, the culture has changed. Most people working in hospitals today wouldn't think of determining admission on the basis of color; insurance, maybe, but not color. Most physician privileges are awarded on the basis of qualification. Minorities supervise white employees all the time. In most settings, it just isn't an issue. And hospital efforts to increase minority representation in the C-suite and the boardroom, and to address racial and ethnic disparities, are ongoing.

I was witness to the beginning of this cultural shift. In 1969, I was the laboratory test slip delivery person in a hospital in Oakland,

(continued)

California. (It was one of several jobs I have had that no longer exist.) I was crazy about the work, because I love hospitals and I got to roam all over the facility, delivering little pieces of paper and pasting them into charts.

One day, there was an incident, and it was the talk of the hospital. An African-American surgical resident was in danger of being dismissed. It certainly wasn't his skill level; he was considered one of the best surgeons ever to set foot in the place. Nor was it his color.

No, it turned out that a lady friend had embroidered flowers on the lapels of his resident's coat, and he was out of compliance with uniform code. The hospital was threatening to take action against him, not because of his race, but because he had embroidered lapels.

Hey, it was the Bay Area in the '60s. The times they were a-changing.

Suggested Readings

Friedman, Emily. "Tapestry." *Hospitals & Health Networks OnLine*. Feb. 9, 2006. Available at www.emilyfriedman.com.

Institute for Diversity in Health Management/Health Research & Educational Trust. *Diversity & Disparities: A Benchmark Study of U.S. Hospitals*. 2011. Available at www.hpoe/diversity-disparities.

Quigley, James. Hospitals and the Civil Rights Act of 1964. *Journal of the National Medical Association*, vol. 57, no. 6, Nov. 1965. (Speech presented to the annual meeting of the American Hospital Association, Sept. 1, 1965.)

Reynolds, P. Preston. "Hospitals and Civil Rights, 1945–1963: The Case of *Simkins v. Moses H. Cone Memorial Hospital*." *Annals of Internal Medicine*, vol. 126, no. 11, June 1, 1997, pp. 898–906.

Reynolds, P. Preston. "The federal government's use of Title VI and Medicare to racially integrate hospitals in the United States, 1963 through 1967." *American Journal of Public Health*, vol. 87, no. 11, Nov. 1997, pp. 1850–1858.

Terry, Luther. Hospitals and Title VI of the Civil Rights Act. *Hospitals*, vol. 39, part 1, Aug. 1, 1968.

Wesley Jr., Nathaniel. *Black Hospitals in America: History, Contributions, and Demise*. Tallahassee, Fla: NRW Publications, 2010.

Source: Friedman (2014). Reprinted with permission.

(continued)

Discussion Questions

1. From the case study, provide one example of each of the forms that public policies can take: laws, rules or regulations, other implementation decisions, and judicial decisions.
2. From the case, provide one example of each of the categories of health policies.
3. Why is the Civil Rights Act a health policy as well as a civil rights policy?
4. What environmental forces influenced enactment of the Civil Rights Act?
5. Discuss the role played by the courts in the Civil Rights Act.
6. Discuss the impact of the Civil Rights Act on American hospitals.
7. Discuss the role of private-sector actors in implementing the Civil Rights Act.
8. Based on the limited information provided in the case, was the Hill-Burton Act effective policy?

References

Association of Academic Health Centers. 2013. *Out of Order, Out of Time: The State of the Nation's Health Workforce, 2013.* Call to action. Accessed January 5, 2014. www.aahcdc.org/Portals/0/Resources/AAHC_OutofTimeCallTo Action_final.pdf.

Bircher, J. 2005. "Towards a Dynamic Definition of Health and Disease." *Medicine, Health Care and Philosophy* 8 (3): 335–41.

Birkland, T. A. 2001. *An Introduction to the Policy Process: Theories, Concepts, and Models of Public Policy Making.* Armonk, NY: M. E. Sharpe.

Blum, H. 1974. *Planning for Health.* New York: Human Sciences Press.

Brook, R. H., and E. A. McGlynn. 1991. "Maintaining Quality of Care." In *Health Services Research: Key to Health Policy*, edited by E. Ginzberg, 284–314. Cambridge, MA: Harvard University Press.

Byrne, D. 2004. *Enabling Good Health for All: A Reflection Process for a New EU Health Strategy.* European Commission report. Accessed April 7, 2015. http://ec .europa.eu/health/ph_overview/Documents/pub_good_health_en.pdf.

Center for Health Workforce Studies. 2012. *Health Care Employment Projections: An Analysis of Bureau of Labor Statistics Occupational Projections, 2010–2020.* Published March. www.healthit.gov/sites/default/files/chws_bls _report_2012.pdf.

Centers for Disease Control and Prevention (CDC). 2014. "Leading Causes of Death." Published July 14. www.cdc.gov/nchs/fastats/lcod.htm.

Chassin, M. R., and J. M. Loeb. 2011. "The Ongoing Quality Improvement Journey: Next Stop, High Reliability." *Health Affairs* 30 (4): 559–68.

Cochran, C. L., and E. F. Malone. 1999. *Public Policy: Perspectives and Choices,* second edition. New York: McGraw-Hill.

Congressional Research Service. 2005. "An Overview of the U.S. Public Health System in the Context of Emergency Preparedness." CRS report for Congress. Updated March 17. www.fas.org/sgp/crs/homesec/RL31719.pdf.

Dahlgren, G., and M. Whitehead. 2006. *European Strategies for Tackling Social Inequities in Health: Levelling Up Part 2.* Reprinted 2007. Accessed January 10, 2014. www.euro.who.int/__data/assets/pdf_file/0018/103824/E89384 .pdf.

Do, D. P., and B. K. Finch. 2008. "The Link Between Neighborhood Poverty and Health: Context or Composition?" *American Journal of Epidemiology* 168 (6): 611–19.

Doran, K. M., E. J. Misa, and N. R. Shah. 2013. "Housing as Health Care—New York's Boundary-Crossing Experiment." *New England Journal of Medicine* 369 (25): 2374–77.

Dubos, R. 1959. *The Mirage of Health.* New York: Harper.

Friedman, E. 2014. "U.S. Hospitals and the Civil Rights Act of 1964." *H&HN Daily.* Published June 3. www.hhnmag.com/display/HHN-news-article .dhtml?dcrPath=/templatedata/HF_Common/NewsArticle/data/HHN /Daily/2014/Jun/060314-friedman-health-equity-diversity.

Garfield, R., and A. Damico. 2012. "Medicaid Expansion Under Health Reform May Increase Service Use and Improve Access for Low-Income Adults with Diabetes." *Health Affairs* 31 (1): 159–67.

Gawande, A. 2009. "Getting There From Here: How Should Obama Reform Health Care?" *The New Yorker,* January 26, 26–33.

Hlatky, M. A., G. D. Sanders, and D. K. Owens. 2005. "Evidence-Based Medicine and Policy: The Case of the Implantable Cardioverter Defibrillator." *Health Affairs* 24 (1): 42–51.

Institute of Medicine (IOM). 2002. *Unequal Treatment: Confronting Racial and Ethnic Disparities in Health Care.* Washington, DC: National Academies Press.

James, C., M. Thomas, M. Lillie-Blanton, and R. Garfield. 2007. *Key Facts: Race, Ethnicity and Medical Care.* Published January. www.kff.org/minorityhealth /upload/6069-02.pdf.

Jost, T. S. 2014. "Implementing Health Reform: Four Years Later." *Health Affairs* 33 (1): 7–10.

————. 2008. "'MetLife v. Glenn': The Court Addresses a Conflict over Conflicts in ERISA Benefit Administration." *Health Affairs* 27 (5): w430–w440.

Liptak, A. 2012. "Supreme Court Upholds Health Care Law, 5–4, in Victory for Obama." *New York Times*, June 28.

Longest, B. B., Jr., and K. Darr. 2014. *Managing Health Services Organizations and Systems*, sixth edition. Baltimore, MD: Health Professions Press.

Luhby, T. 2013. "The New Inequality: Health Care." CNN Money. Published December 18. http://money.cnn.com/2013/12/18/news/economy/health-inequality/index.html.

Murray, J. E. 2007. *Origins of American Health Insurance: A History of Industrial Sickness Funds*. New Haven, CT: Yale University Press.

National Center for Health Statistics. 2013. *Health, United States, 2012*. Department of Health and Human Services Publication No. 2013-1232. Published May. www.cdc.gov/nchs/data/hus/hus12.pdf.

National Institutes of Health (NIH). 2014. "NIH Budget." Accessed January 10. www.nih.gov/about/budget.htm.

Ogden, L. 2012. "Financing and Organization of National Health Systems." In *World Health Systems: Challenges and Perspectives*, second edition, edited by B. J. Fried and L. M. Gaydos, 49–70. Chicago: Health Administration Press.

Organisation for Economic Co-operation and Development (OECD). 2014. "OECD.StatExtracts: Health Expenditure Since 2000." Accessed August 11. http://stats.oecd.org/index.aspx?DataSetCode=SHA.

Partnership for Sustainable Health Care. 2013. "Strengthening Affordability and Quality in America's Health Care System." Published April. www.rwjf.org/content/dam/farm/reports/reports/2013/rwjf405432.

Peters, B. G. 2013. *American Public Policy: Promise and Performance*, ninth edition. Thousand Oaks, CA: CQ Press.

Pharmaceutical Research and Manufacturers of America (PhRMA). 2014. "About PhRMA." Accessed January 10. www.phrma.org/about.

Saracci, R. 1997. "The World Health Organisation Needs to Reconsider Its Definition of Health." *British Medical Journal* 314 (7091): 1409–10.

Schoen, C., D. C. Radley, P. Riley, J. A. Lippa, J. Berenson, C. Dermody, and A. Shih. 2013. "Health Care in the Two Americas: Findings from the Scorecard on State Health System Performance for Low-Income Populations, 2013." Accessed January 5, 2014. www.commonwealthfund.org/Publications/Fund-Reports/2013/Sep/Low-Income-Scorecard.aspx.

Shi, L. 2014. *Introduction to Health Policy*. Chicago: Health Administration Press.

Sisko, A. M., S. P. Keehan, G. A. Cuckler, A. J. Madison, S. D. Smith, C. J. Wolfe, D. A. Stone, J. M. Lizonitz, and J. A. Poisal. 2014. "National Health

Expenditure Projections, 2013–23: Faster Growth Expected with Expanded Coverage and Improving Economy." *Health Affairs* 33 (10): 1841–50.

Smith, M., R. Saunders, L. Stuckhardt, and J. M. McGinnis (eds.). 2012. *Best Care at Lower Cost: The Path to Continuously Learning Health Care in America.* Washington, DC: National Academies Press.

Squires, D. A. 2011. *The U.S. Health System in Perspective: A Comparison of Twelve Industrialized Nations.* Commonwealth Fund. Published July. www.common wealthfund.org/~/media/Files/Publications/Issue%20Brief/2011/Jul /1532_Squires_US_hlt_sys_comparison_12_nations_intl_brief_v2.pdf.

Steinbrook, R. 2009. "Health Care and the American Recovery and Reinvestment Act." *New England Journal of Medicine* 360 (11): 1057–60.

Sterman, J. D. 2006. "Learning from Evidence in a Complex World." *American Journal of Public Health* 96 (3): 505–14.

Taubman, S. L., H. L. Allen, B. J. Wright, K. Baicker, and A. N. Finkelstein. 2014. "Medicaid Increases Emergency-Department Use: Evidence from Oregon's Health Insurance Experiment." *Science* 343 (17): 263–68.

Thompson, F. J. 2013. "Health Reform, Polarization, and Public Administration." *Public Administration Review* 73 (S1): S3–S12.

US Census Bureau. 2014. "USA QuickFacts." Published December 3. http://quick facts.census.gov/qfd/states/00000.html.

US Department of Health and Human Services (HHS). 2014a. "Healthy People 2020." Accessed January 15. www.healthypeople.gov.

———. 2014b. *2013 National Healthcare Disparities Report.* Published May. www .ahrq.gov/research/findings/nhqrdr/nhdr13/2013nhdr.pdf.

US Food and Drug Administration (FDA). 2014. "What We Do." Accessed January 10. www.fda.gov/AboutFDA/WhatWeDo/default.htm.

Vietor, R. H. K., and M. Weinzierl. 2012. "Macroeconomic Policy and U.S. Competitiveness." *Harvard Business Review* 90 (3): 113–16.

Williams, R. A. 2011. *Healthcare Disparities at the Crossroads with Healthcare Reform.* New York: Springer.

World Health Organization. 1946. "Preamble to the Constitution of the World Health Organization." In *Basic Documents,* forty-seventh edition. Geneva, Switzerland: World Health Organization.

THE CONTEXT OF HEALTH POLICYMAKING

After reading this chapter, you should be able to

- describe the legislative, executive, and judicial branches of the federal government;
- describe the legislative, executive, and judicial branches of state governments;
- appreciate the roles of federal and state governments in health policy;
- understand the concept of a policy market and its operation;
- define demanders and suppliers of health policy;
- define interest groups;
- appreciate the role of interest groups in the health policy market; and
- distinguish between the pluralist and elitist perspectives on interest groups.

Whether health policies take the form of laws, rules or regulations, implementation decisions, or judicial decisions, as shown in Exhibit 1.3, all policies are authoritative decisions made in a context through a complicated process. In this chapter, we consider the context. The policymaking process is discussed in the next chapter.

The most basic fact about the context of public-sector health policymaking is that the context includes government. The context is broader than government, but the various levels of government, and the branches within each, as well as the individuals and entities in each level and branch, are a good starting point for understanding the context of public policymaking, including health policymaking. As Peters (2013, 3) has observed, government in the United States is "an immense network of organizations and institutions affecting the daily lives of all citizens in countless ways."

Encompassing all of government and more, the context of health policymaking is large and complex, and well beyond full description in this chapter. However, there is excellent literature on the structure of the US government, including the state and local levels. For example, see Edwards,

Wattenberg, and Lineberry (2014). Brief descriptions of federal, state, and local governments in the United States are provided in the next sections.[1]

Federal Government

Since the Second Continental Congress declared America's independence from Great Britain on July 4, 1776, the federal government has sought to realize the fundamental principle on which the nation was founded: that all people have the right to life, liberty, and the pursuit of happiness. This principle was formalized in 1788 with the ratification of the Constitution. That document became the foundation of a federal government that allowed the several states to act together as one, while protecting the sovereignty of each individual state.

To ensure that no person or group would amass too much power, the founders established a government in which the powers to create, implement, and adjudicate laws were separated into legislative, executive, and judicial branches (see Exhibit 2.1 for an organization chart of the federal government). Each branch of government is balanced by powers in the other two coequal branches: The president can veto the laws of the Congress; the Congress confirms or rejects the president's appointments and can remove the president from office in exceptional circumstances; and the justices of the Supreme Court, who can overturn unconstitutional laws, are appointed by the president and confirmed by the Senate.

Executive Branch

As head of the executive branch, the president is responsible for implementing and enforcing the laws written by Congress and, to that end, appoints the heads of the 15 federal executive departments, who must be confirmed by the Senate. These individuals comprise the president's cabinet. The cabinet departments and other independent federal agencies are responsible for the day-to-day implementation and enforcement of federal laws. These departments and agencies have missions and responsibilities as divergent as those of the Department of Defense, the Department of Health and Human Services (HHS), the Environmental Protection Agency, the Social Security Administration, and the Securities and Exchange Commission.

Among the 15 departments shown in Exhibit 2.1, HHS (www.hhs.gov/about/) is the federal government's principal agency for protecting the health of Americans and providing essential human services, especially for those who are most vulnerable. Agencies of HHS conduct health and social science research, work to prevent disease outbreaks, ensure food and drug safety, and provide health insurance. In addition to administering

EXHIBIT 2.1
The Government of the United States

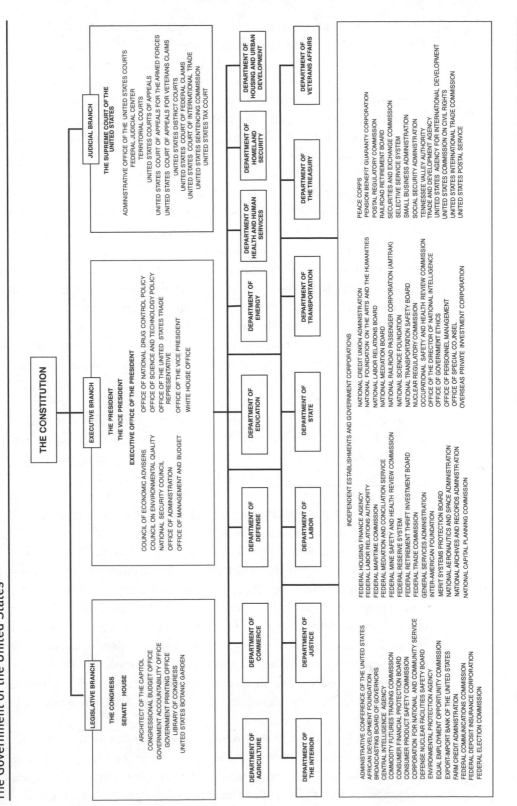

Source: US Government Printing Office (2015).

the Medicare and Medicaid programs and many aspects of the Affordable Care Act (ACA), HHS also includes the National Institutes of Health, the Food and Drug Administration, and the Centers for Disease Control and Prevention. The secretary of health and human services oversees a budget of approximately $760 billion and approximately 65,000 employees. The department's programs are administered by 11 operating divisions, including 8 agencies in the US Public Health Service and 3 human services agencies, and 10 regional offices.

Legislative Branch

The legislative branch of the federal government consists of the House of Representatives and the Senate, which together form the US Congress. (Extensive information about Congress is available at www.congress.gov). The Constitution vests all legislative power at the federal level in Congress, meaning that it is the only part of the federal government that can make new laws or amend existing laws. To pass legislation and send it to the president for signature, both the House and the Senate must pass the same bill by majority vote. If the president vetoes a bill, they may override the veto by passing the bill again in each chamber with at least two-thirds of each body voting in favor.

Although the legislative process will be covered more fully in Chapter 6, the process is outlined here. Additional information on this complex process is available at www.congress.gov/legislative-process. The first step in the legislative process is the introduction of a bill—which is a piece of proposed legislation—to Congress. Bills can be introduced in either chamber of Congress, and sometimes are introduced in both simultaneously. Anyone can draft a bill, but only members of Congress can introduce bills.

After being introduced, whether in the House of Representatives, the Senate, or both, a bill is referred to the appropriate committee or committees for review. The role of the legislative committees in this process is critical. There are 16 Senate committees, with many subcommittees, and 20 House committees, also with many subcommittees. The committees are not set in stone, but change in number and form with each new Congress as required for the efficient consideration of legislation. Each committee oversees a specific policy area, and the subcommittees take on more specialized policy areas. For example, the House Committee on Ways and Means (http://waysandmeans .house.gov) includes subcommittees on Health, Social Security and Trade, and others.

A bill is first considered in a subcommittee, where it may be accepted, amended, or rejected entirely. If the members of the subcommittee agree to move a bill forward, it is reported to the full committee, where the process is repeated again. Throughout this stage of the process, the committees and subcommittees call hearings to investigate the merits and flaws of the pro-posal. They invite experts, advocates, and opponents to appear before the committee and provide testimony.

If the full committee votes to approve the bill, it is reported to the floor of the House or Senate, and the majority party leadership decides when to place the bill on the calendar for consideration. If a bill is particularly press-ing, it may be considered right away. Others may wait for months or never be scheduled. When a bill is approved in one chamber or the other, it is referred to the other chamber for consideration. A bill must pass in both chambers of Congress before it goes to the president for consideration. Though the Con-stitution requires that the two bills have the exact same wording, this rarely happens in practice. To bring the bills into alignment, a conference commit-tee is convened, consisting of members from both chambers. The members of the committee produce a conference report, intended as the final version of the bill. Each chamber then votes again to approve the conference report. Depending on where the bill originated, the final text is then enrolled by either the clerk of the House or the secretary of the Senate, and presented to the speaker of the House and the president of the Senate for their signatures. The bill is then sent to the president.

Upon receiving a bill from Congress, the president may substantially agree with it and sign it into law. If the president believes the law to be bad policy, it can be vetoed and sent back to Congress. Congress may override the veto with a two-thirds vote of each chamber, at which point the bill becomes law. (Appendix 5 shows an example of a law.)

Part of Congress's exercise of legislative authority is the establishment of an annual federal budget. To this end, Congress levies taxes and tariffs to provide funding for essential government services. If enough money cannot be raised to fund the government, then Congress may also authorize borrow-ing to make up the difference.

Oversight of the executive branch is an important congressional check on the president's power and a balance against the president's discretion in implementing laws and making rules and regulations. A major way that Congress conducts oversight is through hearings. The House Committee on Oversight and Government Reform and the Senate Committee on Home-land Security and Government Affairs are both devoted to overseeing gov-ernment operations. Congress also maintains an investigative organization, the Government Accountability Office (www.gao.gov), which audits and generates reports on every aspect of the government.

Structurally, the House of Representatives is made up of 435 elected members, divided among the 50 states in proportion to their total popula-tion. In addition, there are 6 nonvoting members, representing the District of Columbia, the Commonwealth of Puerto Rico, and four other territories of the United States. The presiding officer of the chamber is the Speaker of the House, elected by the representatives. Members or representatives are elected every 2 years and must be 25 years of age, a US citizen for at least 7 years, and a resident of the state they represent. The House has several powers assigned exclusively to it, including the power to initiate revenue bills, impeach federal officials, and elect the president in the case of an Electoral College tie.

Structurally, the Senate is composed of 100 senators, 2 for each state. Senators are elected to six-year terms by the people of each state. The vice president of the United States serves as president of the Senate and may cast the decisive vote in the event of a tie in the Senate. Senators' terms are staggered so that about one-third of the Senate is up for reelection every 2 years. Senators must be 30 years of age, a US citizen for at least 9 years, and a resident of the state they represent. The Senate has the sole power to confirm those of the president's appointments that require consent, and to ratify treaties.

Judicial Branch

Although the role of the judicial branch in health policymaking is discussed much more extensively in Chapter 4, the basic structure of the federal court system in the United States is outlined here as part of our discussion of the context of policymaking. Unlike the executive and legislative branches of the federal government, which are elected by the people, members of the judicial branch are nominated by the president and confirmed by the Senate. Federal judges hold their offices under life tenure. Because federal judges do not have to run or campaign for reelection, they have the opportunity to be insulated from political pressure when deciding cases. Justices may remain in office until they resign, die, or are impeached and convicted by Congress.

The Constitution leaves Congress significant discretion to determine the shape and structure of the federal judiciary. Even the number of Supreme Court justices is left to Congress. The Constitution also grants Congress the power to establish courts inferior to the Supreme Court, and to that end Congress has established the US district courts, which try most federal cases, and 13 US courts of appeals, which review appealed district court cases.

Federal courts enjoy the sole power to interpret the law, determine the constitutionality of the law, and apply it to individual cases. The courts, like Congress, can compel the production of evidence and testimony through the use of a subpoena. The inferior courts are constrained by the decisions of the Supreme Court—once the Supreme Court interprets a law, inferior courts must apply the Supreme Court's interpretation to the facts of particular cases.

The Supreme Court of the United States is the highest court in the land and the only part of the federal judicial branch specifically required by the Constitution. The Court's caseload is almost entirely appellate in nature, and the Court's decisions cannot be appealed to any authority, as it is the final judicial arbiter in the United States on matters of federal law.

In almost all instances, the Supreme Court does not hear appeals as a matter of right; instead, parties must petition the Court for a writ of certiorari. A litigant who loses in a federal court of appeals, or in the highest court of a state, may file such a petition asking the Supreme Court to review the case. The Court typically will agree to hear a case only when it involves a new and important legal principle, or when two or more federal appellate courts have interpreted a law differently. Of the approximately 7,500 requests for certiorari filed each year, the Court usually responds positively to fewer than 150. As noted in Chapter 1, the Supreme Court's ruling in 2012 that the ACA was constitutional was a crucial milestone for the law, permitting it to proceed (Liptak 2012), and is an example of the type of cases the Court chooses to hear.

If the Supreme Court grants certiorari, justices accept legal briefs from the parties to the case, as well as from *amicus curiae,* or "friends of the court." These can include industry trade groups, academics, or even the US government itself. Before issuing a ruling, the Court usually hears oral arguments, where the various parties to the case present their arguments and the justices ask them questions. If the case involves the federal government, the solicitor general of the United States presents arguments on behalf of the United States. The justices then hold private conferences, make their decision, and issue the Court's opinion, along with any dissenting arguments that may have been written.

State Government

In the United States, each state is a sovereign government unto itself (Carruth and Goldstein 2014). Under the Tenth Amendment to the US Constitution, all powers not granted to the federal government are reserved for the states and the people. Each state has a constitution and a bill of rights. These documents set forth the structure and function of the state government and of the local governments within their boundaries. State constitutions tend to be as elaborate as their federal counterpart. Some are even more so. The Alabama Constitution, for example, contains 310,296 words—more than 40 times as many as the US Constitution.

Each state has three branches of government, and the duties of each branch are essentially the same as those in the federal government. The legislative branch passes laws and oversees the executive branch, which implements the laws. The judicial branch determines the constitutionality of laws and adjudicates violations of them.

Executive Branch

In every state, the executive branch is headed by a governor who is directly elected by the people. In most states, the other leaders in the executive branch are also directly elected, including the lieutenant governor, the attorney general, the secretary of state, and auditors and commissioners. States reserve the right to organize in any way, so they often vary greatly with regard to executive structure. No two state executive organizations are identical.

Legislative Branch

All 50 states have legislatures made up of elected representatives, who consider matters brought forth by the governor or introduced by its members to create legislation that can become law. The legislature also approves a state's budget and initiates tax legislation.

Except for Nebraska, all states have a bicameral legislature made up of two chambers: a smaller upper house and a larger lower house. Together the two chambers make state laws and fulfill other governing responsibilities. The smaller upper chamber is always called the Senate, and its members generally serve longer terms, usually four years. The larger lower chamber is most often called the House of Representatives, but some states call it the Assembly or the House of Delegates. Its members usually serve shorter terms, often two years.

Judicial Branch

State judicial branches are usually led by the state supreme court, which hears appeals from lower-level state courts. Court structures and judicial appointments/elections are determined either by legislation or the state constitution. Most states have a three-tiered judicial structure: trial courts, intermediate appellate courts, and a state supreme court. The supreme court of each state focuses on correcting errors made in lower courts and therefore holds no trials. Rulings made in state supreme courts are normally binding; however, when questions are raised regarding consistency with the US Constitution, matters may be appealed directly to the US Supreme Court.

Local Government

Local governments generally include two tiers: counties, also known as boroughs in Alaska and parishes in Louisiana, and municipalities, or cities and towns. In some states, counties are divided into townships. Municipalities can be structured in many ways, as defined by state constitutions, and are called townships, villages, boroughs, cities, or towns. Various kinds of districts also provide functions in local government outside county or municipal boundaries, such as school districts or fire protection districts.

Municipal governments—those defined as cities, towns, boroughs (except in Alaska), villages, and townships—are generally organized around a population center and in most cases correspond to the geographic designations used by the US Census Bureau for reporting housing and population statistics. Municipalities vary greatly in size, from the millions of residents of New York City and Los Angeles to the 287 people who live in Jenkins, Minnesota.

Municipalities generally take responsibility for parks and recreation services, police and fire departments, housing services, emergency medical services, municipal courts, public transportation, and public works such as streets, sewers, snow removal, and signage. Local governments often play important environmental protection roles through such activities as zoning, planning, and issuance of building permits.

Whereas the federal government and state governments are constitutionally based sovereign governments, which share power in countless ways, local governments must be granted power by the states in which they are located. In general, mayors, city councils, and other governing bodies are directly elected by the people.

Governments at All Three Levels Make Health Policy

In the United States, governments at the federal, state, and local levels make health policy. A debate over the appropriate distribution of health policy responsibilities between the levels of government dates from the nation's founding and remains unsettled. Government's responsibility for health rests primarily at the federal and state levels, but also to a more limited degree with local governments.

The term for the arrangement of shared responsibility among levels of government is *federalism*, especially pertaining to how responsibilities and powers are distributed between the states and the national government. Federalism is any system of government with both a national, or central, authority and autonomous constituent jurisdictions like states (Bovbjerg, Wiener, and Houseman 2003). In practical terms, federalism means that responsibility for health policy is shared between the federal government and the states, and to a limited degree with local governments, with each level playing important roles. Sometimes these roles overlap. For example, the federal government is largely responsible for the ACA and Medicare, but federal and state governments share responsibility for Medicaid and certain operational aspects of the ACA. All three levels of government are responsible for the health and well-being of their citizens, and all levels can use policy in the pursuit of health. Their policy tools include the ability to regulate, raise and

An important source of state-level health policy information is available at this Kaiser Family Foundation website: http://kff.org/statedata/.

spend funds, confer benefits, and contract with private entities in pursuit of public purposes. Some of the key responsibilities at each level are described in the following sections.

Federal Government's Role in Health Policy

Over the years since the enactment of Medicare and Medicaid and culminating with passage of the ACA, the federal government plays an increasingly dominant role in health policy. Other aspects of its role include maintenance of massive healthcare delivery programs for the Departments of Veterans Affairs, Defense, and HHS through which services are provided directly to veterans, the military and their dependents, and American Indians and Alaska Natives. In addition, the federal role in health policy includes regulation of food and drugs, support for medical research, prevention of diseases, and homeland security.

State Government's Role in Health Policy

States play several important health policy roles (King 2005; Leichter 2008), which are summarized in Exhibit 2.2. Medicaid, in which the states play a critical role, is the largest health insurance program in the United States. States also play a major role in maintaining public health and in financing and providing services for individuals who are elderly, chronically mentally ill, and in substance abuse prevention and treatment.

A salient feature of health policy in the United States is the wide variability from state to state in the approach to health policy and in the related health status of the citizenry. This variability across states can be seen in data reported in *The Commonwealth Fund's Scorecard on State Health System Performance, 2014* (Radley et al. 2014). This study assesses performance in the states on 42 key indicators grouped into four categories as follows:

1. Access and Affordability, using 6 indicators such as rates of insurance coverage and cost-related barriers to receiving care
2. Prevention and Treatment, using 16 indicators such as measures of receiving preventive care and the quality of care in various settings
3. Potentially Avoidable Hospital Use and Cost, using 9 indicators such as hospital use that might have been reduced with timely and effective care and follow-up
4. Healthy Lives, using 11 indicators such as measures of premature death and health risk behaviors

Guardians of the Public's Health

States have constitutional authority to establish laws that protect the public's health and welfare, including protecting against the consequences of natural and human-caused disasters; dealing with environmental challenges; ensuring safe practices in workplaces and food service establishments; mounting programs to prevent injuries and promote healthy behaviors; and providing health services such as public health nursing and communicable disease control.

Purchasers of Healthcare Services

In addition to their Medicaid funding roles, states also typically provide health insurance benefits to state employees and their dependents and, in many states, to other public-sector workers, such as teachers.

Regulators

States have legal authority to license and regulate health professionals and health-related organizations. States also establish and monitor compliance with environmental quality standards. A particularly important aspect of the role of states in health-related regulation is their responsibility for the health insurance industry as it operates within their boundaries. States control the content, marketing, and pricing of health insurance products and health plans, although the ACA established a larger federal role in regulation of the health insurance industry.

Safety Net Providers

States provide safety nets—although these are often porous—through their support for community-based providers, hospitals that provide charity care, local health departments and clinics that serve low-income people, and other programs that ensure access to appropriate healthcare services.

Educators

States subsidize medical education and graduate medical education through Medicaid payments to teaching hospitals, state appropriations, and scholarship and loan programs. More broadly, states provide funding and expertise for large-scale health education campaigns to improve population health through such educational programs as informing parents about immunization benefits and requirements or encouraging the general public to use seat belts and motorcycle helmets.

Laboratories

States are viewed as laboratories in which experimentation with new policy takes place. For example, Massachusetts enacted a health reform law, An Act Providing Access to Affordable, Quality, Accountable Health Care, in 2006. Many features of this state law presaged features of the federal ACA.

EXHIBIT 2.2
State Government's Multifaceted Role in Health Policy

The Commonwealth Fund study found twofold to eightfold differences between the best-performing and worst-performing states on multiple indicators. Because the study was conducted as a time series, it also showed variation in rates of change in performance over time. Although this study does not show causation, at least some of the variation in performance across states' healthcare systems likely reflects policy differences among the states.

Local Government's Role in Health Policy

Local governments, especially in larger cities and urbanized counties, are major providers of services for the indigent through operation of public hospitals and clinics. They also play roles in regulating smoking and maintaining cleanliness standards for restaurants.

Indeed, as noted at the outset of this discussion of the levels and branches of government, the context of public-sector health policymaking is large and complex because it encompasses all of government. Expanding and complicating the context even more is the fact that the context includes all those variables outside the policymaking process that affect or are affected by the authoritative decisions made in the policymaking process. These variables include the situations and preferences of individuals, organizations, and groups, as well as biological, biomedical, cultural, demographic, ecological, economic, ethical, psychological, science, social, and technological variables in the larger society. A useful way to consider the context of health policy is to view the context as a market.

The Health Policy Market

There is a market for health policies. In this market, some people provide the authoritative decisions that comprise health policy and other people seek particular decisions. The market for health policies has characteristics in common with a traditional economic market. Many different products and services are bought and sold in the context of economic markets. In these markets, willing buyers and sellers enter into economic exchanges in which each party attains something of value. One party demands, and the other supplies. By dealing with one another through market transactions, individuals and organizations buy needed resources and sell their outputs. These relationships are summarized in Exhibit 2.3. Because people are calculative regarding the relative rewards and costs of market exchanges, they negotiate. Negotiation is a key feature of economic markets and policy markets.

Negotiation in Markets

Negotiation, or bargaining, involves two or more parties attempting to settle what each will give and take (or perform and receive) in an economic transaction. In the negotiations that take place in an economic market, the parties

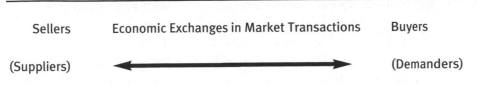

EXHIBIT 2.3
Relationships in Economic Markets

seek a mutually acceptable outcome in a situation where their preferences are usually negatively related (e.g., buyers prefer lower prices, while sellers prefer higher prices). Indeed, if the preferences for outcomes are positively related, an agreement can be reached almost automatically.

More typically, at least two types of issues must be resolved through the negotiations. One type involves the division of resources—the so-called tangibles of the negotiation, such as who will receive how much money and what products or services. Another type centers on the resolution of the psychological dynamics and the satisfaction of personal motivations of the negotiating parties. These issues are the intangibles of the negotiation and can include such notions as appearing to win or lose, to compete effectively, and to cooperate fairly.

Negotiations in economic exchanges usually follow one of two strategic approaches: cooperative (win–win) or competitive (win–lose) strategies. The better negotiating strategy in a particular situation is a function of the interaction of several variables (Wheeler 2013). For example, according to Greenberger and colleagues (1988) cooperative negotiating strategies work best when

- the tangible goal of both negotiators is to attain a specific settlement that is fair and reasonable;
- sufficient resources are available in the environment such that both negotiators can attain their tangible goal, more resources can be attained, or the situation can be redefined so that both negotiators can "win";
- each negotiator thinks it is possible for both to attain their goals through the negotiation process; or
- the intangible goals of both negotiators are to establish a cooperative relationship and to work together toward a settlement that maximizes their joint outcomes.

In contrast, competitive negotiating strategies work best when

- the tangible goal of both negotiators is to attain a specific settlement or to get as much as they possibly can;

- the available resources are not sufficient for both negotiators to attain their goals, or their desire to get as much as possible makes it impossible for one or both to attain their goals;
- both negotiators think it is impossible for both to attain their goals simultaneously; or
- the intangible goal of each negotiator is to beat the other.

The Operation of Policy Markets

Health policies—indeed, all public policies—are made in the context of policy markets that, as noted earlier, operate like traditional economic markets in many ways. However, there are notable differences. The most fundamental difference is that buyers or demanders in economic markets express their preferences by spending their own money. That is, they reap the benefits of their choices, and they directly bear the costs of those choices. In policy markets, on the other hand, the link between who receives benefits and who bears costs is less direct. Often, this link is especially indirect in health policy markets.

Many decisions made by contemporary policymakers are influenced by the preferences of current voters, perhaps to the detriment of future generations of citizens. Feldstein (2006) observes that public policies that impose costs on future generations are routinely established. Allocative policies such as Medicare and Social Security are examples of this phenomenon. In the case of Social Security, outlays began to exceed annual tax revenues in 2010, and the trust funds supporting this program could be exhausted in 2031 (Congressional Budget Office 2013).

There are a limited number of ways to close Social Security's outlay–revenue gap, each of which has substantial drawbacks:

1. The benefits that are scheduled to be paid to future recipients under current law could be reduced.
2. The taxes that fund Social Security could be raised.
3. The resources consumed by other federal programs could be reduced to cover the gap.
4. The federal government's borrowing could be increased to cover the gap.

Of course, Social Security is not the only source of pressure on the federal budget. The financial crisis that engulfed the United States and most of the world beginning in late 2008 caused an unprecedented increase in the federal deficit as government worked through the crisis. In addition, the aging of the US population—which is the main cause of the projected increase in Social Security spending—will raise costs for other entitlement programs. In particular, the Congressional Budget Office (www.cbo.gov) projects that Medicare and Medicaid expenditures will grow even faster than Social Security outlays because of rising healthcare costs, which continue to rise, albeit at a slower rate of increase in recent years (Martin et al. 2014). Unless taxation reaches much higher levels in the United States, current spending policies are likely to prove financially unsustainable over the long term. The resulting burden of federal debt will have a corrosive and potentially contractionary effect on the economy.

Feldstein (2006) also points out that decision makers in policy markets use different criteria from those used in traditional economic markets. In both markets, thoughtful decision makers take benefits and costs into account. In policy markets, however, decision makers may use different time frames. Because legislators stand for periodic reelection, they typically favor policies that provide immediate benefits to their constituencies, and they tend to weigh only, or certainly more highly, immediate costs. Unlike most decision makers in economic markets, who consider costs and benefits over the long run, decision makers in policy markets are more likely to base decisions on immediate costs and benefits. An obvious consequence of such decisions is policies with immediate benefits but burdensome future costs.

In policy markets, suppliers and demanders stand to reap benefits and incur costs because of the authoritative decisions called policies. Policies are therefore valued commodities in these markets. These relationships are shown in Exhibit 2.4.

Given that demanders and suppliers will enter into exchanges involving policies, knowledge of who the demanders and suppliers are and what motivates their decisions and actions in policy markets is helpful.

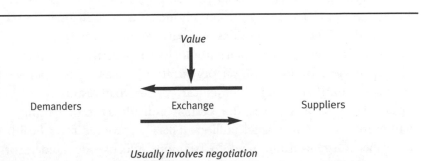

EXHIBIT 2.4
The Operation
of Policy
Markets

Demanders and Suppliers of Health Policies

As we noted earlier, policy markets operate much like typical economic markets. In both markets, something of value is exchanged between suppliers and demanders. Considering policy markets in this way permits us to view public policies as a means of satisfying certain demanders' wants and needs in much the same way that products and services produced and sold in economic markets serve to satisfy demanders (or, in an economic context, consumers). In commercial markets, demanders seek products and services that satisfy them. In policy markets, demanders seek public policies that satisfy their preferences. Policymakers are in a position to supply the public policies that demanders seek.

The Demanders of Health Policies

Broadly, the demanders of health policies can include (1) individuals who consider such policies relevant to the pursuit of their own health or that of others about whom they care and (2) individuals who consider such policies a means to some other desired end, such as economic advantage. These desires motivate participation in policy markets, just as desires motivate participation in economic markets.

For individuals, however, effective participation in a policy market presents certain problems and limitations. To participate effectively, individuals must acquire substantial policy-relevant information, which can require considerable time and money. Beyond this, individual participants or demanders often must be prepared to expend additional time and money in support of achieving desired policies. Any particular health policy might have significant, or even noticeable, benefits for only a few individuals. Consequently, individual demander participation is limited in the markets for policies.

Organizations—such as large health systems, health plans, and technology suppliers—have a significant advantage over individuals in the health policy market. These large entities may have the necessary resources to garner needed policy-relevant information and to support their efforts to achieve desired policies. In addition, an organization's health policy interests may be concentrated. A change in Medicare policy that results in an increased deductible of $100 per year for certain individuals is one thing; a policy change that results in several million dollars of revenue for a health system is another. Organizations tend to be more effective demanders of health policies than individuals because they have more resources and the stakes for them tend to be higher.

The most effective demanders of policies, however, are well-organized interest groups. These are groups of people or organizations with similar policy goals that enter the policymaking process to try to achieve their goals. By combining and concentrating the resources of their members, interest groups can have a much greater impact than individuals or organizations alone.

In effect, interest groups provide their members—whether individuals or organizations—with greater opportunities to participate effectively in the policy market (Cigler and Loomis 2011). The American Nurses Association (www.nursingworld.org) provides such opportunities for individual nurses, the American Association of Retired Persons (www.aarp.org) does so for older individuals, and the Pharmaceutical Research and Manufacturers of America does so for its member companies. Because of their power in policy markets, interest groups, as demanders of health policy, are described more fully in the next section.

Interest Groups in the Policy Market

Interest groups (also called advocacy groups, lobby groups, pressure groups, or special interest groups) arise in democratic societies because the opportunities to achieve particular outcomes are enhanced through collective action in the policy market, specifically through influencing the public policymaking process. They are ubiquitous in the United States, more in the health sector than any other sector of the economy. In 2013, lobbyists in the health sector spent almost $360 million seeking to influence health policy. The only other sector spending approximately as much was the finance/insurance/real estate sector, with the communications/electronics sector and the energy/natural resources sector spending $70 to $100 million less in their attempts to influence policy in their domains (Center for Responsive Politics 2014).

The First Amendment to the US Constitution guarantees the American people the right "peaceably to assemble, and to petition the Government for a redress of grievances." However, constitutional guarantees notwithstanding, political theorists from the nation's beginning to the present day have disagreed about whether interest groups play positive or negative roles in public policymaking (Cigler and Loomis 2011; Edwards, Wattenberg, and Lineberry 2014; Gray, Lowery, and Benz 2013; Peters 2013).

James Madison, writing in the *Federalist Papers* in 1787, discusses the relationship of groups, which he called "factions," to democratic government. In *Federalist* Number 10, he defines a *faction* as "a number of citizens, whether amounting to a majority or a minority of the whole, who are united and actuated by some common impulse of passion, or of interest, adverse to the rights of citizens, or to the permanent and aggregate interests of the community." Madison felt strongly that factions, or interest groups, were inherently bad. He also believed, however, that the formation of such groups was a natural outgrowth of human nature (he writes in *Federalist* Number 10 that "the latent causes of faction are sown into the nature of man") and that government should not seek to check this activity. Madison felt that what he called the "mischiefs of faction" could and should be contained by setting the "ambition" of one faction against the selfish preferences and behaviors of others. So began the uncertainty about and ambiguity toward the role of interest groups in public policymaking in the United States.

One point about which there is neither uncertainty nor ambiguity, however, is that interest groups play an active role in the public policymaking process. Reflecting widely divergent views on the manner in which interest groups play their role in this process, two distinct perspectives on ways in which groups influence policymaking have emerged: the pluralist and the elitist models.

The Pluralist Perspective

People who hold the pluralist perspective on the role of interest groups in policymaking believe that because so many interest groups are operating, everyone's interests can be represented by one or more of them. Adherents to the pluralist model usually maintain that interest groups play an essentially positive role in public policymaking. They argue that various interest groups compete with and counterbalance each other in the policy marketplace. Pluralists do not question that some groups are stronger than others. However, they contend that as groups seek their preferred outcomes, power is widely dispersed among competing groups, with each group winning some of the time and losing some of the time.

Pluralist theory about how the policymaking process works includes several interconnected arguments that, taken together, constitute what has come to be called a group theory of politics (Edwards, Wattenberg, and Lineberry 2014). The central tenets of the group theory include the following:

- Interest groups provide essential links between people and their government.
- Interest groups compete among themselves for outcomes, with the interests of some groups counterbalanced by the interests of others.
- No group is likely to become too dominant in the competition; as groups become powerful, other countervailing interests organize or existing groups intensify their efforts. An important mechanism for maintaining balance among the groups is their ability to rely on various sources of power. Groups representing concentrated economic interests may have money, but consumer groups may have more members.
- The competition among interest groups is basically fair. Although there are exceptions, groups typically play by the rules of the game.

There are critics of the pluralist approach, claiming that it is dysfunctional and out of control. The pluralist critics make two key points:

1. Interest groups have become too influential in the policymaking process. Satisfying their multiple and often conflicting demands seems to drive government, rather than government being driven by a desire to base policy decisions on considerations of what is best for the nation as a whole—that is, on the public interest.

2. Seeking to satisfy the multiple and often conflicting demands of various interest groups leads to confusion, contradiction, and even paralysis in the policymaking process. Rather than making a difficult choice between satisfying X or Y, government seems frequently to pretend that there is no need to make the choice and seeks to satisfy both X and Y.

Some pluralist critics believe that the perspective itself is misguided, even wrong. Some people believe that, instead of everyone having a chance to influence the policymaking process through one group or another, such influence actually resides only in the hands of an elite few. This belief gives rise to a second perspective on the ways groups influence policymaking.

The Elitist Perspective

Whereas pluralists point with pride to the large number of organized groups actively and aggressively participating in the American process of public policymaking, elitists point out how most groups are fairly powerless and ineffectual. The elitist perspective on the role of interest groups, which is the opposite of the pluralist viewpoint, grows out of a power elite model of American society.

This model is based on the idea that real political power in the United States is concentrated in the hands of the small proportion of the population that controls the nation's key institutions and organizations and much of its wealth. In the elitist perspective, these so-called big interests look out for themselves in part by disproportionately influencing, if not controlling, the public policymaking process. Whether this model accurately reflects American policy markets is debatable, but the model does represent the opinions of a growing majority of Americans concerning which members of the society have the most influence.

The elitist theory holds that a power elite, often referred to as "the establishment," acts as a gatekeeper to the public policymaking process. Unless the power elite considers an issue important, the issue does not get much attention in policymaking circles. Furthermore, the theory holds, once an issue is on the policy agenda, public policies made in response reflect the values, ideologies, and preferences of this governing elite (Dye 2012). Thus, the power elite dominates public policymaking through its superior position in society. Its powerful role in the nation's economic and social systems allows the elite to shape the formulation of policies and control their implementation. It has been argued that the nation's social and economic systems depend on the power elite's consensus regarding the system's fundamental values, and the only policy alternatives that receive serious consideration are those that fall within the shared consensus (Dye 2002).

The central tenets of the power elite theory stand in stark contrast to the pluralist perspective. These tenets are as follows (Dye, Zeigler, and Schubert 2012; Edwards, Wattenberg, and Lineberry 2014):

- Real political power resides in a small number of groups; the large number of interest groups is practically meaningless because the power differentials among them are so great. Other groups may win minor policy victories, but the power elite always prevails on significant policy issues.

- Members of the power elite share a consensus or near consensus on the basic values that should guide public policymaking: private property rights, the preeminence of markets and private enterprise as the best way to organize the economy, limited government, and the importance of individual liberty and individualism.

- Members of the power elite have a strong preference for incremental changes in public policies. Incrementalism in policymaking permits time for the economic and social systems to adjust to changes without feeling threatened, with minimal economic dislocation or disruption and with minimal alteration in the social system's status quo.

- Elites protect their power bases. Some limited movement of non-elites into elite positions is permitted to maintain social stability, but only after non-elites clearly accept the elites' consensus values.

Which Perspective Is Correct?

Those who hold the power elitist perspective challenge those who hold the pluralist perspective by pointing to the highly concentrated and interlocked power centers in American society. Studies of the concentration of power do find that many of the top leadership positions in the United States—on corporate, foundation, and university governing boards, for example—are held by people who occupy more than one such position (Domhoff 2013).

Those who prefer the pluralist perspective, however, are equally quick to cite numerous examples in which those who traditionally have been grossly underrepresented in the inner circles of the power elite have succeeded in their collective efforts to significantly influence the public policymaking process.

African Americans, women, and consumers in general provide examples of the ability of groups once ignored by policymakers to organize as effective interest groups and redirect the course of the public policymaking process.

Neither the pluralist nor the elitist perspective alone fully explains how the interests of individuals or organizations relate to the public policymaking process. The results of that process affect the interests of all individuals and all organizations to varying degrees. Many, if not all, individuals and organizations with interests can influence the policymaking process, although, again, not to equal degrees. The elitist and pluralist approaches each have something to contribute to an understanding of the roles interest groups play in the markets for public policies. Whether such groups work proactively, by seeking to stimulate new policies that serve the interests of their members, or reactively, by seeking to block policy changes that they do not believe serve their members' best interests, they are intrinsic to the public policymaking process. Interest groups provide their members with a way to link their policy preferences into a more powerful, collective voice that greatly increases the likelihood of a significant influence on policymaking.

The Suppliers of Health Policies

Because policies are made in the executive, legislative, and judicial branches of government, the list of potential policymakers is lengthy. Members of each branch of government supply policies in the political market, although each branch plays its role differently.

Legislators as Suppliers

One important group of public policy suppliers is elected legislators, whether members of the US Congress, state legislatures, or city councils. Few aspects of the policy marketplace are as interesting, or as widely observed and studied, as the decision-making behaviors of legislators and the motives and incentives behind those behaviors. To a large extent, this intense interest in the motivations of policy suppliers reflects the desire of policy demanders to exert influence over the suppliers.

Although neither extreme fully reflects the motivations of legislators, the end points on a continuum of behaviors that policymakers might exhibit can be represented by those who seek to maximize the public interest on one end and by those who seek to maximize self-interest on the other end. A legislator at the public interest extreme would always seek policies—that is, would make authoritative decisions—that maximize the public interest, although the true public interest might not always be easy to identify. A legislator whose motivations lie at the self-interest extreme would always behave in a manner that maximizes self-interest, whether that interest is reelection, money, prestige, power, or whatever appeals to the self-serving person.

In policy markets, legislators can be found all along the continuum between extreme public-interest and extreme self-interest motivations. Although some people incorrectly ascribe dominant self-interest motives to all legislators, the actions and decisions of most legislators reflect a complex mixture of the two motivations, with exclusively self-interested or public-interested motives only rarely dominating decisions.

Motives aside, legislators at all levels of government are key policy suppliers, especially of policies in the form of laws. For example, only Congress can enact new or amend existing public laws. In policy markets, legislators constantly calculate the benefits and costs of their policymaking decisions and consider who will reap these benefits and bear these costs. Factoring in the interests they choose to serve, they make their decisions accordingly. Their calculations are complicated by the fact that the costs and benefits of a particular decision often affect many people in different ways.

In effect, policies typically create winners and losers. The gains some people enjoy come at the financial expense of others, or at least at the expense of having someone's problems ignored or someone's preferred solutions postponed. Most of the time, most legislators seek to maximize their own net political gains through their policy-related decisions, because reelection is an abiding objective.

In view of the reality of most policies creating winners and losers, legislators may find that their best strategy is to permit the winners their victory, but not by a huge margin, and in so doing cushion the impact on the losers. For example, suppose a legislator is considering a policy that would increase health services for an underserved population but at the expense of higher taxes on others. Options include various policies with the following outcomes: (1) few services at relatively low cost, (2) more services at higher cost, and (3) many services at high cost. Facing such a decision, and applying the concept of net political gain, policymakers might opt for the provision of a meaningful level of services, but one far below what could have been provided and at a cost below what would have been required for a higher level of services. The "winners" receive more services, but the expense for the "losers," who have to pay for the new services, is not as great as it might have been. Through such calculations and determinations, legislators routinely seek to maximize their net political gains.

Executives and Bureaucrats as Suppliers

At all levels of government, members of the executive branch are important policy suppliers, although their role differs from that of legislators (see Exhibit 1.2). Presidents, governors, mayors, and other senior public-sector executives offer policies in the form of legislative proposals and seek to have legislators enact their preferred policies. Chief executives and those in charge of government departments and agencies are directly responsible for policies in the form of rules or regulations used to guide the implementation of laws and operational protocols and procedures for the policies they implement. Career bureaucrats who participate in these activities and thus become suppliers of policies in the policy markets join elected and appointed executives and managers in their rulemaking and other policy implementation duties.

Elected and appointed officials of the executive branch are often affected by the same self-interest/public-interest dichotomy that affects legislators; reelection concerns, in particular, often influence their decisions. Like legislators, elected and appointed members of executive branches are apt to calculate the net political gains of their policy-related decisions and actions. As a result, their motivations and behaviors in policy markets can be similar to those of legislators. However, the behaviors of members of the executive branch of a government and members of its legislative branch show some important differences.

The most fundamental difference derives from the fact that the executive branch generally bears greater responsibility than the legislative branch for the state of the economy, and it is widely perceived to bear even more responsibility than it actually does. Presidents, governors, and mayors, along with their top appointees, are held accountable for economic conditions much more explicitly than are Congress, state legislatures, or city councils. Although legislators do not escape this responsibility altogether, the public typically lays most of the responsibility at the feet of the executive branch. When people do blame the legislative branch, they tend to hold the entire Congress or the state or city legislature collectively responsible rather than to blame individual legislators.

The concentration of responsibility for the economy in the executive branch influences the decision making that takes place there. Because of the close connection between government's budget and the state of the economy, the budget implications of policy decisions are carefully weighed in the executive branch. Not infrequently, the legislative and executive branches will hold different positions on health policies because members in the two branches give different weight to the budget implications of the policies they are considering.

Career bureaucrats, or civil servants, in the executive branch also participate in policymaking in the legislative branch when they collect, analyze, and transmit information about policy options and initiate policy proposals in their areas of expertise. However, the motivations and behaviors of career bureaucrats tend to differ from those of legislators and those of members of executive branches.

The behaviors and motivations of career bureaucrats in the public sector are often analogous to those of employees in the private sector. Workers in both settings typically seek to satisfy certain personal needs and desires through their work. Behaviors and motivations can obviously be categorized as self-serving in both cases. But government employees are no more likely to be totally motivated by self-interests than are private-sector workers. Most workers in both sectors are motivated by blends of self-interest and interest in what is good for the larger society.

However, most career bureaucrats watch a constantly changing mix of elected and senior government officials—with an equally dynamic set of policy preferences—parade past, while they remain as the most permanent human feature of government. It should surprise no one that career bureaucrats develop a strong sense of identification with their home department or agency or that they become protective of it. This protectiveness is most visible in the relationships between government agencies or departments and those with legislative oversight of them, including authorization, appropriation, and performance review responsibilities. Many career bureaucrats equate the well-being of their agencies, in terms of their size, budgets, and prestige, with the public interest. Obviously, this is not always the case.

The Judiciary as Supplier

The judicial branch of government is also a supplier of policies. This role is discussed in more depth in Chapter 4. For example, whenever a court interprets an ambiguous law, establishes judicial procedure, or interprets the US Constitution, it makes a policy. These activities are conceptually no different from those involved when legislators enact public laws or when members of the executive branch establish rules and regulations to guide implementation of laws or make operational decisions regarding their implementation. All of these activities are policymaking, because they lead to authoritative decisions made in government to influence or direct the actions, behaviors, and decisions of others.

Policymaking in the judicial branch, however, differs from that in the legislative and executive branches, not only in focus but in operation. The responsibilities of courts require them to focus narrowly on the issues involved in specific cases or situations. This narrow focus stands in stark contrast to the wide-open political arena in which most other public policymaking occurs.

The courts are involved in numerous and diverse aspects of health policy, reflecting the entire range of health determinants (i.e., physical environment, behavior and genetics, social factors, and health services). For example, in a 1980 opinion in what is called the "Benzene Case," the US Supreme Court invalidated an Occupational Safety and Health Administration (OSHA; www.osha.gov) rule limiting benzene to no more than one part per million parts in the air in workplaces. In the Court's view, OSHA had not found a significant risk to workers' health before issuing the rule.

In a 1905 landmark ruling in *Jacobson v. Massachusetts*, the US Supreme Court upheld compulsory vaccination as an appropriate use of state police power to protect the health, welfare, and safety of a state's citizens. Police powers granted to the states by the US Constitution provide the legal basis for state authority in the field of public health. This case involved a compulsory vaccination regulation of the Cambridge, Massachusetts, Board of Health. Defendant Jacobson refused to be vaccinated and contended that the requirement invaded his liberty. The Court held, however, that

> the liberty secured by the Constitution to every person . . . does not import an absolute right in each person to be at all times and in all circumstances wholly freed from restraint . . . It was the duty of the constituted authorities primarily to keep in view the welfare, comfort and safety of the many, and not permit the interests of the many to be subordinated to the wishes or convenience of the few.

Furthermore, the Court stated that

> it is equally true that in every well-ordered society charged with the duty of conserving the safety of its members the rights of the individual in respect of his liberty may at times, under the pressure of great dangers, be subjected to such restraint, to be enforced by reasonable regulations, as the safety of the general public may demand.

The heart of the judiciary's ability to supply policies lies in its interpretative role. The courts can exercise the powers of nullification, interpretation, and application to the rules and regulations established by the executive branch in carrying out its implementation responsibilities. The courts also have the power to declare federal and state laws unconstitutional—that is, to declare laws enacted by the legislative branch to be null and void. This role of the courts is clearly illustrated in a ruling by the Ninth US Circuit Court of Appeals that overturned Arizona legislation requiring abortion clinics in that state to submit to warrantless searches and to make patient files available to state regulators. These onerous state regulations had been established following the death of a patient having a clinic abortion. The appeals court based its ruling on an interpretation that the regulations violated constitutional restrictions on searches and seizures and that requiring the clinics to submit patient files to state regulators on demand violated the patients' privacy rights (Kravets 2004).

Another example of the interpretative role of the courts in health policymaking is the ruling by the US Supreme Court in April 1995 that the Employee Retirement Income Security Act (ERISA; P.L. 93-406) does not preclude states from setting hospital rates. The case that resulted in this ruling arose out of New York's practice of adding a surcharge to certain hospital bills to help pay for health services for some of the state's low-income citizens. The state's practice was challenged by a group of commercial insurers and health maintenance organizations and by New York City (Green 1995). A number of health-related interest groups filed a joint *amicus curiae* (friend of the court) brief in which they asserted that Congress, in enacting ERISA, never intended for it to be used to challenge state health reform plans and initiatives. The Supreme Court's ruling is generally seen as supportive of state efforts to broaden access to health services for their poorer residents through various reforms and initiatives.

Health policymaking in the judicial branch is far more prevalent in state courts and lower federal courts than in the US Supreme Court. A state-level example of courts making important health policy can be seen in Pennsylvania cases involving the tax-exempt status of healthcare organizations. In one 1995 case, for example, the Indiana County, Pennsylvania, Court of Common Pleas rebuffed the leaders of Indiana Hospital in their appeal to have the hospital's tax-exempt status restored after the exemption had been revoked by the county. In making its ruling, the court held that the hospital failed to adequately meet one of the state's tests through which an organization qualifies for tax exemption. Among other criteria, at the time of this case the state required a tax-exempt organization "to donate or render gratuitously a substantial portion of its services."

In making its ruling, the Indiana County court took note of the fact that Indiana Hospital's uncompensated charity care in the prior year had amounted to approximately 2 percent of its total expected compensation and contrasted this amount with that in an earlier case resulting from the revocation of the tax-exempt status of a nursing home in the state. The state supreme court decision in the St. Margaret Seneca Place nursing home case (*St. Margaret Seneca Place v. Board of Property Assessment Appeals and Review, County of Allegheny, PA*) had been that the nursing home did meet the state's test because it demonstrated that it bore more than one-third of the cost of care for half of its patients.

The variation in these and several other Pennsylvania cases in the courts' interpretation of the state's partial test for tax-exempt status (i.e., the requirement that a tax-exempt organization is "to donate or render gratuitously a substantial portion of its services") led to enactment in 1997 of clarifying legislation on this and other points regarding the determination of tax-exempt status. Late in that year, the governor of Pennsylvania signed into law House Bill 55, known as the Institutions of Purely Public Charity Act, or Act 55. This act permits an institution to meet the charitable purpose test and qualify for tax exemption if it has a charitable mission, is free of private profit motive, is designated a 501(c)(3) by the federal government, and is organized for any of the following reasons:

- Relief of poverty
- Advancement and provision of education, including secondary education
- Advancement of religion
- Prevention and treatment of disease or injury, including mental retardation and mental illness
- Government or municipal purposes
- Accomplishment of a purpose that is recognized as important and beneficial to the public and that advances social, moral, or physical objectives

The act specifically clarified, quite liberally, how an institution could meet the requirement for donating or rendering gratuitously a substantial portion of its services. Act 55 established 3 percent of an institution's total operating expenses as the necessary contribution of charitable goods or services. In this instance, court decisions were policies themselves, and the impact of the decisions eventually led to a significant change in Pennsylvania's public laws.

It is generally acknowledged that, because the pursuit of health in the United States is so heavily influenced by laws and regulations, the courts are a major factor in the development and implementation of health policies (Gostin 2008; Jost 2014). The courts include not only the federal court system but also the court systems of the states and the territories. Each of these systems has developed in idiosyncratic ways, and each has a constitution to guide it, specific legislation to contend with, and its own history of judicial decisions. A great deal of information on the structure and operation of the US legal system can be found in the outline of the legal system provided by the US Department of State (2004).

Although the federal and state courts play significant roles as policy suppliers, their behaviors, motivations, and roles differ significantly from those of participants in the legislative and executive branches. In their wisdom, the drafters of the US Constitution created the three branches, and Article III ensured the judicial branch's independence, at least mostly so, from the other branches.

An independent judiciary facilitates adherence to the rules all participants in the policymaking process must follow. Federal judges are appointed rather than elected, and the appointments are for life. Consequently, federal judges are not subject to the same self-interest concerns related to reelection that many other policymakers face. This characteristic enhances their ability to act in the public interest, although judges, like all policymakers, vary in their personal commitments to this objective (Sunstein et al. 2006).

Interplay Among Demanders and Suppliers in Policy Markets

In the policy marketplace, demanders and suppliers of policies seek to further their objectives. These objectives can be based on self-interest or they can be based on what is best for the public, or at least some subset of society, such as individuals who are elderly, poor, or medically underserved. In either case, the outcome depends on the relative abilities of some participants in policy markets to influence the actions, behaviors, and decisions of other participants.

Influence in Policy Markets

Influence in policy markets is the power to shape or help determine policy. Such power can derive from several sources. The classic categories for sources of interpersonal power include legitimate, reward, coercive, expert, and referent (French and Raven 1959). These bases of interpersonal power apply to individuals, organizations, and interest groups in policy markets.

Legitimate power, for example, derives from one's relative position in a social system, organization, or group; this form of power is also called formal power or authority. It exists because assigning or ascribing certain powers to individuals, organizations, or groups better enables them to fulfill their duties or perform their work effectively. Elected officials, appointed executives, judges, health professionals, corporation executives, union leaders, and many other individual participants in policy markets possess certain legitimate power that accompanies their social or organizational positions. Suppliers and demanders of policies possess legitimate power. That is, they can exert influence in the policymaking process because they are recognized as legitimate in the process.

Reward power is based on the ability of one person, organization, or group to reward others for their decisions and actions. Reward power stems in part from legitimate power. It comes from many sources and takes many forms. In organizations, it includes the obvious: control over pay increases, promotions, work and vacation schedules, recognition of accomplishments, and such status symbols or perks as club memberships and office size and location. In economic markets, the buying power of consumers is a form of reward power. In policy markets, reward power is more likely to take the form of favors that can be provided or exchanged, specific influence with particular individuals or groups, and whatever influence can be stored for later use. Coercive power is the opposite of reward power and is based on the capacity to withhold or to prevent someone from obtaining desired rewards.

Expert power tends to reside in individuals but can also reside in a group or organization. It derives from possessing expertise valued in policy markets, such as expertise in solving problems or performing crucial tasks. People with expert power often occupy formal positions of authority, transferring some of the expert power to the organization or group. People who can exercise their expert power in the policymaking arena may also be trusted advisers or associates of other participants in policy markets.

Referent power derives from the influence resulting from the ability of some people, organizations, and interest groups to engender admiration, loyalty, and emulation from others. In the markets for policies, this form of power, when it pertains to individuals, is also called charismatic power. Charismatic power usually belongs to a select few people who typically have strong convictions about the correctness of their preferences, have great self-confidence in their own abilities, and are widely perceived to be legitimate agents of change. Rarely does a person, organization, or interest group gain sufficient power to heavily influence policymaking simply from referent or charismatic power, even in policy markets where charisma is highly valued. But it can certainly give the other sources of power in a policy market a boost.

The bases of power in policy markets are interdependent. They can and do complement and conflict with each other. For example, people, organizations, or groups that are in a position to use reward power and who do so wisely can strengthen their referent power. Conversely, those who abuse coercive power might quickly weaken or lose their referent power. Effective participants in the marketplace for policies—those individuals, organizations, and groups that succeed at influencing policymaking—tend to be fully aware of the sources of their power and to act accordingly. They seem to understand intuitively the costs and benefits of using each kind of power and can draw on them appropriately in different situations and with various people they wish to influence.

Influence of Interest Groups: Breaking the Iron Triangles

Some interest groups, including several in the health domain, are extraordinarily influential in public policymaking. Yet these groups are not as influential as they once were. At the height of their influence, certain interest groups formed part of what were called iron triangles. The iron triangle was a model of the relationships that sometimes existed among participating individuals, organizations, and groups in policy markets.

Any policy domain attracts a set of participating individuals, organizations, and groups. Each participant has some stake in policies affecting the domain and thus seeks to influence policymaking. Some of the participants, or stakeholders, in a domain demand policies; others supply policies. Collectively, these stakeholders form a *policy community*.

Traditionally, the policy community formed around a particular policy domain (such as health) has included legislators with focused interest in a domain, usually serving on legislative committees with jurisdiction in the domain, the executive branch agencies responsible for implementing public laws in the domain, and the private-sector interest groups involved in the domain. The first two categories are suppliers of the policies demanded by the third category. This triad of organized interests has been called an *iron triangle* because when all three sides are in accord, the resulting stability allows the triad to withstand attempts to make undesired changes.

A policy community that could be appropriately characterized as a strong and stable iron triangle dominated the health policy domain until the early 1960s, when battle lines began to be drawn over the eventual shape of the Medicare program. This triangle featured a few powerful interest groups with concordant views that, for the most part, found sympathetic partners among members of the legislative committees and in the relevant implementing agencies of government.

During this period, the private-sector interest group members of the iron triangle that dominated health policy, notably the American Medical Association (AMA; www.ama-assn.org) and the American Hospital Association (AHA; www.aha.org), joined later by the American College of Physicians (ACP; www.acponline.org) and the American College of Surgeons (www.facs.org), generally held a consistent view of the appropriate policies in this domain. Their shared view of optimal health policy was that government should protect the interests of health services providers and not intervene in the financing or delivery of health services (Peterson 1993). Under the conditions and expectations extant in these largely straightforward relationships, it was relatively simple for the suppliers and demanders of policies to satisfy each other. This triangle was unbreakable into the second half of the twentieth century.

The dynamics of the situation began to change dramatically with the policy battles over Medicare, and they worsened with the addition of Medicaid to the debate. Fundamental differences emerged among the participants in the health policy community in terms of their views of optimal health policy. Today, there is rarely a solid block of concordant private-sector interests driving health policy decisions. For example, differences over questions of optimal policy shattered the accord between AMA and AHA. Splintering within the memberships of these groups caused even more damage. For example, the medical profession no longer speaks through the single voice of AMA; organizations such as ACP and the American Academy of Family

Physicians (www.aafp.org) can and sometimes do support different policy choices. Similarly, AHA is now joined in policy debates by organizations with diverse preferences representing the specific interests of teaching hospitals, public hospitals, for-profit hospitals, and other hospital subsets. These changes have eroded the solidarity among private-sector interest groups and the public-sector members of the health policy community. This phenomenon has recently been seen clearly in the formulation and implementation of the ACA. A large number of active groups, with divergent views, are participating in policymaking and influencing policymaking in this area.

Rather than an iron triangle, the contemporary health policy community is far more heterogeneous in its membership and much more loosely structured. At most, this community can be thought of as a group of members whose commonality stems from the fact that they pay attention to issues in the health policy domain. There is an important difference, however, between shared attentiveness to health policy issues and shared positions on optimal health policy or related issues. The loss of concordance among the members of the old iron triangle has diminished the power of certain interest groups. Nevertheless, they remain highly influential, and other interest groups have also been able to assume influential roles in health policymaking.

Having considered the context in which health policies are made, especially the structure and operations of policy markets, and having identified the demanders and suppliers who interact in these markets and the important operational aspects of these interactions, it is now possible to consider the intricate process through which public policies are made. The consideration is the focus of the next chapter, which will begin at the conceptual level and include a schematic model of the policymaking process; applied discussions of the component parts of the policymaking process follow in subsequent chapters.

Summary

Health policies, like those in other domains, are made in the context of policy markets, where demanders for and suppliers of policies interact. The federal, state, and, to a lesser extent, local governments have important health policy roles.

The demanders of policies include those who view public policies as a mechanism for meeting their health-related objectives or other objectives, such as economic advantage. Although individuals alone can demand public policies, the far more effective demand emanates from organizations and especially from organized interest groups. The suppliers of health policy include elected and appointed members of all three branches of government and the civil servants who staff the government.

The interests of the various demanders and suppliers in this market cannot be completely coincident—often, they are in open conflict—and the decisions and activities of any participant always affect and are affected by the activities of other participants.

Review Questions

1. Discuss the roles of federal and state governments in health policy.
2. Compare and contrast the operation of traditional economic markets with that of policy markets.
3. Who are demanders and suppliers of health policies? What motivates each in the policy marketplace?
4. Compare and contrast the pluralist and elitist perspectives on interest groups in policy markets.
5. Define *power* and *influence*. What are the sources of power in policy markets?

Note

1. The sections describing the federal, state, and local levels of government in the United States are adapted from the White House website's "Our Government" pages, accessed January 8, 2014 (www.whitehouse.gov/our-government). Additional descriptive information about the federal judicial branch can be found at the United States Courts website (www.uscourts.gov/Home.aspx). Additional information about the federal legislative branch, including the legislative process, can be found at the US Congress website (www.congress.gov).

References

Bovbjerg, R. R., J. M. Wiener, and M. Houseman. 2003. "State and Federal Roles in Health Care: Rationales for Allocating Responsibilities." In *Federalism and Health Policy*, edited by J. Holahan, A. Weil, and J. M. Wiener, 25–57. Washington, DC: Urban Institute Press.

Carruth, R. S., and B. D. Goldstein. 2014. *Environmental Health Law*. San Francisco: Jossey-Bass.

Center for Responsive Politics. 2014. "Ranked Sectors." Accessed January 8. www.opensecrets.org/lobby/top.php?indexType=c&showYear=2013.

Cigler, A. J., and B. A. Loomis (eds.). 2011. *Interest Group Politics*, eighth edition. Washington, DC: CQ Press.

Congressional Budget Office. 2013. "The 2013 Long-Term Projections for Social Security: Additional Information." Published December. www.cbo.gov/sites /default/files/cbofiles/attachments/44972-SocialSecurity.pdf.

Domhoff, G. W. 2013. *Who Rules America? The Triumph of the Corporate Rich*, seventh edition. Hightstown, NJ: McGraw-Hill.

Dye, T. R. 2012. *Understanding Public Policy*, fourteenth edition. New York: Pearson.

———. 2002. *Who's Running America? The Bush Restoration*, seventh edition. White Plains, NY: Pearson Longman.

Dye, T. R., H. Zeigler, and L. Schubert. 2012. *The Irony of Democracy: An Uncommon Introduction to American Politics*, fifteenth edition. Boston: Wadsworth Cengage Learning.

Edwards, G. C., M. P. Wattenberg, and R. L. Lineberry. 2014. *Government in America: People, Politics, and Policy*, sixteenth edition. Upper Saddle River, NJ: Pearson.

Feldstein, P. J. 2006. *The Politics of Health Legislation: An Economic Perspective*, third edition. Chicago: Health Administration Press.

French, J. R. P., and B. H. Raven. 1959. "The Basis of Social Power." In *Studies of Social Power*, edited by D. Cartwright, 150–67. Ann Arbor, MI: Institute for Social Research.

Gostin, L. O. 2008. *Public Health Law: Power, Duty, Restraint*, second edition. Berkeley, CA: University of California Press.

Gray, V., D. Lowery, and J. K. Benz. 2013. *Interest Groups and Health Care Reform Across the United States*. Washington, DC: Georgetown University Press.

Green, J. 1995. "High-Court Ruling Protects Hospital-Bill Surcharges." *AHA News* 31 (18): 1.

Greenberger, D., S. Strasser, R. J. Lewicki, and T. S. Bateman. 1988. "Perception, Motivation, and Negotiation." In *Health Care Management: A Text in Organization Theory and Behavior*, second edition, edited by S. M. Shortell and A. D. Kaluzny, 81–141. New York: Wiley.

Jost, T. 2014. "The Courts." In *Health Politics and Policy*, fifth edition, edited by J. A. Morone and D. C. Ehlke, 76–93. Stamford, CT: Cengage Learning.

King, M. P. 2005. *State Roles in Health: A Snapshot for State Legislators*. Denver, CO: National Conference of State Legislatures.

Kravets, D. 2004. "Arizona Abortion Regulation Invades Privacy, Appeals Court Says." Associated Press, June 19.

Leichter, H. M. 2008. "State Governments: E Pluribus Multa." In *Health Politics and Policy*, fourth edition, edited by J. A. Morone, T. J. Litman, and L. S. Robins, 173–95. Clifton Park, NY: Delmar Cengage Learning.

Liptak, A. 2012. "Supreme Court Upholds Health Care Law, 5–4, in Victory for Obama." *New York Times*, June 28.

Madison, J. 1787. "The Same Subject Continued: The Union as a Safeguard Against Domestic Faction and Insurrection." *Federalist Papers* No. 10. Accessed January 14, 2015. www.ourdocuments.gov/doc.php?flash=true&doc=10.

Martin, A. B., M. Hartman, L. Whittle, A. Catlin, and the National Health Expenditure Accounts Team. 2014. "National Health Spending in 2012: Rate of Health Spending Growth Remained Low for the Fourth Consecutive Year." *Health Affairs* 33 (1): 67–77.

Peters, B. G. 2013. *American Public Policy: Promise and Performance*, ninth edition. Thousand Oaks, CA: CQ Press.

Peterson, M. A. 1993. "Political Influence in the 1990s: From Iron Triangles to Policy Networks." *Journal of Health Politics, Policy and Law* 18 (2): 395–438.

Radley, D. C., D. McCarthy, J. A. Lippa, S. L. Hayes, and C. Schoen. 2014. *Aiming Higher: Results from a Scorecard on State Health System Performance, 2014.* Commonwealth Fund report. Published April 30. www.commonwealthfund .org/publications/fund-reports/2014/apr/2014-state-scorecard.

Sunstein, C. R., D. Schkade, L. M. Ellman, and A. Sawicki. 2006. *Are Judges Political? An Empirical Analysis of the Federal Judiciary*. Washington, DC: Brookings Institution Press.

US Department of State. 2004. *Outline of the U.S. Legal System*. Accessed April 12, 2015. www.america.gov/media/pdf/books/legalotln.pdf#popup.

US Government Printing Office. 2015. "The United States Government Manual." Accessed January 6. www.usgovernmentmanual.gov.

Wheeler, M. 2013. *The Art of Negotiation: How to Improvise Agreement*. New York: Simon & Schuster.

THE PROCESS OF HEALTH POLICYMAKING

Learning Objectives

After reading this chapter, you should be able to

- appreciate some of the important frameworks and theories about policymaking;
- define the stages heuristic policymaking framework;
- draw a schematic model of the phases of the policymaking process;
- understand the relationship between the policymaking process and its external environment;
- discuss the agenda setting and development of legislation activities of policy formulation;
- discuss the designing, rulemaking, operating, and evaluating activities of policy implementation;
- discuss the modification phase of policymaking;
- discuss how the phases of policymaking interact with one another; and
- appreciate the political nature of policymaking.

Whether health policies take the form of laws, rules or regulations, implementation decisions, or judicial decisions, all policies are authoritative decisions made through a complex process. The most important thing to understand about policymaking is that it is a decision-making process. This chapter describes this process. As we will see, with certain variations policies at the federal, state, and local levels of government are made through similar decision-making processes (Bovbjerg, Wiener, and Houseman 2003).

Having considered the context in which health policies are made in the previous chapter (in particular the structure and operations of policy markets), and having identified the demanders and suppliers who interact in these markets and the important operational aspects of these interactions, consideration of the intricate process through which public policies are made is now possible. The discussion begins in this chapter at the conceptual level and includes a schematic model of the core policymaking process; applied discussions of the component parts of the policymaking process follow in subsequent chapters.

Conceptual Frameworks and Theories of Policymaking

As a precursor to discussing any model of the public policymaking process, consideration of some of the important frameworks and theories that have guided inquiry about how the process works will be useful. *Frameworks* guide inquiry by organizing elements and relationships among elements that may lead to theory development (Ostrum, Cox, and Schlager 2014). *Theories*, which are more specific than frameworks, postulate testable relationships between variables (Walt et al. 2008).

Both frameworks and theories are useful devices, but it must be admitted at the outset that there is no universally agreed-upon framework or theory about how the public policymaking process works. Instead, there are many frameworks of and theories about the process (Sabatier and Weible 2014), each offering only a partial explanation of public policymaking. We will review some of the most important and enduring ones and select relevant and workable frameworks and theories around which to structure a model of the policymaking process.

Stages Heuristic

The best known of the policymaking frameworks is the *stages heuristic,* which is attributable to early work by Lasswell (1956). The policymaking process model presented later in this chapter is heavily influenced by this framework. The framework essentially views policymaking as occurring in four stages: agenda setting, formulation, implementation, and evaluation. The framework has been legitimately criticized for oversimplifying reality but remains useful for thinking about the policymaking process.

Among alternatives to the stages heuristic, Walt and Gilson (1994) developed the *policy triangle framework*, which considers how actors, context, and processes interact to produce policy. Another framework, *networks*, evolved to help explain the way growing numbers of actors interact around policy issues (Sabatier and Weible 2014). Policy communities, described in Chapter 2, are simply tightly knit networks.

Multiple-Streams and Punctuated-Equilibrium Theories

Theories, which as noted earlier are more focused than frameworks, have been developed to explain certain aspects of the policymaking process. Among the most important policymaking theories are Kingdon's (2010) *multiple-streams theory* and Baumgartner and Jones's (1993) *punctuated-equilibrium theory*. The multiple-streams theory, which focuses on agenda setting, postulates that problems, possible solutions, and politics flow along in separate streams in our society. Sometimes the streams merge and the confluence creates a *window of opportunity* for government to engage in policymaking. The punctuated-equilibrium theory postulates that policymaking typically proceeds in small incremental steps that can be disrupted by bursts of rapid transformation. The enactment of Medicare and Medicaid in 1965 and the passage of the Affordable Care Act (ACA) decades later are examples of the phenomenon of punctuated-equilibrium in the health domain.

A Core Model of the Public Policymaking Process

Incorporating some of the frameworks and theories noted previously and adding other components, we can diagram the complex and intricate process through which public policymaking occurs. Remember, the most important attribute of this process is that it is a decision-making process. Although such schematic models tend to be oversimplifications, they can accurately reflect the component parts of the process and their interrelationships. Exhibit 3.1 is a model of the public policymaking process in the United States. This model depicts the policymaking process as it occurs at federal, state, and local levels of government. We discuss the component parts of the model in the following sections and then in greater detail in subsequent chapters. As can be seen in the model, policymaking occurs in three interrelated and cyclical phases: formulation, implementation, and modification. Each of these phases of policymaking at the federal level is described in the following sections.

Formulation Phase

The formulation phase of health policymaking is made up of two distinct and sequential parts: agenda setting and development of legislation. Each part involves a set of activities in which policymakers and those who would influence their decisions and actions engage. The formulation phase results in policy in the specific form of new public laws or the far more likely result of amendments to existing laws. In other phases of the process, policies emerge in the forms of rules and regulations and other implementation decisions; policies in the form of judicial decisions can emerge from throughout the entire process.

EXHIBIT 3.1
Three Phases of the Policymaking Process

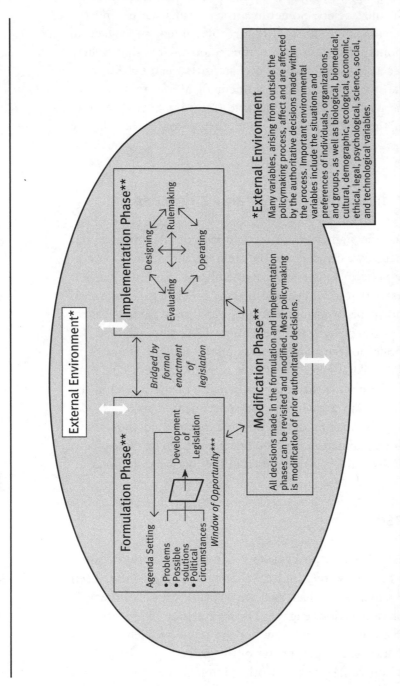

External Environment*

Formulation Phase**

Agenda Setting
- Problems
- Possible solutions
- Political circumstances

Development of Legislation

Window of Opportunity***

Bridged by formal enactment of legislation

Implementation Phase**

Designing ↔ Rulemaking

Evaluating ↔ Operating

Modification Phase**

All decisions made in the formulation and implementation phases can be revisited and modified. Most policymaking is modification of prior authoritative decisions.

*External Environment
Many variables, arising from outside the policymaking process, affect and are affected by the authoritative decisions made within the process. Important environmental variables include the situations and preferences of individuals, organizations, and groups, as well as biological, biomedical, cultural, demographic, ecological, economic, ethical, legal, psychological, science, social, and technological variables.

Policymakers in all three branches of government make policy in the form of position-appropriate, or authoritative, decisions. Their decisions differ in that the **legislative branch is primarily involved in formulation, the **executive branch** is primarily involved in implementation, and both are involved in modification of prior decisions or policies. The **judicial branch** interprets and assesses the legality of decisions made within all three phases of the policymaking process.

***A window of opportunity opens for possible progression of issues through formulation, enactment, implementation, and modification when there is a favorable confluence of problems, possible solutions, and political circumstances.

Agenda Setting

The public laws or amendments pertaining to health are initiated by the inter-actions of diverse health-related problems, possible solutions, and dynamic political circumstances that relate to the problems and to their potential solutions. Before the policymaking process can progress, some mechanism must initiate the emergence of certain problem–solution combinations and their subsequent movement through the development-of-legislation process. In essence, this step is deciding what to make decisions about within the policymaking process.

At any given time, there are many problems or issues related to health. Many of them have possible solutions that are apparent to policymakers. Often these problems have alternative solutions, each of which has its sup-porters and detractors. Diverse political circumstances surround the actual problems and potential solutions. *Agenda setting*, a crucial initial step in the policymaking process, describes the ways in which particular combinations of problems, possible solutions, and political circumstances emerge and advance to the next stage. Agenda setting is discussed in depth in Chapter 5.

Development of Legislation

Once a problem or issue that might be addressed through public policy rises to a prominent, possibly actionable place on the policy agenda—through the confluence of the problem's identification, the existence of possible policy solutions, and the political circumstances surrounding the problem and its potential solutions—it can, but does not necessarily, proceed to the next point in the policy formulation phase, *development of legislation*. Kingdon (2010) describes the point at which problems, potential solutions to them, and political circumstances converge to stimulate legislation development as a *window of opportunity* (see Exhibit 3.1).

At this second step in policy formulation, policymakers propose spe-cific legislation. One can think of these proposals, or bills as they are techni-cally called, as hypothetical or unproven solutions to the problems they are intended to address. The proposals then go through carefully prescribed steps that can, but do not always, lead to policies in the form of new public laws or, more often, amendments to previously enacted laws. The steps in the develop-ment of legislation, also called the *legislative process*, are listed in Exhibit 3.2.

Only a small fraction of the problems, health-related or otherwise, that might be addressed through public policy ever emerge from agenda setting with sufficient impetus to advance them to legislation development. And even when they do, only some of the attempts to enact legislation are success-ful. The path of legislation—that is, of policy in the form of new public laws or amendments to existing laws—can be long and arduous (Hacker 1997). The details of this path that pertain to agenda setting are described more fully

EXHIBIT 3.2
The
Development of
Legislation or
the Legislative
Process at the
Federal Level

Introduction

Anyone may draft a bill; however, only members of Congress can introduce legislation, and by doing so become the sponsor(s). There are four basic types of legislation: bills, joint resolutions, concurrent resolutions, and simple resolutions. The official legislative process begins when a bill or resolution is numbered— *H.R.* signifies a House bill and *S.* a Senate bill—referred to a committee and printed by the Government Printing Office.

Step 1. Referral to Committee

With few exceptions, bills are referred to standing committees in the House or Senate according to carefully delineated rules of procedure.

Step 2. Committee Action

When a bill reaches a committee it is placed on the committee's calendar. A bill can be referred to a subcommittee or considered by the committee as a whole. At this point, a bill is examined carefully and its chances for passage are determined. The committee not acting on the bill is the equivalent of killing it.

Step 3. Subcommittee Review

Often, bills are referred to a subcommittee for study and hearings. Hearings provide the opportunity to put on the record the views of the executive branch, experts, other public officials, supporters and opponents of the legislation. Testimony can be given in person or submitted as a written statement.

Step 4. Mark Up

When the hearings are completed, the subcommittee may meet to "mark up" the bill, that is, make changes and amendments prior to recommending the bill to the full committee. If a subcommittee votes not to report legislation to the full committee, the bill dies.

Step 5. Committee Action to Report a Bill

After receiving a subcommittee's report on a bill, the full committee can conduct further study and hearings, or it can vote on the subcommittee's recommendations and any proposed amendments. The full committee then votes on its recommendation to the House or Senate. This procedure is called "ordering a bill reported."

Step 6. Publication of a Written Report

After a committee votes to have a bill reported, the committee chairman instructs staff to prepare a written report on the bill. This report describes the intent and scope of the legislation, impact on existing laws and programs, position of the executive branch, and views of dissenting members of the committee.

Step 7. Scheduling Floor Action

After a bill is reported back to the chamber where it originated, it is placed in chronological order on the calendar. In the House there are several different

(continued)

legislative calendars, and the Speaker and majority leader largely determine if, when, and in what order bills come up. In the Senate there is only one legislative calendar.

Step 8. Debate

When a bill reaches the floor of the House or Senate, there are rules or procedures governing the debate on legislation. These rules determine the conditions and amount of time allocated for general debate.

Step 9. Voting

After the debate and the approval of any amendments, the bill is passed or defeated by the members voting.

Step 10. Referral to Other Chamber

When a bill is passed by the House or the Senate, it is referred to the other chamber, where it usually follows the same route through committee and floor action. This chamber may approve the bill as received, reject it, ignore it, or change it.

Step 11. Conference Committee Action

If only minor changes are made to a bill by the other chamber, the legislation commonly goes back to the first chamber for concurrence. However, when the actions of the other chamber significantly alter the bill, a conference committee is formed to reconcile the differences between the House and Senate versions. If the conferees are unable to reach agreement, the legislation dies. If agreement is reached, a conference report is prepared describing the committee members' recommendations for changes. Both the House and the Senate must approve of the conference report.

Step 12. Final Actions

After a bill has been approved by the House and Senate in identical form, it is sent to the President. If the President approves of the legislation he/she signs it and it becomes law. Or, the President can take no action for ten days, while Congress is in session, and it automatically becomes law. If the President opposes the bill he/she can veto it; or, if he/she takes no action after the Congress has adjourned its second session, it is a "pocket veto" and the legislation dies.

Step 13. Overriding a Veto

If the President vetoes a bill, Congress may attempt to "override the veto." To override the veto requires a two-thirds roll call vote of the members who are present in sufficient numbers for a quorum. See more at congress.org/advocacy-101/the-legislative-process.

Source: Congress.org (2014). Reprinted with permission.

EXHIBIT 3.2
The Development of Legislation or the Legislative Process at the Federal Level *(continued)*

in Chapter 5, and those that pertain to the development of legislation are discussed more fully in Chapter 6.

Implementation Phase

When the formulation phase of policymaking yields a new or amended public law, *enactment of legislation* marks a transition from formulation to implementation, although the boundary between the two phases is porous. The bridge connecting formulation and implementation in the center of Exhibit 3.1 is intentionally shown as a two-way connector.

The implementation phase of policymaking, including a discussion of the responsibility for implementation, is described here and in more depth in Chapters 7 and 8. As can be seen in Exhibit 3.1, policy implementation unfolds in a series of interrelated steps: designing, rulemaking, operating, and evaluating. These steps are briefly described in this section. First, however, a few words about responsibility for implementation.

Implementing organizations, primarily the departments and agencies in the executive branch of federal and state governments, are established and maintained and the people within them employed to carry out the intent of public laws as enacted by the legislative branch. Legislators rely on implementers to bring their legislation to life. Thus, the relationship between those who formulate policies and those who implement them is symbiotic.

In short, health policies must be implemented effectively if they are to affect the determinants of health. Otherwise, policies are only so much paper and rhetoric. An implemented law can change the physical or social environment in which people live and work, affect their behavior and even their biology, and an implemented law can certainly influence the availability and accessibility of health services.

The implementation phase of public policymaking involves managing human, financial, and other resources in ways that facilitate achievement of the goals and objectives embodied in enacted legislation. Policy implementation is primarily a management undertaking. That is, policy implementation in its essence is the use of resources to pursue the objectives inherent in public laws. This type of management is typically called public administration (Abramson and Lawrence 2014).

Depending on the scope of policies being implemented, the managerial tasks involved can be simple and straightforward, or they can require massive effort. For example, President Johnson, who played a major role in both formulation and implementation of Medicare, observed that implementing the Medicare program represented "the largest managerial effort the nation

[had] undertaken since the Normandy invasion" (Iglehart 1992, 1468). More recently, implementation of the ACA is proving to be a monumental management undertaking (Jacobs and Skocpol 2012; Thompson 2013). No matter the scale, however, the implementation of public laws always involves the set of interrelated activities shown in Exhibit 3.1: designing, rulemaking, operating, and evaluating.

Designing

The relationship among the activities in the implementation phase is essentially cyclical and interactive. As shown in Exhibit 3.1, implementation begins with *designing*, which entails establishing the working agenda of an implementing organization (e.g., the Food and Drug Administration), planning how to accomplish the work, and organizing the agency to perform the work. This activity is rather straightforward management, which is defined as "the process, composed of interrelated social and technical functions and activities, occurring within a formal organizational setting for the purpose of helping establish objectives and accomplishing the predetermined objectives through the use of human and other resources" (Longest and Darr 2014, 255).

More detail about the designing activity is provided in Chapter 8, but suffice to say here that this implementation activity entails the traditional management functions: planning, organizing, staffing, directing (motivating, leading, and communicating), controlling, and decision making (Daft 2014). These interrelated functions, including how decision making intertwines with all the other functions, are shown and briefly described in Exhibit 3.3.

Rulemaking

Again following Exhibit 3.1, the next step in the implementation phase of policymaking is *rulemaking*. Rules, which may also be called regulations, are specific detailed directives developed by implementing organizations in the executive branch. Rules are themselves policies because they are authoritative decisions made in the executive branch to implement laws and amendments. Recall from Chapter 1 that authoritative decisions refer to those made anywhere within the three branches of government that are under the legitimate purview (i.e., within the official roles, responsibilities, and authorities) of those making the decisions. For example, rules promulgated to implement a law are as much policies as are the laws they support. Similarly, operational decisions made by implementing organizations, to the extent that they require or influence particular behaviors, actions, or decisions by others, are policies. Furthermore, decisions made in the judicial branch regarding the applicability of laws to specific situations or the appropriateness of the actions of implementing organizations are policies. By definition, policies

EXHIBIT 3.3
The Management
Functions in an
Implementing
Organization

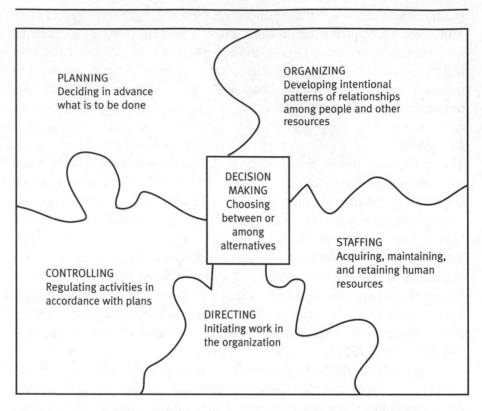

PLANNING
Deciding in advance
what is to be done

ORGANIZING
Developing intentional
patterns of relationships
among people and other
resources

DECISION
MAKING
Choosing
between or
among
alternatives

STAFFING
Acquiring, maintaining,
and retaining human
resources

CONTROLLING
Regulating activities in
accordance with plans

DIRECTING
Initiating work in
the organization

Source: Longest, B. B., Jr., and K. Darr. 2014. *Managing Health Services Organizations and Systems*, sixth edition. Baltimore, MD: Health Professions Press, 259. © 2014 by Beaufort B. Longest, Jr., and Kurt Darr. Reprinted by permission of Health Professions Press, Inc.

are established in both the formulation and implementation phases of the policymaking process.

The Clean Air Act, the Food and Drug Act, the Civil Rights Act, and, more recently, the ACA are all examples of landmark legislation requiring extensive rulemaking to guide their implementation. The rules promulgated to implement laws and amendments can undergo revision—sometimes extensive and continual revision—and new rules can be adopted as experience dictates. This characteristic of policymaking tends to make the process more dynamic than it would be otherwise.

The promulgation of rules is itself guided by certain rules and protocols set forth in legislation. Key among the rules of rulemaking is the requirement that implementing agencies publish *proposed* rules, which gives those with interests in the issue an opportunity to participate in the rulemaking prior to the adoption of a *final* rule. Proposed and final rules are published in the *Federal Register*, a daily publication of important official documents. The rulemaking process is discussed in more detail in Chapter 8.

Operating

Continuing to follow the diagram presented in the implementation phase of Exhibit 3.1, implementation eventually requires those responsible to actually operationalize policies. If a policy in the form of a public law or an amendment to one is intended to protect people from exposure to toxic substances in their environments, for example, its operation entails the activities involved in actually providing such protection. Such activities would include measuring and assessing dangers from substances in the environment and imposing sanctions, such as against polluters. If the intent of legislation is to expand Medicaid enrollment, as is the case with the ACA, successful operation of this policy requires enrolling new people in the program.

The essence of the implementation phase of policymaking is that one or more organizations or agencies undertake the operation of enacted legislation in accord with the design of how to do so and the rules established to guide operating the policy. As will be discussed more fully in Chapter 8, the operation of policies is affected by a number of variables, including the fit between implementing organizations and a policy's objectives as well as the capabilities of the managers in the implementing organizations.

Evaluating

The fourth core activity in implementing policy is *evaluating* (again, see Exhibit 3.1). This activity brings the other elements of implementation full circle and can lead to new rounds of designing, rulemaking, and operating policy. Evaluating, and using the results of evaluation, is an important activity in effective policy implementation.

Fundamentally, evaluating something means determining "its merit, worth, value, or significance" (Patton 2012, 2). Managers of implementing organizations approach this determination by asking questions such as: How effective is the policy, or some component of it? Were the policy's objectives achieved? Do the benefits of the policy justify its costs?

Policy evaluation is defined as systematically collecting, analyzing, and using information to answer basic questions about a policy. There are numerous types of evaluations, including process and outcome evaluations, formative and summative evaluations, and cost–benefit and cost-effectiveness evaluations. Each of these types of evaluations has specific characteristics and uses, which are described more fully in Chapter 8.

The legislative and executive branches of government are involved in policy evaluation and other forms of analysis because they are interested in the performance of the policies they enact and implement. A number of agencies support the evaluation activity at the federal level, including the Agency for Healthcare Research and Quality, which is currently involved in evaluating the ACA's coverage expansions, and the Center for Medicare and Medicaid Innovation, which was established by the ACA to test innovative payment and service delivery models for Medicare, Medicaid, and the Children's Health Insurance Program.

Modification Phase

As we have noted, policymaking is an intricate process. It is not a perfect process. Mistakes of omission and commission are routinely made in the formulation and implementation phases. The policymaking process model presented in Exhibit 3.1 is brought full circle by the third phase of the process, modification. This phase is necessary because perfection eludes policymakers in the formulation and implementation phases. Even policy decisions that are correct when they are made must adjust to accommodate changing circumstances.

In a hypothetical policymaking process without a modification phase, policies would be formulated in their original version and then implemented, and that would be the end of the process—except, of course, for the policies' consequences. In practice, however, policymaking does not work this way. The consequences of policies—including consequences for those who formulate and implement the policies and for the individuals, organizations, and interest groups outside the process but affected by policies—cause people to seek modification. They do so continually throughout the life of many policies.

At a minimum, individuals, organizations, or interest groups that benefit from a particular policy may seek modifications that increase or maintain these benefits over time. Similarly, those who are negatively affected by a policy will seek to modify it to minimize the negative consequences. In addition, when the policymakers who formulate and implement a public policy observe it in operation, they will evaluate it against their objectives for that policy. When preferences and reality do not match, efforts to modify the policy typically ensue.

Policies have histories. An initial version is formulated and then evolves as it is implemented, either through amendments to the original legislation or through new or revised rules and other implementation decisions. Some policies eventually die—they are repealed by the legislative branch—but most have long and dynamic lives during which they are continually modified in various ways. Chapter 9 addresses the policy modification phase of public policymaking in more detail.

Key Features of the Policymaking Process

Having brought the policymaking process full circle, we can now turn our attention to several key features of the policymaking process that are especially helpful in understanding this complicated process. The first of these features is the fact that policymaking does not take place in a vacuum. It occurs in the context of a dynamic external environment with which the process interacts in many ways. We will explore this feature, along with several others, in the following sections.

Policymaking Occurs in the Context of a Dynamic External Environment

An important feature of the public policymaking process is the impact of factors external to the process on policymaking and, in turn, the impact of the process on the larger environment. The impact of external factors is depicted in Exhibit 3.1 by the large double-headed arrows connecting each phase of the process to the external environment. The impact of external factors means the policymaking process is an *open system*, one in which the process interacts with—affects and is affected by—factors in its external environment.

The external environment in Exhibit 3.1 is shown to contain a number of important variables, including the situations and preferences of individuals, organizations, and groups, as well as biological, biomedical, cultural, demographic, ecological, economic, ethical, legal, psychological, science, social, and technological variables. These environmental variables affect the policymaking process and are affected by the policies produced by the process. Technology provides an example of an environmental variable that illustrates the two-way relationship between policymaking and the processes' external environment.

The United States is the world's major producer and consumer of health-related technology. As Exhibit 3.1 shows, technology variables flow into and out of the policymaking process. Technology is produced in part through public funding, and the policies that determine funding levels and priorities, and once in place various technologies must be factored into public and private insurance programs including Medicare and Medicaid. Medical technologies can be cost-increasing, neutral, or cost-saving but must be taken into account in establishing funding for publicly financed health services (Congressional Budget Office 2014; Sorenson, Drummond, and Bhuiyan Khan 2013).

Legal variables provide another example of the two-way relationship between policymaking and its external environment. As we discussed briefly in Chapter 1 and will discuss more fully in Chapter 4, authoritative decisions made within judicial branches of governments are themselves policies. In addition, however, decisions made within the legal system influence other decisions made within the larger policymaking process. Legal variables may help shape all other policy decisions, including by reversing them when they are unconstitutional.

The Phases of the Policymaking Process Are Interactive and Interdependent

While the policymaking model shown in Exhibit 3.1 emphasizes the phases of the policymaking process, it also shows that they are highly interactive and interdependent. Exhibit 3.4 illustrates the interactive and interdependent nature of the three phases of policymaking in a different way.

Furthermore, within the phases, much of the activity is also interactive and interdependent. Designing for implementation—planning, organizing, staffing, directing (motivating, leading, and communicating), controlling, and decision making—leads to rulemaking, which in turn guides the operation of policies, which can be evaluated and may lead to new rounds of designing, rulemaking, and operating.

The public policymaking process modeled in Exhibit 3.1 includes the following three interconnected phases:

1. Policy formulation, which incorporates activities associated with setting the policy agenda and, subsequently, with the development of legislation
2. Policy implementation, which incorporates activities associated with designing for implementation, rulemaking that helps guide the

EXHIBIT 3.4
The Interactive and Interdependent Relationships Among the Policy Formulation, Implementation, and Modification Phases of Policymaking

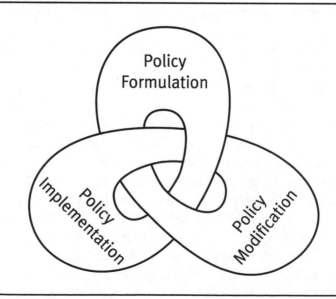

implementation of policies, the actual operationalization of policies, and evaluation, which may lead to subsequent rounds of these activities

3. Policy modification, which allows for all prior decisions made within the process to be revisited and perhaps changed

Once enacted as laws, policies remain to be implemented. The formulation phase (making the decisions that lead to or amend public laws) and the implementation phase (taking actions and making additional decisions necessary to implement public laws) are bridged by the formal enactment of legislation, which shifts the cycle from the formulation to the implementation phase.

Implementation responsibility rests mostly with the executive branch, which includes the Department of Health and Human Services (www.hhs.gov) and the Department of Justice (www.usdoj.gov), and independent federal agencies such as the Environmental Protection Agency (EPA; www.epa.gov) and the Consumer Product Safety Commission (www.cpsc.gov). These and many other departments and agencies in the executive branch exist primarily to implement the policies formulated in the legislative branch. This relationship between policy formulation and implementation is illustrated by the list of major federal laws that the EPA is responsible for implementing (see Appendix 9).

Authoritative decisions made in the course of policy implementation become policies themselves. Rules and regulations promulgated to implement a law and operational protocols and procedures developed to support a law's implementation are policies as surely as is the law itself. Similarly, judicial decisions regarding the applicability of laws to specific situations or regarding the appropriateness of the actions of implementing organizations are public policies. Policies are routinely established within the formulation and the implementation phases of the overall process.

The policy modification phase exists because perfection cannot be achieved in the other phases and because policies are established and exist in a dynamic world. Suitable policies made today may become inadequate with future biological, biomedical, cultural, demographic, ecological, economic, ethical, legal, psychological, science, social, and technological changes. Pressure to change established policies may come from new priorities or the perceived needs of individuals, organizations, and interest groups affected by the policies.

Policy modification, which is shown as two-direction arrows in Exhibit 3.1, may entail only minor adjustments in the implementation phase or modest amendments to existing public laws. In some instances, however, the consequences of implementing certain policies can feed all the way back to the agenda-setting stage. For example, formulating policies to contain the costs of providing health services—a continuing challenge facing policymakers today—is to a large extent an outgrowth of previous policies that expanded access and increased the supply of human resources and advanced technologies to be used in providing health services.

Policymaking Is a Cyclical Process

As Exhibit 3.1 illustrates, the policymaking process is a continuous cycle in which all decisions are subject to modification. Public policymaking is a process in which numerous decisions are reached and then revisited as circumstances change. The continuously cyclical nature of health policymaking can be seen in the pattern of Medicare policy presented in Appendix 10, in which Medicare policy is revisited and modified on a regular basis.

Policymaking occurs in each of the three phases of interconnected activity. In reality, of course, all three phases are active simultaneously. At any point in time, in all levels of governments it is possible to find multiple policies in the form of authoritative decisions being made in each of the three phases. The essence of the flow of these decisions, however, is cyclical: Policy in the form of laws and amendments is formulated, then implemented—which involves more policymaking in the form of designing, rulemaking, operating, and evaluating decisions, and finally, all decisions made in the formulation and implementation phases can be revisited and possibly modified. It helps all involved in the process or affected by the decisions resulting from policymaking to know of the cyclical nature of the process. There is comfort to be taken from the fact that the decisions made in the policymaking process are not final. There is always at least the potential to change unsatisfactory policies.

Policymaking Is a Highly Political Process

One feature of the public policymaking process that the model presented in Exhibit 3.1 cannot adequately represent—but one that is crucial to understanding the policymaking process—is the political nature of the process in operation (Weissert and Weissert 2012). In this process, all decisions are made by humans. Thus, various mixes of altruism and egoism influence what takes place. Human control of the public policymaking process means that its operation, outcomes, and consequences are directly affected by the ethics of those who participate in the process. Ethical considerations help shape and guide the development of new policies by contributing to definitions of problems and the structure of policy solutions.

While many people believe—and still others naively hope—that public policymaking is a predominantly rational decision-making process, this is not the case. The process would no doubt be simpler and better if it were driven exclusively by fully informed consideration of the best ways for policy to support the nation's pursuit of health, by open and comprehensive debate about potential policies, and by rational selection from among policy choices strictly on the basis of ability to contribute to the pursuit of health, and all done by ethical decision makers.

Those who are familiar with the policymaking process, however, know that a wide range of other factors and considerations influence the process. The preferences and influence of interest groups, political bargaining and vote trading, and ideological biases are among the most important of these factors. This is not to say that rationality plays no part in health policymaking. However, it is, at best, only one of many considerations involved in the complex decision making that leads to policy.

The political nature of the policymaking process in the United States accounts for competing theories about how this process plays out. At the opposite ends of a continuum sit strictly public-interest and strictly self-interest theories of how policymakers behave. Policies made entirely in the public interest would be the result of all participants acting according to what they believe to be the public's interest. Alternatively, policies made entirely through a process driven by self-interests would reflect the interplay of the various self-interests of the diverse participants. Policies resulting from these two hypothetical extremes would indeed be different.

In reality, however, health policies always reflect a mix of public-interest and self-interest influences. The balance between public- and self-interests being served is important to the ultimate shape of health policies. For example, the present coexistence of the extremes of excess (the exorbitant incomes of some physicians and health plan managers, esoteric technologies, and various overcapacities in the healthcare system) and deprivation (lack of insurance for millions of people and inadequate access to basic health services for millions more) resulting from or permitted by some of the nation's existing health policies suggests that the balance has been tipped too often toward the service of self-interests. As the ACA is more fully implemented, some of the disparities and gaps in access may be diminished. However, that is unlikely to take place on a large scale for years to come.

Public- and self-interest influences aside, public policymaking in the US health domain is a remarkably complex process, although clearly an imperfect one. The intricacies of the process are explored more thoroughly in subsequent chapters. In general, policymaking is a highly political process, it is continual and cyclical in its operation, it is heavily influenced by factors external to the process, and the component phases and the activities within the phases of the process are highly interactive and interdependent.

Summary

Health policies, like those in other domains, are made in the context of policy markets, where demanders for and suppliers of policies interact, as was described in Chapter 2. The federal, state, and to a lesser extent local governments have important health policy roles, and their policymaking processes are similar.

Public policymaking in the health domain is a human process, a fact with great significance for the outcomes and consequences of the process and one that argues for ethical behavior and good judgment by all involved in the process.

The policymaking process itself, as depicted in Exhibit 3.1, is a highly complex, interactive, and cyclical process that incorporates formulation, implementation, and modification phases. These phases are outlined in this chapter and discussed in greater detail in subsequent chapters.

Review Questions

1. Draw a schematic model of the three phases of the public policymaking process.
2. Describe the general features of the model drawn in question 1.
3. Discuss the formulation phase of policymaking.
4. Discuss the implementation phase of policymaking.
5. Discuss the modification phase of policymaking.

References

Abramson, M. A., and P. Lawrence. 2014. *What Government Does: How Political Executives Manage.* Lanham, MD: Rowman and Littlefield.

Baumgartner, F. R., and B. D. Jones. 1993. *Agendas and Instability in American Politics.* Chicago: University of Chicago Press.

Bovbjerg, R. R., J. M. Wiener, and M. Houseman. 2003. "State and Federal Roles in Health Care: Rationales for Allocating Responsibilities." In *Federalism and Health Policy*, edited by J. Holahan, A. Weil, and J. M. Wiener, 25–57. Washington, DC: Urban Institute Press.

Congress.org. 2014. "The Legislative Process." Accessed February 16. http://congress.org/advocacy-101/the-legislative-process/.

Congressional Budget Office. 2014. "The Budget and Economic Outlook: 2014–2024." Published February. www.cbo.gov/publication/45010.

Daft, R. L. 2014. *Management,* eleventh edition. Mason, OH: South-Western Cengage Learning.

Hacker, J. S. 1997. *The Road to Nowhere.* Princeton, NJ: Princeton University Press.

Iglehart, J. K. 1992. "The American Health Care System: Medicare." *New England Journal of Medicine* 327 (20): 1467–72.

Jacobs, L. R., and T. Skocpol. 2012. *Health Care Reform and American Politics,* second edition. New York: Oxford University Press.

Kingdon, J. W. 2010. *Agendas, Alternatives, and Public Policies,* updated second edition. Upper Saddle River, NJ: Pearson Education, Longman.

Lasswell, H. 1956. *The Decision Process.* College Park, MD: University of Maryland Press.

Longest, B. B., Jr., and K. Darr. 2014. *Managing Health Services Organizations and Systems,* sixth edition. Baltimore, MD: Health Professions Press.

Ostrum, E., M. Cox, and E. Schlager. 2014. "An Assessment of the Institutional Analysis and Development Framework and Introduction of the Socio-Ecological Systems Framework." In *Theories of the Policy Process,* third edition, edited by P. A. Sabatier and C. Weible, 267–306. Boulder, CO: Westview Press.

Patton, M. Q. 2012. *Essentials of Utilization-Focused Evaluation.* Thousand Oaks, CA: Sage.

Sabatier, P. A., and C. Weible (eds.). 2014. *Theories of the Policy Process,* third edition. Boulder, CO: Westview Press.

Sorenson, C., M. Drummond, and B. Bhuiyan Khan. 2013. "Medical Technology as a Key Driver of Rising Health Expenditure: Disentangling the Relationship." *ClinicoEconomics and Outcomes Research* 5: 223–34.

Thompson, F. J. 2013. "Health Reform, Polarization, and Public Administration." *Public Administration Review* 73 (S1): S3–S12.

Walt, G., and L. Gilson. 1994. "Reforming the Health Sector in Developing Countries: The Central Role of Policy Analysis." *Health Policy and Planning* 9 (4): 353–70.

Walt, G., J. Shiffman, H. Schneider, S. F. Murray, R. Brugha, and L. Gilson. 2008. "'Doing' Health Policy Analysis: Methodological and Conceptual Reflections and Challenges." *Health Policy and Planning* 23 (5): 308–17.

Weissert, C. S., and W. G. Weissert. 2012. *Governing Health: The Politics of Health Policy,* fourth edition. Baltimore, MD: Johns Hopkins University Press.

THE ROLE OF COURTS IN HEALTH POLICY AND POLICYMAKING

Learning Objectives

After reading this chapter, you should be able to

- understand how the role of the judicial branch in policymaking differs from the roles of the legislative and executive branches;
- understand the three core roles played by courts in policymaking: constitutional referee, meaning giver, and rights protector;
- understand critical structural features of the judicial branch;
- understand the structure of federal and state court systems;
- understand the concepts of separation of powers, judicial review, and institutional competence;
- appreciate the importance of the states' police power in health policymaking;
- define the Constitution's supremacy clause;
- identify the three most common areas of disputes requiring courts to act as referees; and
- appreciate the importance of *NFIB v. Sebelius*.

As noted in Chapter 1, health policies established in the public sector take the form of laws, rules or regulations, other implementation decisions, and judicial decisions. All are authoritative decisions and, thus, policies. The nation's constitutionally determined structure (see Exhibit 2.1 for the resulting organization chart of the federal government) requires that the legislative branch enact laws, that the executive branch make additional policy to implement the laws, and that the judicial branch, especially through the courts, play a different and less direct part in policymaking (Anderson 1992; Teitelbaum and Wilensky 2013). This chapter explores the vital part the courts play in health policymaking.

This chapter was written by Mary Crossley, professor of law, University of Pittsburgh School of Law.

As we begin to examine how decisions rendered by courts—judicial decisions—are themselves health policy and, more important, how these decisions may significantly affect other health policies and policymaking, it should be acknowledged that some people take a restrictive view of the part courts should play in policymaking. Often using the pejorative phrase "judicial activism," some people assert that courts should not make new law (a job properly handled by the legislative or, to a more limited degree, executive branches), but instead should only apply existing law and interpret any unclear provisions of existing law, all as needed to resolve legal disputes between parties.

This limited view of the judicial role in policymaking reasons that, because judges are not politically accountable (at least in the federal court system where judges are appointed and have life tenure), they should not actually make policy. As this chapter will demonstrate, however, concerns about judicial activism or about judges "making law" are not relevant as applied to the impact that judicial decisions have on health policy and policymaking in the United States (Jacobson, Selvin, and Pomfret 2001). As we will see, even political conservatives, historically identified as critics of activist judges, sanction an important role for courts and invoke courts' authority in ways that affect health policy and policymaking.

This chapter focuses on the traditional core roles or functions of courts in the United States' constitutional scheme of government (see Appendix 11 for additional information on the constitutional scheme of government), how courts performing those roles in individual cases make policy in the form of authoritative judicial decisions, and how those decisions affect other health policies and the policymaking process. We begin our exploration of the unique part courts play in health policymaking by considering the three core roles of courts.

The Core Roles of Courts

This section provides a brief overview of three core roles of the courts. Later sections will more fully describe these roles and provide specific case examples in which courts have played these roles in ways that affect health policy and policymaking.

A long-standing core role of courts in the United States' constitutional scheme of checks and balances among the branches of government is deciding disputes regarding the extent of authority enjoyed by each of the three branches. In performing this role, courts act as *constitutional referees*, making decisions about whether a branch of government has acted within the scope of its constitutional authority or has somehow overreached.

A second core role for courts is interpreting laws whose meaning or application to a particular dispute is somehow unclear. In performing this role, courts act as *meaning givers* in that they clarify the meaning of a law.

A third core role for courts is vindicating (or rejecting) the legal or constitutional rights of parties who come to court alleging a violation of their rights. In performing this role, courts act as *rights protectors* (or rights limiters).

Although these initial descriptions of core judicial roles are brief, much of this chapter is devoted to fleshing out some of their nuances and complicating aspects, as well as examining how each of these core roles of courts affects health policy and policymaking. The judicial branch of government, through the courts, plays a significant part in policymaking by serving as referee, meaning giver, and rights protector.

Premised on the fact that courts have no formal institutional role in either formulating policy (as the legislative branch does) or in implementing policy (as the executive branch does), the central question we examine in this chapter is: How do courts—acting as constitutional referees, meaning givers, and rights protectors—affect health policy and policymaking? What we will see is that, as they decide the cases brought to them by litigants, courts may sometimes play an important role in constraining and shaping policies relating to health, and—more rarely—even in creating them. We will also see how the judicial branch may supplement the work of the other branches, be in tension with what they do, or even have to fill gaps left by the other branches' failure to act.

Before examining these core roles more closely, two general points must be made about them. First, the three roles of courts are not mutually exclusive. In other words, a single lawsuit may call on a court to play more than one role simultaneously. For example, if an individual claims a government action violates one of her constitutional rights, the court hearing the case may have to decide on the existence and scope of the asserted constitutional right (its meaning-giver role) and then determine whether the government's action impermissibly infringes on that right (its rights-protector role).

In thinking about the three core roles that courts play in policymaking, it may be helpful to visualize a simple Venn diagram consisting of three overlapping circles, one for each of the judicial roles outlined previously and as shown in Exhibit 4.1. The diagram reflects that some cases potentially represent a point where the court must play two of its core roles to resolve the parties' dispute; some cases (those represented by the space where all three circles intersect) would require a court to perform all three roles simultaneously.

A second important general point about the three core roles of courts and their impact on health policy and policymaking is the fact that judicial

EXHIBIT 4.1
The Roles
of Courts in
Policymaking

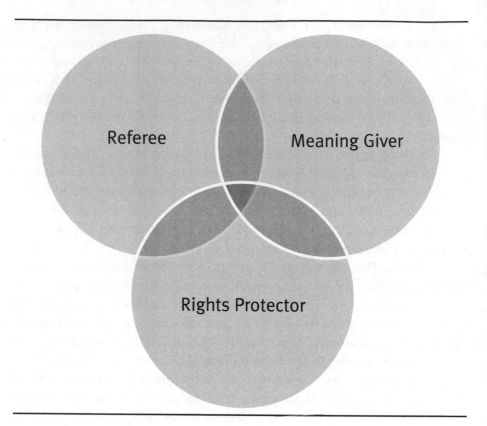

Referee   Meaning Giver

Rights Protector

decisions have effects in the public and private sectors. Recall from our discussion in Chapter 1 that policy is made in both of these sectors. The judicial decisions made by courts affect decisions made by actors in both sectors. This point is important because of the United States' heavy reliance on the private sector for healthcare financing and delivery.

Many decisions that affect the cost and quality of and access to healthcare are decentralized and privatized. For example, until the national health reform accomplished by the Affordable Care Act (ACA), employers had complete discretion to decide whether to provide insurance coverage for their employees, and insurers (whether traditional insurance companies or managed care plans) had great latitude in deciding what benefits to provide as part of their plans. In effect, the aggregated decisions by private-sector actors have provided the answers to many questions that might have been addressed through public policy, but were not.

These private-sector decisions may direct or influence the actions, behaviors, or decisions of others in important matters relating to health. A good example of how judicial decisions constrain or influence private-sector policymaking related to health can be seen in how the courts have interpreted the Employee Retirement Income Security Act (ERISA), a law that Congress passed in 1974 to establish rules for employer pension and benefit plans.

By interpreting how ERISA applies in numerous cases, judicial decisions have played a critical role in establishing the balance of power among employers, health insurers, and employees in health benefits disputes. Later discussion in this chapter will show how specific cases invoking ERISA have required courts to play each of their traditional roles—referee, meaning giver, and rights enforcer.

Before providing a more in-depth discussion of the three core roles the courts play in health policy and policymaking, we will consider as background some key features of the structure and functioning of the judicial system in the United States. This background description includes the division of authority among the three branches of government and between the federal and state governments. It also explains several concepts specific to the judicial system: judicial review, the sources of law that courts rely on, and precedent. After this background discussion on the structure and function of the judicial branch, we will return to a closer examination of how judicial decisions affect health policy and policymaking.

Structure of the Judicial Branch

Two structural features of the judiciary are critical to appreciating how court decisions can affect health policy: (1) the judiciary's existence in a tripartite system of government, where government power is shared among three branches: executive, legislative, and judicial; and (2) the judiciary's existence in a federal system of government, where the authority to make policy is shared between the federal and state governments.

The extensive sharing of power in government, across branches and between levels, gives rise to disputes about whether a particular exercise of power is legitimate or overreaching, or is correctly exercised at the federal or state level. Deciding those disputes is the essence of the core refereeing role of the courts. For example, in this chapter we will discuss court cases that decided whether regulations promulgated by an implementing organization or agency in the executive branch (referred to in this chapter simply as *administrative agencies*) improperly usurped the legislative authority to make laws, as well as cases that considered whether state legislative attempts to enact health reform were invalid because an act of Congress had "preempted" state authority in a particular area.

The Courts in a Tripartite System of Government

As we have noted, under the US Constitution the judiciary is one of three coequal branches of government, each with its own responsibilities and authority. Article III of the Constitution vests the nation's judicial power in the Supreme Court and authorizes Congress to create lower federal courts. Congress has done so, establishing a system of federal district (trial) courts and intermediate courts of appeal, which are divided geographically into 13 federal circuits.

The federal courts have jurisdiction (the legal authority to make decisions or, technically, to enter judgments) over certain types of cases and controversies, including cases involving the federal Constitution or a federal law (also called a statute), as well as certain high-value cases where the parties reside in different states. Although more than 300,000 cases are filed in federal district courts each year, most lawsuits cannot be filed in a federal court because of the courts' limited jurisdiction.

Each state also has its own system of courts to adjudicate legal disputes. Each state judicial system is established by its state constitution and, like the federal courts, the state courts operate within a tripartite system of state government. Unlike federal courts, however, state court systems have "general jurisdiction" over a wide range of cases—basically all cases except a narrow range that can be brought only in federal court (e.g., cases against the United States or cases brought under certain federal laws or statutes). As a result, the large majority of lawsuits are filed in state courts.

Several concepts vital to understanding how the courts operate in a tripartite system of government are discussed in the following sections. These concepts are separation of powers, judicial review, and institutional competence.

Separation of Powers

As noted earlier, at both the federal and state levels the court system shares governmental authority with the legislative and executive branches of government. Under the Constitution's framework, these branches are separate from one another and equally powerful in different ways. Through this *separation of powers*, each branch exercises distinctive but limited powers, a feature the Constitution's framers at the federal level meant to prevent the tyranny that can flow from the concentration of power.

No branch is truly independent of the others, however, because each one's power is limited or "checked" by powers that the Constitution assigns to the other branches. For example, the Constitution gives the legislative branch the power to enact laws, but the president can veto a law that Congress passes and the judicial branch can determine that an act of Congress violates the Constitution. Similarly, while the president has the authority to appoint federal judges, the federal courts can judicially review the constitutionality of executive branch actions. These are only examples of a broader set of constitutional "checks" that seek to strike a "balance" of governmental power among the three branches.

Judicial Review

The judicial branch has the exclusive power of *judicial review*—the power to interpret the Constitution to determine whether an act by a legislative body or an executive official exceeds constitutional limits. This power of judicial review is not expressly granted in the Constitution's text; instead, it is itself the product of judicial decision making in a landmark case (*Marbury v. Madison*) decided in 1803. While lower federal courts interpret the Constitution to assess a law's constitutionality, as a practical matter decisions invalidating laws typically are appealed to the Supreme Court, leaving it the final say on the question.

A court's power to interpret the Constitution to strike down laws enacted by Congress or an executive branch action is potentially enormous. Over the decades, however, the Supreme Court has prudently fashioned limits on when it will engage in judicial review, and the other branches have acquiesced in the Court's exercise of this power. Nonetheless, Supreme Court decisions holding a law unconstitutional are often cited in the political realm as prime examples of judicial activism (or policymaking by the courts). Engaging in judicial review is an important way that courts shape or constrain health policy by limiting (or validating) another branch's formulation or implementation of health policy.

Institutional Competence

Although the division of authority was constitutionally established as a means of protecting against a concentration of governmental power, it also is in accord with the concept that each branch of government has its own particular *institutional competence*. As Gostin (1995) suggests, each branch of government possesses particular strengths and weaknesses relevant to making policy generally and to health policymaking in particular. For example, through the legislative process involving agenda setting and legislation development, the legislative branch can investigate broadly the real-world conditions that require a policy response, including tapping into relevant expertise when needed.

In theory, the legislature can examine the "big picture" to determine whether new policy is needed and what form it should take. Because its members must regularly stand for election, they are publicly accountable, which helps ensure that policies do not deviate substantially from the popular will.

Once the legislature has formulated a new policy, the executive branch is responsible for implementing and enforcing it. In the case of many health policies dealing with complicated financing or delivery systems or scientifically complex health risks, for example, the administrative agencies in the executive branch house the expertise necessary to flesh out policy details through the rulemaking process and perhaps to ensure policy compliance through enforcement actions.

By contrast, courts are not institutionally well suited to formulate or implement policy. Rather than looking at the larger picture of health policy problems and possible solutions, courts must focus on the lawsuit immediately in front of them. A judge's or jury's understanding of the facts is shaped by the parties' presenting evidence in an adversarial process—facts that may be highly germane to the parties' dispute, but may not shed light on social, economic, or health conditions more broadly. Moreover, while judges hearing cases have considerable expertise in interpreting and applying the law, they typically do not have training that would permit a sophisticated evaluation of the scientific, economic, or ethical questions inherent in policymaking in general.

Thus, the division of labor among the three branches of government, each with particular competence, is not only constitutionally mandated, it arguably is also efficient in allocating to each branch the policy-related tasks it is best equipped to handle effectively. Of course, these theories about how things should work don't always play out in the messy arena of real-life governing. The judgment of legislators, which in theory should be focused on the public interest, may be compromised by ideological commitments or by the influence of politically powerful interest groups. Administrative agencies similarly may be subject to powerful interest group pressure or ideological direction. Even the courts themselves are not immune from political pressures. Although recognizing that no system of government is perfect or always lives up to ideal standards, the United States' system of government, featuring its checks and balances, has stood the test of time.

Courts in a Federal System of Government

Because governmental power in the United States is shared between the national and state governments, the power-sharing relationships existing in the levels of government should be addressed. These relationships affect the functioning of courts, and judicial decisions affect the boundaries of these relationships. As was discussed briefly in Chapter 2, in our federal system of government, the term *federalism* refers to the Constitution's division between the national (federal) government and the governments of the states of the authority to govern, including the ability to formulate and implement policy.

The Constitution lists a number of powers that the federal government can exercise (e.g., the powers to tax and spend funds to provide for the nation's defense and general welfare, to regulate interstate and foreign commerce, and to regulate immigration), and that list establishes the boundaries of federal authority. In short, the federal government is often said to be one of "limited powers."

In contrast, the Tenth Amendment of the Constitution makes clear that all governmental powers not accorded to the federal government are "reserved to the States." In other words, the states keep all the powers to govern and regulate that the Constitution does not give to the federal government. This broad scope of governmental power includes the states' "police power," which is their ability to regulate a wide range of areas to protect the common good of their citizens.

This division of governmental authority is evident in health policy. For example, many public health measures enacted by state governments, such as laws requiring vaccination or newborn screening, represent exercises of the police power. The states also retain the power to regulate the practice of medicine, the provision of healthcare services, and insurance, including health insurance. The federal government, by contrast, has used its spending authority to establish federal health insurance programs such as Medicaid and Medicare, its taxing power to fund those programs, and its power to regulate interstate commerce to regulate the marketing of tobacco and prescription drugs.

Questions about whether a particular matter can properly be addressed by Congress or is properly reserved to the states, however, can be contentious politically and legally and typically require judicial resolution. A prominent recent example, discussed in more detail later, is the politically charged question about Congress's constitutional authority to require individuals to purchase health insurance as part of the ACA, a question that the Supreme Court ultimately decided in 2012.

Another important aspect of federalism is the Constitution's supremacy clause, which states that the Constitution and federal laws authorized by the Constitution are the "supreme law of the land." The supremacy clause's effect is that federal laws may be found to preempt any state laws regulating the same subject. As we will see in later discussion, when some states sought to enact health reform measures in the 1990s and 2000s, they found their ability to do so to be constrained and limited by judicial applications of federal preemption under the supremacy clause. Federal preemption also has limited state courts' ability to apply state tort law as a mechanism for compensating consumers harmed by unsafe products, such as pharmaceuticals, regulated by federal law.

In summary, the Constitution creates a system in which the power to govern is shared—shared among the legislative, executive, and judicial branches of government and shared between the federal and state governments. But in any system premised on sharing, situations arise when one participant claims that another is taking more than its allotted share. When these questions arise in our constitutional democracy (e.g., when a state asserts that the federal government is encroaching on rights reserved to the states or when Congress asserts that the president is overreaching his or her authority), the courts are responsible for settling them. In a later section of this chapter, which discusses courts as referees, we will explore several examples of how courts' resolutions of disputes regarding the reach of governmental authority have shaped health policy.

Functioning of the Courts

Beyond the discussion of the structure of the judicial branch and the description of how the courts operate in the federal system of government under the US Constitution, several aspects of how courts function will help us understand how courts make decisions that are by definition health policy and how their decisions in turn may affect other health policy and policymaking. In effect, we want to consider what courts actually do and how they do it.

What Courts Do: Resolving Cases and Controversies

Unlike legislatures, which can identify a problem and affirmatively initiate the policy formulation process in response, courts function in a reactive mode. They act only in response to lawsuits properly filed and subject to their jurisdiction. Only parties who have some stake in the outcome of a dispute or controversy are permitted to pursue litigation. As a result, except in the rare situations when a court is authorized to declare its opinion on a legal question in the absence of a live controversy (by issuing a "declaratory judgment" or "advisory opinion"), courts address legal questions in concrete disputes, not in the abstract or in anticipation of possible future disputes.

Courts resolve those legal questions in an adversarial system where attorneys advocate for their parties' positions, arguing legal authority and factual evidence particular to the case. The trial court (which in some, but not all, cases relies on a jury to determine what version of disputed facts is true) renders a decision resolving the dispute between the parties. If one or both parties disagree with the trial court's resolution and can point to an error in how it reached that resolution, they may choose to appeal the decision to an appellate court.

The federal judicial system has two levels of appellate courts. District (trial) court decisions can be appealed to a federal circuit court of appeals. A party disappointed by the decision of the circuit court of appeals can petition the US Supreme Court to hear its case, but the Court hears argument in and decides only a small percentage of cases in which petitions are filed. As a result, the circuit court of appeals will have the final word in most federal cases where a party appeals. Similarly, most state court systems have two layers of appellate courts, and the states vary in how they address parties' ability to appeal beyond the first appellate level.

Understanding how courts decide cases is important to appreciating courts' role in shaping health policy. While far from a complete description of how courts function, the following discussion highlights several pertinent points about how they work.

How Courts Decide Cases: Identifying, Interpreting, and Applying "the Law"

The central function of the judicial system in the United States is to apply "the law" to the facts of a particular case to resolve a dispute between the parties involved. That dispute may be as mundane as whether a landlord violated the terms of a residential lease, or it may be as momentous as whether an act of Congress violated an individual's constitutional rights. In any case, the court must identify which law applies, what that law means, and how it applies to the particular case's facts.

The law to which the courts look in deciding a dispute derives from multiple sources of potentially binding legal authority. These sources of law include constitutions (federal and state), laws or statutes passed by legislative bodies, rules and regulations issued by implementing organizations and agencies, and the common law (a term referring to the body of judge-made law). In addition, in contract disputes between private litigants, a court is called on to enforce terms that parties have themselves agreed to; in these cases, the court is effectively applying the parties' "private law."

A common misconception is that the "law on the books" provides a clear answer to decide legal disputes. As a practical matter, however, in cases where a statute, regulation, common-law ruling, or contract provides a clear answer, it is rarely in the parties' interest to devote resources to litigating a dispute; these cases typically settle out of court. Consequently, many of the cases that courts are called on to decide raise legal questions for which the law's answer is uncertain.

In many cases this uncertainty reflects the difficulty of determining what general language used in a constitution or statute (or other source of law) means when applied to a specific case. The federal Constitution is itself fairly short and written mostly in general terms, a circumstance that has produced endless controversy over how courts should interpret its terms, with judges and scholars divided on which interpretive method is appropriate.

Statutes, or laws enacted by legislatures, tend to be longer and more specific, with rules and regulations written by administrative agencies being even more detailed and definite. Even so, it is probably beyond the ability of any policymaker to anticipate and provide for every situation that may possibly arise. As a result, courts regularly must give meaning to a source of law that is ambiguous or vague, so that it can then apply the law to resolve the dispute at hand. In the later discussion on courts as meaning givers, we will explore several examples of how courts' interpretations of the law have shaped health policy.

How Courts Decide Cases: The Conservative Influence of Precedent

Given the inherent imprecision of language, the need frequently arises for courts to give meaning to a source of law. As a result, courts exercise significant power in interpreting the law. That power, however, is subject to a restraint found in judicial adherence to the principle of *stare decisis* (meaning "to stand by a decision"). This principle dictates that a court should decide legal questions (like a law's meaning) consistently with how the question has been decided previously by the same court or any court superior to it in the judicial hierarchy. For example, a federal district court follows the precedent of its own prior decisions, decisions of the circuit court of appeals for its federal judicial circuit, and decisions of the US Supreme Court. Reliance on precedent means that a court deciding a new case will be guided by how courts have decided previous, similar cases, thus ensuring some level of stability, predictability, and consistency in the law and satisfying the basic precept of justice that "like cases should be treated alike."

The power of precedent is not absolute, however, and the Supreme Court may overrule a prior decision if a majority of the Court becomes convinced that the prior case was wrongly decided and has produced a rule that is unworkable, particularly in light of changes in society. A notable example of such overruling was the Court's 2003 decision in *Lawrence v. Texas*, which declared unconstitutional Texas's criminal antisodomy statute and overruled the Court's prior decision in another case, *Bowers v. Hardwick*.

With this discussion of the structure and functioning of courts as background, we can return to a fuller consideration of the three roles courts play in health policy and policymaking: refereeing, meaning giving, and rights protecting. Specific cases are noted that illustrate each role.

Courts Acting as Referees

When the complexity of the policymaking process depicted in Exhibit 3.1 and discussed in Chapter 3 is considered, the frequent need for refereeing disputes among various parties is apparent. These disputes arise primarily in three areas: (1) questions of the extent of congressional authority, (2) questions of the power of implementing agencies, and (3) questions of federalism pertaining to federal and state levels of government. Each of these areas is considered in the following sections, with actual case examples.

Courts Refereeing Questions of Congressional Authority

Our discussion of how courts act as constitutional referees to affect health policy begins with one of the most celebrated or reviled, depending on one's opinion about the ACA, Supreme Court decisions in recent times: *National Federation of Independent Businesses (NFIB) v. Sebelius*. This lawsuit challenged the constitutional authority of Congress to enact, as part of the ACA, a requirement that individuals have health insurance or pay a fine to the federal government. This so-called individual mandate is a crucial piece in the ACA's attempt to ensure near-universal health coverage for Americans.

As we have discussed previously, the ACA builds on the nation's existing structure of private health insurance, but restricts insurers' ability to limit or deny coverage or charge higher premiums for persons with pre-existing health conditions. With those changes, the cost of health insurance could be expected to rise sharply unless people who are relatively healthy and young also enroll in health plans. The individual mandate, coupled with tax subsidies for low-income persons, supplied the mechanism to get those young and healthy "good risks" to purchase health insurance. Conceptually, this mechanism would satisfy the concerns of health insurance companies to create larger risk pools and increase access to care for millions of formerly uninsured Americans.

The law's opponents, however, objected that Congress did not have the constitutional authority to enact the individual mandate as part of the ACA. As discussed, the Constitution limits Congress's powers to legislate, and in *NFIB v. Sebelius* the Supreme Court considered the constitutionality of the individual mandate. Proponents of the ACA argued that the power to regulate interstate commerce (articulated in the commerce clause of the Constitution) extended to Congress's ability to mandate the purchase of health insurance as part of a comprehensive regulatory scheme affecting the financing and delivery of healthcare.

The Supreme Court historically has interpreted the commerce clause expansively, permitting Congress to regulate any economic activity that substantially affects interstate commerce. Because of the scope and economic importance of the healthcare and health insurance industries, this expansive reading of the commerce clause has supported a broad exercise of congressional power in health-related fields.

As for the individual mandate, proponents asserted that the failure of millions of Americans to have health insurance undoubtedly affected interstate commerce. The Supreme Court, however, disagreed and held that the individual mandate did not regulate existing commercial activity; instead, it compelled individuals to engage in the activity of purchasing insurance. The Court was unwilling to extend Congress's commerce clause authority to permit regulation of individuals not already acting in the market, fearing that to do so, in the Court's words, "would open a new and potentially vast domain to congressional authority."

Many Court-watchers had assumed that if the Supreme Court held that the individual mandate was not authorized under the commerce clause, it would strike down this linchpin of the ACA, thus crippling the health reform law. To their surprise, the Court proceeded to consider other sources of constitutional authority for the individual mandate and ultimately upheld it as an exercise of Congress's constitutionally based taxing power. Although the law itself refers to the payment that persons who do not have health insurance must make to the government as a "penalty," the Court reasoned that Congress did not mean for the payment to punish persons for failing to purchase insurance, but instead to induce people to purchase coverage and to raise revenue—both of which are characteristic of taxes. Thus, the Court framed the individual mandate as a tax on persons who do not purchase health insurance and therefore within the scope of Congress's taxing powers. As a result, the Court judged the individual mandate to be constitutional.

NFIB v. Sebelius vividly illustrates how courts can affect health policy through their refereeing role. Although the Supreme Court's decision neither formulated nor implemented policy, through the process of judicial review the Court validated a crucial piece of the most sweeping health reform legislation in a generation. A Court decision striking down the individual mandate as beyond Congress's constitutional authority would have severely weakened the ACA.

As referees, courts have the power to rein in legislative policymaking by deciding a policy exceeds constitutional bounds. And although the Supreme Court upheld the individual mandate under the taxing power, many commentators suggest that its commerce clause holding augurs future limitations on congressional power. Finally, as discussed later in the section on courts as federalism referees, judicial decisions regarding the scope of congressional authority also may have implications for the federal government and states' sharing of power to make health policy.

Courts Refereeing Questions of the Power of Administrative Agencies

As we saw in Chapter 3, when Congress (or a state legislature) enacts a policy, it expects certain agencies in the executive branch to implement them. In formal terms, Congress delegates implementation authority to administrative agencies in the executive branch. This authority includes the ability, indeed the responsibility, to write and issue rules and regulations that flesh out the details of a legislatively enacted policy and establish specific standards for regulated parties' compliance with the legislation.

Agencies also enforce those standards and, when a dispute arises about an agency's implementation and enforcement activities (e.g., when an individual disputes the Social Security Administration's determination that the individual is not disabled enough to receive Social Security disability benefits), the agency may adjudicate those disputes. However, when a dispute arises about an agency's authority to act in a particular way, the courts resolve those disputes.

Judicial decisions concerning the validity of an agency's exercise of authority can have an important impact on health policy. Although they all address whether an agency has somehow exceeded its proper authority, three types of challenges can arise. First, a party may challenge an agency's rule or regulation as an unreasonable interpretation of what Congress charged it to do and therefore invalid. A second type of challenge is similar, but goes further in asserting that the agency's promulgation of rules and regulations exceeds the scope of the authority Congress delegated to it. Third, a rule or regulation may be challenged as essentially legislative in nature. In these situations the claim is that the agency has usurped the legislative role by going beyond its role in implementing or enforcing the legislature's policy. Specific case examples illustrate each type of challenge in the following sections.

A Challenge Asserting an Unreasonable Interpretation of Authority: The IRS and Tax Subsidies Under the ACA

Even when Congress clearly delegates to an agency responsibility for issuing rules or regulations on a particular matter, questions may arise about whether the resulting rules or regulations legitimately interpret the authorizing statute. A core precept of administrative law, established by the Supreme Court, is that courts ordinarily should uphold an agency's reading of a law it is responsible for implementing, as long as that reading is permissible (Jost 2004; Richards 2007). This so-called *rule of deference* to agency judgment applies when a law being implemented is silent or ambiguous on some implementation issue. If the law speaks specifically to the issue, the rule does not apply. The rule of deference gives agencies a good deal of leeway in interpreting ambiguous language and filling gaps in laws and prevents courts from simply substituting their own judgment about how best to fulfill the legislature's policy objectives for the agency's judgment.

A contemporary example of this type of dispute can be found in *King v. Burwell*. At issue is the validity of Internal Revenue Service (IRS) rules and regulations making tax subsidies available to persons purchasing health insurance on the federally run health insurance exchanges created under the ACA (Gluck 2014).

The lawsuit asserts that the rules and regulations are inconsistent with the ACA provision providing for tax subsidies, which refers only to exchanges "established by a State." In defending its rules and regulations, the IRS, as the agency with implementation responsibility, takes the position that, viewed in context, the ACA language is unclear and that providing subsidies to purchasers regardless of whether they buy health plans from federally run or state-run exchanges is consistent with the ACA's overall scheme and legislative history. The challengers, by contrast, argue that the particular statutory section's omission of any mention of federal exchanges is clear and unambiguous, so that the IRS interpretation should receive no deference and be struck down. Several lawsuits presenting this challenge have been litigated in the lower federal courts, producing conflicting conclusions, and the Supreme Court has agreed to decide *King v. Burwell* in 2015.

Both sides of the lawsuit agree that if the challenge succeeds, it could potentially hobble the ACA's implementation. In probing the courts' willingness to defer to agency interpretation of a statute, *King v. Burwell* addresses a core question of administrative law and illustrates how critical court decisions can be to the implementation of health policies.

A Challenge Asserting Agency Action Exceeding the Scope of Delegated Authority: The FDA and Tobacco Regulation

Sometimes the judicial challenge to an agency's implementation of a health policy considers whether the organization or agency has overstepped its delegated authority. In the 1938 Food, Drug, and Cosmetic Act (FDCA), Congress delegated to the Food and Drug Administration (FDA) the authority to regulate drugs and medical devices to make sure they are "safe and effective."

In 1996, after decades of mounting evidence regarding the health risks of tobacco and new revelations of tobacco industry deception and efforts to manipulate cigarettes' nicotine levels to enhance addictiveness, the FDA issued regulations designed to restrict the marketing and accessibility of tobacco products to children and adolescents (Gostin 2009). The FDA's rationale was that new evidence confirmed that nicotine was a "drug" and that cigarettes and other tobacco products were "devices" delivering it to users. Thus, the FDA viewed the development and issuance of these rules and regulations as properly within the scope of its authority as granted by the FDCA.

Tobacco companies challenged the rules in court, arguing that they exceeded the FDA's delegated authority under the FDCA. The case ultimately reached the Supreme Court, which in 2000 held in *FDA v. Brown & Williamson Tobacco Corporation* that the FDA lacked any authority to regulate tobacco products.

To reach this conclusion, the Court relied on the interplay of the FDCA's regulatory goal of ensuring that marketed drugs and devices are safe and Congress's passage of other laws specifically regulating tobacco. In short, the Court reasoned that Congress had made clear in other legislation that tobacco products could continue to be sold in the United States, but that regulating tobacco to ensure safety would actually require its removal from the market. Based on this reasoning, the Court found that Congress, in enacting the FDCA, did not intend to give the FDA the authority to regulate tobacco. In this case, the conclusion was not simply that *how* the FDA had regulated tobacco was inconsistent with Congress's policy directives; instead, the Court concluded that any FDA regulation of tobacco was out of bounds.

A Challenge Asserting an Agency's Exercise of Legislative Authority: New York City's Portion Cap Rule for Sugary Drinks

A third type of challenge to administrative agency authority arises from questions as to whether an agency has gone beyond developing and issuing rules and regulations intended to implement the legislature's policy and is instead itself exercising authority that is legislative in nature. Challenges asserting this type of misuse of authority more often arise at the state level. Although the legislative branch at either level of government can delegate to an executive branch agency the authority to interpret and implement a health policy the legislature has enacted, it cannot constitutionally delegate responsibility for making the broad policy judgments inherent in legislating. Any attempt by an agency to make policy judgments that are legislative in nature will be invalid.

When a lower state court, in *NY Statewide Coalition v. NYC Department of Health*, struck down in 2012 the New York City Board of Health's partial ban on the sale of sugary drinks larger than 16 ounces, a judicial determination that the board had made a policy decision reserved for the legislative branch lay at the center of the decision (Mariner and Annas 2013). The Board of Health, which is part of the city's Department of Health and Mental Hygiene, adopted the rule—officially known as the Portion Cap Rule, but popularly referred to as the "Big Gulp Ban"—as part of a broad effort to combat obesity. But the court decided that the City Charter's grant of authority to the Board of Health did not permit the board to ban the sale of a legal item as a means of combatting a chronic disease.

According to the court, any decision to take such a step (and to create a complex set of exceptions to the rule, as the board had done) belongs properly to the legislature, in this case the New York City Council. By this reasoning, when the board adopted the rule, it overreached and acted like a legislature, violating the constitutional separation of powers. According to the judge, such a ban could be made only by an elected city council, not by a board appointed by the mayor. In June 2014, the highest court in New York State affirmed that decision.

The foregoing cases illustrate several ways that courts can affect health policy by functioning as a constitutional referee that establishes the boundaries for how the legislative and executive branches carry out their respective policymaking roles. As the next section describes, the courts, in their referee roles, also may settle disputes about how the power to make health policy is shared between the federal government and the states.

Courts Refereeing Federalism Questions

As noted earlier and discussed extensively in Chapter 2, both the federal and state governments have constitutional authority to make health policy, although the scope of their authority differs. Congress's authority is limited to its exercise of its enumerated constitutional powers, while all other powers are reserved to the states. This section explores how court decisions settling conflicts between federal and state exercises of authority can affect health policy. As we will see, in some cases the existence and exercise of federal power limits states' ability to make health policy relating to a particular concern, but in other instances state interests may constrain the exercise of federal power. In yet other situations, both the federal and state governments can make policy in a certain area, as long as their policies (often in the form of rules or regulations) do not conflict.

"Cooperative Federalism" and Federal Coercion

In the constitutional scheme of government in the United States, the federal government cannot constitutionally compel a state to enact a particular policy, nor can it "commandeer" state employees to implement policies adopted by Congress. Pursuant to its constitutional spending power, however, Congress can provide the states with financial incentives to pursue certain policy objectives. An example of the use of this motivational power was Congress's conditioning the disbursement of federal highway funds on each state's raising its legal drinking age to 21 years.

Another health-related example of Congress's power to incentivize states' behaviors was the enactment of the Medicaid program. As we have discussed, the federal government provides substantial matching funds for state-administered health insurance programs for poor people, as long as the state program meets certain federal standards.

The label "cooperative federalism" is sometimes applied to the federal government's use of financial incentives to encourage state-level implementation of federal policies. In such an approach, the federal and state governments act autonomously, but their policy interventions are cooperative. While largely positive, cooperative federalism does raise the possibility that the federal government's financial inducement to a state—if extremely strong—could effectively override the state's autonomy in formulating policy.

Implementation of the ACA, for example, relies heavily on cooperative federalism, but one aspect of the law was judged to violate federalism principles. We noted in earlier discussion that the Supreme Court played a crucial role by determining the constitutionality of the individual mandate provision of the ACA. In the same case, *NFIB v. Sebelius*, a second important question arose, a federalism question dealing with a challenge to the constitutionality of the ACA's Medicaid expansion provision (Kaiser Family Foundation 2012).

The ACA originally conditioned continued federal Medicaid matching funds on each state's expanding its Medicaid eligibility criteria. The change in criteria would have expanded Medicaid from a program providing health coverage only to certain categories of poor people (e.g., children, pregnant women, people with disabilities, elderly individuals) to a program covering all persons with income below a certain threshold. According to the ACA, a state that chose not to expand coverage would lose all federal matching funds from its Medicaid program.

Opponents of the ACA argued that when Congress induced the states to expand Medicaid eligibility by threatening the loss of all their federal Medicaid funding, it acted coercively, not cooperatively, and thus exceeded its spending power authority. A majority of the Supreme Court in *NFIB v. Sebelius* agreed. According to Chief Justice Roberts, the amount of federal funding that states stood to lose if they did not expand their Medicaid eligibility criteria was so large that the law left states with no real choice—instead, the threatened loss of funding was like a "gun to the head" of the states. From this perspective, Congress was unconstitutionally compelling states to expand Medicaid under the guise of making a constitutionally valid conditional grant of federal funds.

Once the Court found that the ACA's expansion of Medicaid represented an unconstitutional compulsion of state action, though, the question became what effect that finding of unconstitutionality would have on the health reform law. One possibility (which four dissenting justices endorsed) was that the unconstitutionality justified striking down the entire law. Another, less drastic result could have been to sever from the rest of the ACA all provisions of the law relating to the Medicaid expansion and to strike down only the expansion provisions as unconstitutional. That result would have left in force the health insurance market reforms, the individual mandate, and numerous other provisions of the ACA, but no state would expand Medicaid, meaning that the approximately 17 million uninsured low-income persons expected to benefit from the expansion would not receive coverage.

Instead, a majority of the Court concluded that it could remedy the unconstitutionally coercive nature of the Medicaid expansion simply by removing the coercion; their remedy was to deny the federal government's ability to withhold *all* Medicaid matching funds from states choosing not to expand. This remedy left states able to choose *either* to expand their Medicaid population as called for by the ACA and receive federal funding for the expanded population *or* to maintain their Medicaid program at pre-ACA coverage levels, without losing their existing funding.

The Medicaid expansion part of the *NFIB v. Sebelius* decision dramatically demonstrates the Court's power to affect health policy. As with the question of the individual mandate's constitutionality, it was within the scope of the Court's judicial review powers to strike down the health reform law entirely as unconstitutional, which would have rendered moot all the legislative and executive branch efforts to enact and implement the law. But even though it found that Congress exceeded its constitutional authority by attempting to coerce states to expand their Medicaid programs, the Court adopted its more modest remedy so that it could avoid unnecessary judicial intrusion on the legislative authority to formulate policy. In effect, the Court's decision permitted Congress to adopt the Medicaid expansion as a way to increase insurance coverage in states that cooperated, but denied its ability to compel states to go along with that policy.

The Supremacy Clause and Federal Preemption

The Supreme Court's decision in *NFIB v. Sebelius* regarding the Medicaid expansion used the spending clause of the Constitution to constrain Congress's ability to induce states' compliance with federal health policy objectives, but the more typical power-sharing disputes between the federal government and states involve the supremacy clause of the Constitution.

As noted earlier, the supremacy clause declares the Constitution and federal laws authorized by the Constitution to be the "supreme law of the land." Its effect is to permit Congress, by enacting a law on a particular topic, to preempt state laws in that area. The preemption may extend to state common-law actions (e.g., negligence or product liability lawsuits), as well as to statutory law. As a result, questions have arisen about the validity of state health policy initiatives in areas as diverse as a state-mandated hospital budget review for cost-containment purposes (not preempted), a state law prohibiting a particular form of hazardous waste disposal (not preempted), and a state law imposing burdensome requirements on "navigators" charged by the ACA to help consumers use insurance exchanges to enroll in health plans (preempted).

As these examples suggest, federal laws do not always preempt state laws or rules and regulations, and part of the courts' role as constitutional referees is to determine when the supremacy clause and federal preemption apply. The central issue in determining preemption is whether the federal policymakers intended that the federal law displace state laws on the same subject. If a federal law explicitly includes a stated purpose of preempting state laws on the same subject, then a court simply interprets the statute's preemption language to determine whether the particular state law being challenged falls within the scope of preemption. The courts had to make such a decision, for example, when the Massachusetts attorney general issued regulations prohibiting retailers from using self-service displays of cigarettes and banning outdoor advertising of cigarettes in any location within 1,000 feet of a school. Cigarette manufacturers and retailers challenged the regulations as preempted by the Federal Cigarette Labeling and Advertising Act (FCLAA).

The FCLAA prescribes mandatory health warnings for cigarette packaging and advertising and contains an express preemption of state prohibitions "based on smoking and health" relating to cigarette advertising. Massachusetts argued that this preemption did not extend to state regulation of the location of cigarette advertising, as opposed to the content of cigarette advertising, an argument that some lower federal courts accepted. The Supreme Court, however, held in *Lorillard Tobacco Company v. Reilly* that Congress intended to preempt all health-motivated state regulation targeting cigarette advertising, including location restrictions. According to the Court, Congress's decision in the FCLAA to require health warnings on cigarette packaging and advertising and to include a broad preemption clause meant that Massachusetts could not implement its own policy to decrease youth exposure to cigarette advertising by regulating its location.

Even when Congress does not expressly state its intent to preempt state law, a court may find that preemptive intent is implicit in a federal policy. Perhaps the easiest case for finding preemption is when a state law directly conflicts with a federal law. If it would be physically impossible to comply with both the federal and state requirements, a court will invoke the supremacy clause to invalidate the state law. In sum, judicial decisions determining the existence and scope of federal preemption of state law in health-related areas establish a balance of authority between the states and the federal government.

Courts Acting as Meaning Givers

As we noted earlier, a second core role for courts is interpreting laws whose meaning or application to a particular dispute is somehow unclear. In this role, courts function as meaning givers, by clarifying the meaning of laws. In this section, we examine more extensively how courts performing their role as interpreters of the law—meaning givers—can shape the direction or evolution of health policies. There are of course situations in which the law is entirely clear and needs no interpretation, but the facts are in dispute. For example, in a personal injury lawsuit it may be perfectly clear that the defendant will be liable to the plaintiff for injuries sustained in a car accident if he ran a red light before hitting her, but a factual dispute may exist about whether or not the light was red when the defendant went through the intersection. In that case, the court's primary role is that of fact-finder. Often, however, interpretation or meaning giving is needed.

It bears noting that courts actually play the meaning-giver role in most lawsuits. In each of the cases discussed in the previous section, for example, a court had to interpret the Constitution or a law to make a decision about whether a branch of government had acted within the bounds of its constitutional authority or how power should be shared between the federal and state governments.

The cases examined in this section, however, highlight how courts' interpretation of the language of laws can determine the language's policy impact. We will see that court decisions sometimes play an important role in establishing the effects of legislative action. The cases in this section also will preview the final section's discussion of cases in which courts' predominant role is to enforce rights claimed pursuant to contracts, statutes, or the Constitution. In those cases, courts may first have to interpret the relevant source of law to determine the existence and scope of the right claimed.

In particular, this suggests different scenarios where court decisions giving meaning to laws effectively delineate the policy implications of Congress's handiwork. First, in looking again at how broadly to interpret preemptive language in a federal law, we will see how courts' parsing of the preemption clause in a law having little to do with health has substantially affected states' ability to pursue state-level healthcare reforms. The discussion will then turn to judicial interpretations of statutes that regulate the conduct of actors in the healthcare marketplace and create rights on the part of healthcare consumers.

ERISA Preemption and State Health Reform

When Congress enacted ERISA in 1974, its main goal was to create a federal regulatory scheme for employer-sponsored pension plans to make sure they met certain standards for protecting employees. Congress, however, drafted the law to apply to employee benefit plans more broadly, including healthcare benefit plans. The law does not require employers to offer any particular benefit, but instead sets up uniform standards for administering whatever benefits are offered. Congress wanted to encourage employers to establish plans by displacing all state regulation of employee benefit plans; this preemption of state law would permit large multistate employers to avoid having to comply with varying and potentially conflicting plan regulations in different states.

To that end, ERISA includes a broadly worded preemption clause stating that it preempts all state laws that "relate to" employee benefit plans covered by ERISA. Although it wanted to establish the regulation of employee benefit plans—and particularly pensions—as an area of exclusive federal concern, Congress was concerned about unduly intruding on areas of traditional state regulation. So it qualified ERISA's preemption clause with a "savings" clause, which effectively saves from preemption any state law that "regulates insurance." Thus, in essence, state laws that relate to employment benefit plans are preempted, *but* a state can regulate insurance companies.

This gets even more complicated in a situation in which an employer provides health coverage for its employees by self-insuring (i.e., by acting as the insurer itself), rather than by purchasing contracts of insurance from an insurance company. ERISA anticipated this possibility. The statute includes an exception to the savings clause that provides an employee benefit plan shall not be deemed to be in the business of insurance for purposes of applying the savings clause. The simple effect of this "deemer clause" is to qualify the description provided earlier, as follows: State laws that relate to employment benefit plans are preempted, *but* a state can regulate insurance companies, *except for* an employee benefit plan that self-insures to provide health benefits. Language like this and complex legal provisions including exceptions to exceptions ensure a continuing vital role as meaning givers or interpreters for the courts!

For several decades following its enactment, the combination of ERISA's preemption clause, its savings clause, and its deemer clause produced a steady stream of lawsuits probing the precise scope of ERISA's preemption of state health policies. Typically, employers or insurance companies filed these lawsuits to argue that a state law could not be enforced against them because it was preempted by ERISA. The lawsuits required courts to interpret ERISA's statutory language to make decisions with important implications for states' ability to enforce their health policies.

Complicating matters, some of the language in this law that courts had to give meaning to is vague. (What does it mean for a state law to "relate to" an employee benefit plan? What kinds of state laws "regulate insurance"?) This vagueness left courts with a good deal of interpretive latitude. Indeed, numerous decisions by courts, including the Supreme Court, about how to interpret ERISA's preemption provisions over time have swung from an expansive understanding of ERISA's preemptive effect to a more limited one. According to Furrow and colleagues (2013, 370), ERISA preemption lawsuits have included "over twenty Supreme Court decisions and hundreds of state and federal lower court decisions." As a result, states' ability to pursue health policies having any connection to employer-provided health insurance over time has waned and, more recently, waxed.

A few examples help illustrate the role courts have played in disabling or enabling state health policies arguably related to ERISA. For several decades, many state legislatures passed laws requiring health insurers to include in their policies certain types of coverage (e.g., mental health coverage or maternity coverage). Because these "mandated benefit" laws applied to policies purchased as part of an employee benefit plan, insurers argued that the laws were preempted by ERISA. By interpreting the interaction of the preemption clause and the savings clause, the Supreme Court held in a 1985 case, *Metropolitan Life Insurance Company v. Massachusetts*, that a state law mandating coverage of certain mental health benefits did "relate to" employee benefit plans, but was saved from preemption as a law that "regulates insurance." In that case the Court went on to apply the deemer clause to conclude that the mandated benefit law could not be enforced against a self-insured plan providing health coverage to employees. As a result, workers whose employers bought group coverage from an insurance company would receive the benefit, but employees of self-insured employers might not. This result both frustrated the state's policy goal of ensuring coverage of the mental health services and provided additional incentive for employers to self-insure to avoid mandated benefits and other state regulation.

As Jacobson (2009, 88) describes, expansive judicial interpretations of ERISA's preemption provisions at least through the mid-1990s meant that, even as federal policy makers unable to enact comprehensive national health reform encouraged states to pursue their own reforms, a federal law "imperil[ed] aggressive state health coverage experiments." Since the mid-1990s, several Supreme Court decisions have suggested that lower courts should interpret ERISA's "relate to" language in the preemption clause more narrowly (which would shrink the law's preemptive scope) and should interpret the "regulates insurance" language in the savings clause more broadly (which would enlarge states' ability to adopt policies implicating health coverage). For example, in *New York State Conference of Blue Cross and Blue Shield Plans v. Travelers Insurance Company* in 1995, the Supreme Court found that a New York law imposing hospital bill surcharges on most commercial insurers survived preemption. Although the surcharge law had some economic effect on employee benefit plans, the Court read ERISA's "relates to" language as not extending to such an indirect effect.

In 2003, in *Kentucky Association of Health Plans, Inc. v. Miller*, the Supreme Court interpreted the savings clause to uphold a Kentucky "any willing provider" law (requiring health plans to permit any willing provider to join their networks) as a law that "regulates insurance." In that case, the Court adopted a new approach, more permissive of state regulation, to determining whether a state law "regulates insurance" for ERISA savings clause purposes. Thus, evolving judicial interpretations of ERISA's preemption provisions have alternatively constrained and permitted many state health policy initiatives.

Judicial Interpretations of Laws That Regulate the Health Markets and Create Consumer Rights

Besides determining the breadth of federal preemption in the health policy domain, judicial interpretations of the substantive provisions of laws affect health policy and policymaking in other ways. Almost any law can require some judicial explication to clarify its meaning in a particular circumstance. Courts, however, are most likely to be called on to interpret or give meaning when (1) legislative language is vague or ambiguous, with multiple plausible meanings, and (2) a party trying to claim a right or avoid regulation under the statute has enough at stake to litigate its meaning.

When a public entity (e.g., an administrative agency with enforcement authority such as the Centers for Medicare & Medicaid Services or a state attorney general) brings a lawsuit to enforce a law's regulatory provisions, the court's interpretive judgment most obviously determines whether enforcement will succeed in the particular case. It may also signal to the enforcer and other regulated parties the types of conduct that might (or might not) trigger enforcement actions in the future. For example, in a 1982 case, *Arizona v. Maricopa County Medical Society*, the Supreme Court interpreted federal antitrust law (specifically, the Sherman Act's rule against price fixing) to find agreements among physicians setting the maximum fees to be charged to policyholders to be illegal per se. This decision signaled to doctors and other actors in health markets that neither physicians' status as professionals nor the courts' relative inexperience with applying antitrust law to the healthcare industry would immunize them from antitrust liability (Hammer and Sage 2002). From a policy perspective, the court decision also gave a green light to regulators to proceed with enforcement actions in the health field as a way to try to spur competition, efficiency, and cost savings.

Many laws create rights on the part of individuals to enforce the law through private lawsuits (or administrative adjudications). In cases involving such laws, Medicare for example, a court decision interpreting unclear statutory language determines the current plaintiff's ability to prevail, as well as the exposure of regulated parties to future similar suits.

One law in which individual enforcement has been particularly important and where the courts have struggled to give meaning to spare statutory language is the Emergency Medical Treatment and Active Labor Act (EMTALA). Congress enacted EMTALA in 1986 to address the problem of emergency rooms' "dumping" patients (refusing to see them or sending them immediately to a public hospital) because the patient was uninsured and unable to pay potentially large hospital bills (Perez 2007).

In formulating EMTALA as a response to this problem, Congress knew precisely what problem it wanted to address. The language it used in the law, however, failed in several respects to make clear exactly what the law obligated hospitals to do and, by extension, when patients harmed by violations have a right to recover. The most glaring of the law's ambiguities is the requirement that a hospital covered by EMTALA provide an "appropriate medical screening examination" to any person who comes to an emergency room seeking treatment.

EMTALA does not define the phrase "appropriate medical screening examination," and the text of the law provides only a few clues as to what Congress intended the phrase to mean. The law provides only that the screening examination is to be "within the capability of the hospital's emergency department" and that its purpose is "to determine whether or not an emergency medical condition . . . exists." As a result, when patients who suffered some kind of harm after visiting a hospital emergency room sued the hospital for violating EMTALA, it was left to the courts to distinguish an "appropriate medical screening examination" from one that somehow fell short of EMTALA's requirements.

As the court put it in a 1990 case, *Cleland v. Bronson Health Care Group, Inc.*, *appropriate* is "one of the most wonderful weasel words in the dictionary, and a great aid to the resolution of disputed issues in the drafting of legislation." In other words, *appropriate* is a handy term for promoting agreement among legislators, precisely because it sounds good while having no specific meaning.

As plaintiffs filed lawsuits alleging violations of EMTALA, courts had to give some meaning to an "appropriate medical screening examination." In doing so they relied on the clues in the rest of the law, as well as evidence of Congress's intent in enacting the law. It was clear that Congress did not intend to create a new federal cause of action for medical malpractice, or negligent medical care, and accordingly the courts consistently have rejected any argument that an "appropriate screening" requires a nonnegligent screening.

The courts have been less consistent in developing tests for what makes a screening inappropriate. Although most of the federal circuit courts of appeals have adopted the standard that a hospital's screening of a particular patient should be considered "appropriate" as long as it was similar to the screening the hospital typically gives to patients presenting with similar symptoms, some federal circuit courts of appeals have used a slightly different approach. Because the Supreme Court has not addressed this question, no definitive answer exists. The result of Congress's use of vague language in EMTALA is therefore that the standard a hospital is held to in screening an emergency room patient may vary depending on which federal circuit a hospital is located in. Thus, one downside of relying on courts to give meaning to a policy is that—unless the Supreme Court provides a definitive interpretation—judicial interpretations of the legislature's policy objectives may not be consistent.

Courts Acting as Rights Enforcers

The discussion in the previous section of the policy implications of courts' interpretations of EMTALA illustrates how courts can play multiple roles in a single lawsuit. For example, in a patient's lawsuit alleging that a hospital failed to provide an "appropriate medical screening examination," the court must first give meaning to the statutory requirement; then it applies that requirement to the plaintiff's factual scenario. In doing the latter, the court decides whether the hospital violated the plaintiff's statutory right to the required screening, so that the plaintiff is entitled to a monetary judgment against the hospital. Thus, in these cases the court acts as both meaning giver and rights enforcer. Other laws on both the federal and state levels also create health-related rights for patients and providers, and persons who believe their rights have been violated may seek remedies through the courts.

This section, however, will focus primarily on how the courts' enforcement of (or, by contrast, limitation or denial of) common-law rights and constitutional rights can affect health policy. We will first consider how judicial resolution of claims brought by health plan subscribers against their plans can affect health policy. This discussion entails revisiting the subject of ERISA preemption, which has severely limited plan members' ability to sue for a denial of benefits. This section and the chapter will then conclude by considering how court decisions involving constitutional rights of both individuals and corporations have had an important impact on health policy.

Enforcement of Contract and Tort Rights: ERISA Preemption Revisited

Traditionally, a subscriber to a health insurance plan who believed her plan improperly had refused to pay for covered benefits could sue the plan in state court for breach of contract. The lawsuit would require the court to interpret and apply language in the health insurance policy (e.g., whether a particular treatment prescribed for the subscriber fell under the policy's exclusion of "experimental" treatments). And in a managed care setting, if a plan also employed physicians and other providers, a subscriber might file a tort action against the plan if he believed he had suffered injury because his doctor had skimped on his care to save the plan money. That tort action would require the court to decide whether the doctor had acted negligently in making medical decisions or treating the plaintiff.

Over the past several decades, however, courts regularly have found that ERISA preempts contract and tort lawsuits brought by plaintiffs who receive their health coverage through employer-sponsored health plans. As discussed, ERISA preempts state laws—including common-law contract and tort claims—that "relate to" employee benefit plans. Courts have interpreted ERISA's "relate to" preemption language broadly and also have invoked another provision of ERISA that limits remedies for the denial of benefits to a remedy provided by ERISA itself. As a result, courts have kept dissatisfied subscribers from pursuing state law claims, leaving them only the option to go after the remedy provided for in the law itself. The remedy provided by ERISA, however, is limited, permitting a plan member to recover only the value of the benefit that was improperly denied. By contrast, a broader range of remedies (and more generous damages awards) is available to a subscriber who prevails in a contract or tort action. Thus, the preemption of state law claims disadvantaged health plan subscribers who claimed they had been harmed by health plan decisions to limit their care.

Moreover, as Jacobson (2009) points out, these judicial decisions also had important policy implications. Because the preemption decisions limited the remedies available to plan members, they also limited the liability exposure of managed care plans. If the plan got sued and lost, it would have to pay the injured subscriber only the value of the benefit it should have provided to begin with. This judicial application of ERISA to provide plans protection from potential liability for a full range of economic, pain and suffering, and punitive damages effectively gave managed care organizations a green light to employ a variety of techniques to control costs aggressively.

At the same time, however, as news media began covering the plight of injured plan beneficiaries left without a meaningful remedy, the court decisions also prompted state legislatures and Congress to consider possible legislative fixes in the form of a "Patients' Bill of Rights" that would provide some kind of protections to health plan enrollees. Although congressional efforts in the 1990s and early 2000s to enact a federal patients' bill of rights ultimately failed, several states enacted such reforms (Law 2002). Thus, the story of ERISA preemption of health plan subscriber claims illustrates how courts' denial of subscribers' common-law rights catalyzed efforts to enact statutory protections.

Enforcement of Constitutional Rights

In contrast to the common law, which typically creates rights between private parties, the Constitution creates private rights against the exercise of governmental authority. Although state constitutions are also sources of important individual rights, this discussion focuses on the federal Constitution. While the Constitution's separation of powers and federalism provisions prevent the concentration of power in any one branch of government and limit the government's authority to act in the first instance, the Bill of Rights and the Constitution's Fourteenth Amendment guard certain rights of individuals (and in some cases corporations) against governmental intrusion. For health policy purposes, the most important of these constitutional rights are found in the First Amendment (with its protection of free speech and religious freedom) and the Fourteenth Amendment (with its guarantees of equal protection and due process). Persons seeking the vindication of their constitutional rights call on the courts to claim those rights.

As Gostin (1995) points out, the courts have played their most robust—and controversial—role in making policy decisions with respect to constitutional rights in health-related matters. By recognizing constitutional protections of individual rights relating to reproduction (both contraception and abortion rights) and end-of-life decision making, the Supreme Court has addressed issues that are socially divisive and that legislatures had often failed to address. As a result, the "judiciary . . . has sometimes acted as a pathfinder when there was a paucity of established policy" (Gostin 1995, 345).

The effect of the Court's decisions on legislatures' ability to formulate policies in the areas of reproductive and end-of-life rights varies, though. The Court's decisions in the 1960s and 1970s establishing individual rights relating to contraception and abortion limited states' ability to enact policies regulating these areas, but subsequent Court decisions have eroded those limitations, emboldening state legislatures in recent years to enact a plethora of laws regulating abortion. By contrast, while assuming the Constitution provides some protection to individual autonomy in end-of-life decision making, as it did in the 1990 *Cruzan v. Director, Missouri Department of Health* case, the Court has been unwilling to declare that individuals have an absolute right either to terminate medical treatment or to receive physician assistance in dying. This reluctance largely leaves policy decisions about end-of-life care to state legislatures, many of which have enacted laws in the area.

The ability to assert constitutional rights is not limited to individuals; the Supreme Court has recognized that corporations may also claim some constitutional protections. Corporations' success in convincing courts to recognize their First Amendment free speech rights provides a vivid illustration of how court decisions can affect health policy, and in particular the government's ability to protect public health through tobacco policy.

In 2009 (nine years after the Supreme Court held that the FDA did not have delegated authority under the FDCA to regulate tobacco), Congress passed the Family Smoking Prevention and Tobacco Control Act (P.L. 111-31) granting the FDA that authority. One provision of that act mandates that the FDA develop new written health warnings to go on cigarette packages, as well as to select images to accompany those textual warnings (Orentlicher 2013).

In 2011 the FDA made public the nine images it proposed to go on cigarette packages, some of which were quite disturbing. Tobacco companies filed First Amendment challenges to the statutory mandate that the FDA develop graphic warnings for cigarette packages and the actual images the FDA selected. The challenges essentially asserted a violation of the companies' First Amendment right to free speech, arguing that the government did not have a strong enough interest in promulgating the graphic warnings to be able to compel the companies to "speak" against their own interest by including the warnings on their product (Berman 2009; Cortez 2013). Although in 2012 one federal circuit court of appeals upheld Congress's authority to require graphic warnings in *Discount Tobacco City & Lottery, Inc. v. United Sates*, another circuit court of appeals in the same year, in *R.J. Reynolds Tobacco Co. v. FDA*, found that compelling tobacco companies to include the images actually chosen by the FDA on their cigarette packages would violate the companies' First Amendment rights.

What happened next is telling. Normally, when federal courts of appeals from different circuits disagree on the constitutionality of a federal law, the issue is ripe for Supreme Court review. But rather than risk a Supreme Court decision that might establish new precedent broadly limiting the government's ability to protect the public's health by requiring warnings on dangerous products, the FDA chose to withdraw its proposed graphic warnings and announced that it would work on developing new images. As this book goes to press, the FDA is still working on crafting new graphic images deemed more certain to withstand constitutional scrutiny. The tobacco companies' ability to resort to the courts to try to block the FDA's proposed graphic warnings demonstrates how an expansive judicial understanding of corporate First Amendment rights can constrain the government's pursuit of health policy.

Summary

In the drama of policymaking, courts do not typically play the leading role. The cases discussed in this chapter, however, demonstrate that the courts frequently play an important supporting role that may shape or constrain policy formulation and implementation. Courts' traditional roles include performing judicial review of government action, interpreting the law, and applying the law to settle disputes between litigating parties. By acting as constitutional referees, meaning givers, and rights enforcers, courts have affected the development of numerous health policies in areas ranging from national health reform, to tobacco policy, to the regulation of employer-provided health insurance.

Review Questions

1. Discuss the three traditional core roles or functions of courts in the United States' constitutional scheme of government.
2. How do courts affect health policymaking by acting as constitutional referees?
3. How do courts affect health policymaking by acting as meaning givers?
4. How do courts affect health policymaking by acting as rights protectors?
5. What is the supremacy clause of the US Constitution?
6. What are the implications for the courts of existing in a tripartite system of government? Of existing in a federal system of government?
7. What are the concepts of separation of powers, judicial review, and institutional competence?

References

Anderson, G. F. 1992. "The Courts and Health Policy: Strengths and Limitations." *Health Affairs* 11 (4): 95–110.

Berman, M. L. 2009. "Smoking Out the Impact of Tobacco-Related Decisions on Public Health Law." *Brooklyn Law Review* 75 (1): 1–61.

Cortez, N. 2013. "Do Graphic Tobacco Warnings Violate the First Amendment?" *Hastings Law Journal* 64 (5): 1467–1500.

Furrow, B. R., T. L. Greaney, S. H. Johnson, T. S. Jost, and R. L. Schwartz. 2013. *Health Law: Cases, Materials, and Problems*, abridged seventh edition. St. Paul, MN: West Academic.

Gluck, A. R. 2014. "A Legal Victory for Insurance Exchanges." *New England Journal of Medicine* 370 (10): 896–99.

Gostin, L. O. 2009. "FDA Regulation of Tobacco: Politics, Law, and the Public's Health." *Journal of the American Medical Association* 302 (13): 1459–60.

———. 1995. "The Formulation of Health Policy by the Three Branches of Government." In *Society's Choices: Social and Ethical Decision Making in Biomedicine*, edited by F. E. Bulger, E. M. Bobby, and H. V. Fineberg, 335–57. Washington, DC: National Academy Press.

Hammer, P. J., and W. M. Sage. 2002. "Antitrust, Health Care Quality, and the Courts." *Columbia Law Review* 102 (3): 545–649.

Jacobson, P. D. 2009. "The Role of ERISA Preemption in Health Reform: Opportunities and Limits." *Journal of Law, Medicine & Ethics* 37 (Suppl. 2): 86–100.

Jacobson, P. D, E. Selvin, and S. D. Pomfret. 2001. "The Role of the Courts in Shaping Health Policy: An Empirical Analysis." *Journal of Law, Medicine & Ethics* 29 (3–4): 278–89.

Jost, T. S. 2004. "Health Law and Administrative Law: A Marriage Most Convenient." *St. Louis University Law Journal* 49: 1–34.

Kaiser Family Foundation. 2012. *A Guide to the Supreme Court's Decision on the ACA's Medicaid Expansion*. Published August 1. http://kff.org/health-reform /issue-brief/a-guide-to-the-supreme-courts-decision/.

Law, S. A. 2002. "Do We Still Need a Federal Patients' Bill of Rights?" *Yale Journal of Health Policy, Law & Ethics* 3 (1): 1–34.

Mariner, W. K., and G. J. Annas. 2013. "Limiting 'Sugary Drinks' to Reduce Obesity—Who Decides?" *New England Journal of Medicine* 368 (19): 1763–65.

Orentlicher, D. 2013. "The FDA's Graphic Tobacco Warnings and the First Amendment." *New England Journal of Medicine* 369 (3): 204–6.

Perez, V. K. 2007. "EMTALA: Protecting Patients First by Not Deferring to the Final Regulations." *Seton Hall Circuit Review* 4 (1): 149–85.

Richards, E. P. 2007. "Public Health Law as Administrative Law: Example Lessons." *Journal of Health Care Law and Policy* 10 (1): 61–88.

Teitelbaum, J. B., and S. E. Wilensky. 2013. "Law and the Legal System." In *Essentials of Health Law and Policy*, second edition, edited by J. B. Teitelbaum and S. E. Wilensky, 31–44. Burlington, MA: Jones & Bartlett Learning.

POLICY FORMULATION: AGENDA SETTING

Learning Objectives

After reading this chapter, you should be able to

- define agenda setting;
- understand Kingdon's conceptualization of the confluence of problems, possible solutions, and political circumstances in opening a window of opportunity in agenda setting;
- describe how problems emerge for consideration in policymaking;
- appreciate the role of research in selecting among possible solutions to problems;
- describe the role of political circumstances in agenda setting;
- understand the role of interest groups in agenda setting;
- describe the tactics used by interest groups in influencing the policy agenda;
- understand the role of chief executives in agenda setting; and
- describe and explain the nature of the health policy agenda.

This chapter and the four that follow examine in greater detail the three distinct phases of the health policymaking process described and modeled in Chapter 3. This chapter focuses on the agenda setting that occurs in the policy formulation phase. Chapter 6 focuses on the development of legislation that also occurs in that phase. Chapter 7 describes policy implementation and implementing organizations, whereas Chapter 8 describes the policy implementation activities of designing, rulemaking, operating, and evaluating. Chapter 9 discusses the policy modification phase. These chapters apply the model to health policymaking almost exclusively at the national level of government. However, as is true of previous chapters, much of what is said here about the process of public policymaking also applies at the state and local levels. The contexts, participants, and specific mechanisms and procedures obviously differ among the three levels, but the core process is similar.

Remember from the discussion in Chapter 3 that the formulation phase of health policymaking is made up of two distinct and sequential parts: agenda setting and legislation development (see the darkly shaded portion of Exhibit 5.1). Each part involves a complex set of activities in which policymakers and those who would influence their decisions and actions engage, but policy formulation begins with agenda setting.

Agenda Setting

As noted in Chapter 3, agenda setting is deciding what to make decisions about in the policy formulation phase of policymaking. It is the crucial initial step in the process. Kingdon (2010) describes agenda setting in public policymaking as a function of the confluence of three streams of activity: problems, possible solutions to the problems, and political circumstances. According to Kingdon's conceptualization, when problems, possible solutions, and political circumstances flow together in a favorable alignment, a "policy window" or "window of opportunity" opens. When a policy window opens, a problem–potential solution combination that might lead to a new public law or an amendment to an existing one emerges from the set of competing problem–possible solution combinations and moves forward in the policymaking process (see Exhibit 5.2).

Current health policies in the form of public laws—such as those pertaining to environmental protection, licensure of health-related practitioners and organizations, expansion of the Medicaid program, cost containment of the Medicare program, funding for acquired immunodeficiency syndrome (AIDS) research or women's health, and regulation of pharmaceuticals—exist because problems or issues emerged from agenda setting and triggered changes in policy. However, the existence of these problems alone was not sufficient to trigger the development of legislation intended to address them.

The existence of health-related problems, even serious ones such as inadequate health insurance coverage for millions of people or the continuing widespread use of tobacco products, does not always lead to policies intended to solve or ameliorate them. There also must be potential solutions to the problems and the political will to enact specific legislation to implement those solutions. Agenda setting is best understood in the context of its three key variables: problems, possible solutions, and political circumstances.

Problems
The breadth of problems that can initiate agenda setting is reflected in the broad range of health policies. Chapter 1 discussed how health is affected by several determinants: the physical environments in which people live and

EXHIBIT 5.1
Policymaking Process: Agenda Setting in the Formulation Phase

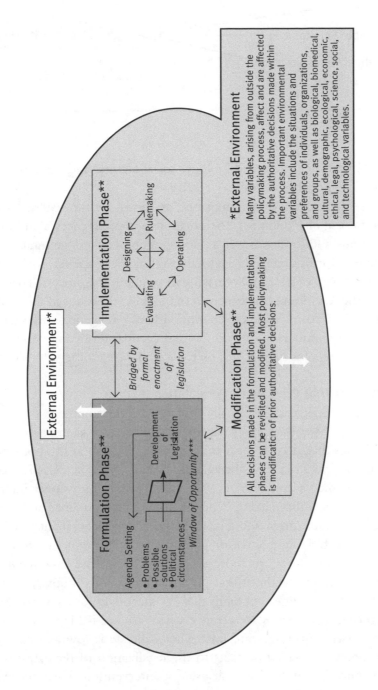

External Environment*

Implementation Phase**

Designing ↔ Rulemaking

Evaluating ↔ Operating

Bridged by formal enactment of legislation

Formulation Phase**

Agenda Setting

Development of Legislation

- Problems
- Possible solutions
- Political circumstances

Window of Opportunity***

Modification Phase**

All decisions made in the formulation and implementation phases can be revisited and modified. Most policymaking is modification of prior authoritative decisions.

*External Environment

Many variables, arising from outside the policymaking process, affect and are affected by the authoritative decisions made within the process. Important environmental variables include the situations and preferences of individuals, organizations, and groups, as well as biological, biomedical, cultural, demographic, ecological, economic, ethical, legal, psychological, science, social, and technological variables.

Policymakers in all three branches of government make policy in the form of position-appropriate, or authoritative, decisions. Their decisions differ in that the **legislative branch is primarily involved in formulation, the **executive branch** is primarily involved in implementation, and both are involved in modification of prior decisions or policies. The **judicial branch** interprets and assesses the legality of decisions made within all three phases of the policymaking process.

***A window of opportunity opens for possible progression of issues through formulation, enactment, implementation, and modification when there is a favorable confluence of problems, possible solutions, and political circumstances.

EXHIBIT 5.2
Agenda
Setting as the
Confluence
of Problems,
Possible
Solutions,
and Political
Circumstances

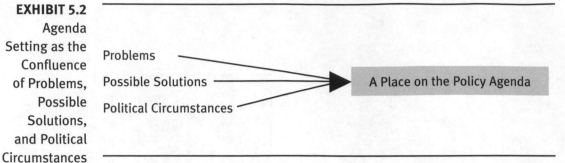

Problems

Possible Solutions

Political Circumstances

A Place on the Policy Agenda

work; their behaviors and biology; social factors; and the type, quality, and timing of health services they receive.

Beyond these determinants, as shown in the external environment component of Exhibit 5.1, the situations and preferences of individuals, organizations, and groups as well as biological, biomedical, cultural, demographic, ecological, economic, ethical, legal, psychological, science, social, and technological variables affect policymaking throughout the process. These inputs join with the results and consequences of the policies produced through the ongoing policymaking process to continuously supply agenda setters with a massive pool of contenders for a place on that agenda. From among the contenders, certain problems find a place on the agenda while others do not.

Problems That Drive Policy Formulation

The problems that eventually lead to the development of legislation are generally those that policymakers broadly identify as important and urgent. Problems that do not meet these criteria languish at the bottom of the list or never find a place on the agenda. Price (1978), in a classic article, argues that whether a problem receives aggressive congressional intervention in the form of policymaking depends on its public salience and the degree of group conflict surrounding it. He defines a publicly salient problem or issue as one with a high actual or potential level of public interest. Conflictive problems or issues are those that stimulate intense disagreements among interest groups or those that pit the interests of groups against the larger public interest. Price contends that the incentives for legislators to intervene in problems or issues are greatest when salience is high and conflict is low. Conversely, incentives are least when salience is low and conflict is high. Appendix 12, which pertains to the legalization of recreational marijuana, illustrates the difficulty of legislative intervention when the conflict surrounding a problem is high.

Problems that lead to attempts at policy solutions find their place on the agenda along one of several paths. Some problems emerge because trends in certain variables eventually reach unacceptable levels—at least, levels unacceptable to some policymakers. Growth in the number of uninsured and cost escalation in the Medicare program are examples of trends that eventually reached levels at which policymakers felt compelled to address the underlying problems through legislation. Both problems are addressed in the Affordable Care Act (ACA).

Problems also can be spotlighted by their widespread applicability (e.g., the high cost of prescription medications to millions of Americans) or by their sharply focused impact on a small but powerful group whose members are directly affected (e.g., the high cost of medical education). Another example of a widespread problem that led to specific legislation was that a large number of people felt locked into their jobs because they feared that preexisting health conditions might prevent them from obtaining health insurance if they changed jobs. In response to this problem, the Health Insurance Portability and Accountability Act of 1996 (P.L. 104-191) significantly enhanced the portability of health insurance coverage when people change jobs. Other provisions in this law guarantee availability and renewability of health insurance coverage for certain employees and individuals and an increase in the tax deduction for health insurance purchased by the self-employed.

Some problems gain their place on the agenda or strengthen their hold on a place because they are closely linked to other problems that already occupy secure places. Efforts by the legislative and executive branches of the federal government to address the nation's budget deficit problem, at least in part through reduced expenditures on the Medicare program, are a recurring example of the link between one problem (cost increases in the Medicare program) and another (growth of the federal deficit). Linking these two problems significantly strengthens prospects for the development of legislation intended to curtail Medicare program expenditures.

Some problems emerge more or less simultaneously along several paths. Typically, problems that emerge this way become prominent on the policy agenda. For example, the problem of the high cost of health services for the private and public sectors has long received attention from policymakers. Even though the rate of growth in health costs has slowed in the past few years, these costs remain high and problematic (Martin et al. 2014). This problem emerged along a number of mutually reinforcing paths. In part, the cost problem has been prominent because the cost trend data disturb many people. The data contribute to and reinforce a widespread acknowledgment of the problem of health costs in public poll after public poll and have attracted the attention of some of those who pay directly for health services through the provision of health insurance benefits, especially the politically powerful business community. Finally, the health cost problem, as it relates to public expenditures—for the Medicare and Medicaid programs especially—has also been linked at times to the need to control the federal budget.

The importance of these variables has been magnified greatly in the context of the global financial crisis engulfing the world beginning in 2008 (Shah 2013). The variables of healthcare costs and the escalating federal budget form a combination of interacting circumstances, which is largely why this problem remains perennially prominent in the minds of many policymakers. The persistence of this problem, and many others, is also related to the difficulty of finding and pursuing potential solutions.

Possible Solutions

The second variable in agenda setting (see Exhibit 5.2) is the existence of possible solutions to problems. Problems themselves—even serious, fully acknowledged ones with widespread implications such as high costs, poor quality, and uneven access to needed health services—do not invariably lead to policies. Potential solutions must accompany them. The availability of possible solutions depends on the generation of ideas and, usually, a period of idea testing and refinement. As Appendix 13, which pertains to the Centers for Medicare & Medicaid Services (CMS) Innovation Center's search for new and better payment and health services delivery models, illustrates, numerous ideas might serve as solutions to problems, either in single application or in various combinations.

While the menus of alternative solutions vary in size and quality, alternative solutions almost always exist. An excessive number of alternatives can slow the problem's advancement through the policymaking process as the relative merits of the competing alternatives are considered. Without at least one solution believed to have the potential to solve it, however, a problem does not advance, except perhaps in some spurious effort to create the illusion that it is being addressed.

When alternative solutions do exist, policymakers must decide whether the potential solutions are worth developing into legislative proposals. Frequently, multiple solutions to a particular problem will be considered worthy of such action, resulting in the simultaneous development of several competing legislative proposals. Competing proposals tend to make agenda setting rather chaotic, although rigorous research and analysis can sometimes provide more clarity.

The Role of Research and Analysis in Defining Problems and Assessing Alternatives

Health services research is "the multidisciplinary field of scientific investigation that studies how social factors, financing systems, organizational structures and processes, health technologies, and personal behaviors affect access to healthcare, the quality and cost of healthcare, and ultimately our health and well-being. Its research domains are individuals, families, organizations, institutions, communities, and populations" (AcademyHealth 2014). It has been defined more succinctly as "scientific inquiry into the ways in which health services are delivered to various constituents" (Forrest et al. 2008). Health services researchers seek to understand how people obtain access to healthcare services, the costs of the services, and the results for patients of using this care. The main goals of this type of research include identifying the most effective ways to organize, manage, finance, and deliver high-quality care and services and, more recently, how to reduce medical errors and improve patient safety. Health services research, along with much biomedical research, contributes to problem identification and specification and the development of possible solutions. Thus, research can help establish the health policy agenda by clarifying problems and potential solutions. Well-conducted health services research provides policymakers with facts that might affect their decisions.

Policymakers value the input of the research community sufficiently to fund much of its work through the National Institutes of Health (NIH), the Agency for Healthcare Research and Quality (AHRQ), and other agencies. AHRQ, the health services research arm of the US Department of Health and Human Services (HHS), complements the biomedical research mission of its sister agency, NIH. AHRQ is the federal government's focal point for research to enhance the quality, appropriateness, and effectiveness of health services and access to those services.

In addition to these traditional research and analysis agencies, the ACA significantly improved the government's ability to use analysis and research in guiding agenda setting. For example, the ACA created the Center for Medicare and Medicaid Innovation (CMI) within CMS, and appropriated $10 billion for the FY2011 to FY2019 period—along with $10 billion for each subsequent ten-year period. The purpose of CMI is to test and implement innovative payment and service delivery models. These models are intended to reduce program expenditures under Medicare, Medicaid, and the Children's Health Insurance Program while preserving or enhancing the quality of care furnished under these programs (Redhead 2014).

The ACA also established and funded an Independent Payment Advisory Board (IPAB) to make recommendations to Congress for achieving specific Medicare spending reductions if costs exceed a target growth rate. IPAB's recommendations are to take effect unless Congress overrides them, in which case Congress would be responsible for achieving the same level of savings.

Further supporting the research and analysis basis for policymaking, the ACA established a trust fund to finance the Patient-Centered Outcomes

Research Institute (PCORI). The main purpose of PCORI (2014) is to support the conduct of comparative clinical effectiveness research. Appropriations to this trust fund were $10 million for FY2010, $50 million for FY2011, and $150 million for each of FY2012 through FY2019, for a total of $1.26 billion over that ten-year period. For each year of FY2013 through FY2019, the trust fund is to receive additional appropriations equal to the net revenues from a new health insurance policy or plan fee, as well as Medicare trust fund transfers. Each fiscal year, 20 percent of the funds in the trust are to be transferred to the secretary of HHS, with 80 percent of the transferred funds provided to AHRQ.

Research and analysis play two especially important roles in agenda setting. First, an important documentation role is played through the gathering, cataloging, and correlating of facts related to health problems and issues. For example, researchers documented the dangers of tobacco smoke; the presence of human immunodeficiency virus (HIV); the numbers of people living with AIDS, a variety of cancers, heart disease, and other diseases; the effect of poverty on health; the number of people who lack health insurance coverage; the existence of health disparities among population segments; and the dangers imposed by exposure to various toxins in people's physical environments. Quantification and documentation of health-related problems give the problems a better chance of finding a place on the policy agenda.

The second way research informs, and thus influences, the health policy agenda is through analyses to determine which policy solutions may work or to compare alternative solutions. Health services research provides valuable information to policymakers as they propose, consider, and prioritize alternative solutions to problems. Often taking the form of demonstration projects intended to provide a basis for determining the feasibility, efficacy, or basic workability of a possible policy intervention, research-based recommendations to policymakers can play an important role in policy agenda setting. Potential solutions that might lead to public policies—even if the policies themselves are formulated mainly on political grounds—must stand the test of plausibility. Research that supports a particular course of action or attests to its likelihood of success—or at least to the probability that the course of action will not embarrass proponents—can make a significant contribution to policymaking by helping shape the policy agenda.

What research cannot do for policymakers, however, is make decisions for them. Every difficult decision regarding the health policy agenda ultimately rests with policymakers.

Making Decisions About Alternative Possible Solutions

Problems that require decisions and alternative possible solutions to them are two prerequisites for using the classical, rational model of decision making outlined in Exhibit 5.3. This model shares the basic pattern of the organizational decision-making process typically followed in the private and public sectors. However, differences between the two sectors in the use of this model typically arise with the introduction of the *criteria* used to evaluate alternative solutions.

Some of the criteria used to evaluate and compare alternative solutions in the private and public sectors are the same or similar. For example, the criteria set in both sectors usually include consideration of whether a particular solution will actually solve the problem, whether it can be implemented using available resources and technologies, its costs and benefits relative to other possible solutions, and the results of an advantage-to-disadvantage analysis of the alternatives.

In both sectors, high-level decisions have scientific or technical, political, and economic dimensions. The scientific or technical aspects can be more difficult to factor into decisions when the evidence is in dispute, as it often is (Atkins, Siegel, and Slutsky 2005; Steinberg and Luce 2005). The most pervasive difference between the criteria sets used in the two sectors, however, is in the roles political concerns and considerations play. Decisions made by public-sector policymakers must reflect greater political sensitivity to the public at large and to the preferences of relevant individuals, organizations, and interest groups. The greater political sensitivity required helps explain the importance of the third variable in agenda setting in the health policymaking process, political circumstances.

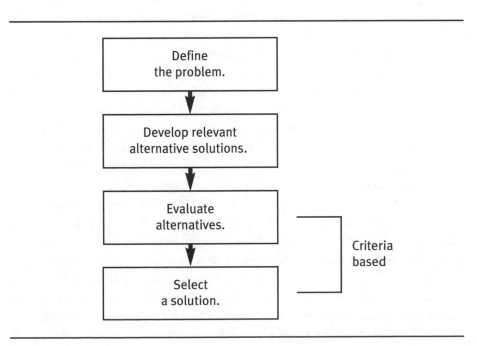

EXHIBIT 5.3
The Rational Model of Decision Making

Political Circumstances

A problem that might be solved or lessened through policy, even in combination with a possible solution to that problem, is not sufficient to move the problem–solution combination forward in the policymaking process. A political force, or what is sometimes called political will, is also necessary.

Thus, the political circumstances surrounding each problem–potential solution form the crucial third variable in creating a window of opportunity through which problems and potential solutions move toward development of legislation. This variable is generally as important as the other two variables in this complex equation (see Exhibit 5.2), and in times of crisis such as the global financial crisis that emerged in 2008, political circumstances can be by far the most significant factor in stimulating policy changes. The American Recovery and Reinvestment Act of 2009 (P.L. 111-5) is an example of this phenomenon.

The establishment of a political thrust forceful enough to move policymakers to act on a health-related problem is often the most challenging variable in the problem's emergence on the policy agenda and progression to legislation development. This variable can be seen clearly in the passage of the ACA in 2010. Following decades of failed attempts to fundamentally reform healthcare in the United States, why did major health reform occur in 2010? The answer to this question is complex, but it certainly involves the political circumstances surrounding the issue. As Hacker suggests (2010, 863), "The obvious answer is the election of a Democratic president, the Democratic capture of Congress in 2006, and the strengthening of the majority in 2008." Hacker goes further to point out that the political circumstances in which the ACA occurred included not only a Democratic majority in Congress, but a more homogeneously liberal composition of members of Congress.

Whether the political circumstances attendant on any problem–potential solution combination are sufficient to actually open a window of opportunity depends on the competing entries on the policy agenda. The array of problems is an important variable in agenda setting. When the nation is involved in serious threats to its national security or its civil order, for example, or when a state is in the midst of a sustained recession, health policy will be treated differently. In fact, health policy, which is often a high priority for the American people, can be pushed to a secondary position at times.

The political circumstances surrounding any problem–potential solution combination include such factors as the relevant public attitudes, concerns, and opinions; the preferences and relative ability to influence political decisions of various groups interested in the problem or the way it is addressed; and the positions of involved key policymakers in the executive and legislative branches of government. Each of these factors can influence whether a problem is addressed through policy and the shape and scope of any policy developed to address the problem. Two factors in particular exert great influence in establishing the policy agenda. These are interest groups and the chief executive (president, governor, or mayor). The role of each in agenda setting is discussed in the next two sections.

Interest Group Involvement in Agenda Setting

As we discussed in Chapter 2, interest groups are ubiquitous in the policy marketplace. Perhaps nowhere in the policymaking process is the influence of interest groups more prevalent than in the agenda-setting activities of the formulation phase (see Exhibit 5.1).

To fully appreciate the role of interest groups in setting the policy agenda, consider the role of individual Americans. In a representative form of government, such as that of the United States, individual members of society, unless they are among the elected representatives, usually do not vote directly on policies. They can, however, vote on policymakers. Thus, policymakers are interested in what individuals, especially voters, want, even when that is not easy to discern.

However, one of the great myths about democratic societies is that their members, when confronted with tough problems such as the high cost of healthcare for everyone, the lack of health insurance for many, or the existence of widespread disparities in health among segments of the society, ponder the problems carefully and express their preferences to their elected officials, who then factor these opinions into their decisions about how to address the problems through policy. Sometimes these steps take place, but even when the public expresses its opinions about an issue, the result is clouded by the fact that the American people are heterogeneous in their views. Opinions are mixed on health-related problems and their solutions. Public opinion polls can help sort out conflicting opinions, but polls are not always straightforward undertakings. In addition, individuals' opinions on many issues are subject to change.

The public's thinking on difficult problems that might be addressed through public policies evolves through predictable stages, beginning with awareness of the problem and ending with judgments about its solution (Yankelovich and Friedman 2010). In between, people explore the problem and alternative solutions with varying degrees of success. The progress of individuals through these stages is related to their views on the problems and solutions.

The diversity among members of society and the fact that individual views on problems and potential solutions evolve over time explain in large part the greater influence of organizations and interest groups in shaping the policy agenda. Interest groups in particular can exert extraordinary influence in policy markets, as we discussed in Chapter 2.

Whether made up of individuals or organizations, interest groups are often able to present a unified position to policymakers on their preferences regarding a particular problem or its solution. A unified position is far easier for policymakers to assess and respond to than the diverse opinions and preferences of many individuals acting alone. Although individuals tend to be keenly interested in their own health and the health of those they care about, their interests in specific health policies tend to be diffuse. These diffused interests stand in contrast to the highly concentrated interests of those who earn their livelihood in the health domain or who stand to gain other benefits there. This phenomenon is not unique to health. In general, the interests of those who earn their livelihood in any industry or economic sector are more concentrated than the interests of those who merely use its outputs.

One result of the concentration of interests is the formation of organized interest groups that seek to influence the formulation, implementation, and modification of policies to some advantage for the group's members. Because all interest groups seek policies that favor their members, their own agendas, behaviors, and preferences regarding the larger public policy agenda are often predictable.

Feldstein (2006) argues, for example, that all interest groups representing health services providers seek through legislation to increase the demand for members' services, limit competitors, permit members to charge the highest possible prices for their services, and lower their members' operating costs as much as possible. Likewise, an interest group representing health services consumers logically seeks policies that minimize the costs of the services to its members, ease their access to the services, increase the availability of the services, and so on. Essentially, interest groups are human nature at work.

As we noted earlier, interest groups frequently play influential roles in setting the nation's health policy agenda, as they subsequently do in the development of legislation and the implementation and modification of health policies. These groups sometimes proactively seek to stimulate new policies that serve the interests of their members. Alternatively, they sometimes reactively seek to block policy changes that they believe do not serve their members' best interests.

Interest Groups Are Ubiquitous in Health Policymaking

A significant feature of the policymaking process in the United States is the presence of interest groups that exist to serve the collective interests of their members. These groups analyze the policymaking process to discern policy changes that might affect their members and inform them about such changes. They also seek to influence the process to provide the group's members with some advantage. The interests of their constituent members define the health policy interests of these groups.

Health services providers rely heavily on interest groups to influence policymaking to their advantage, as do other types of health-related organizations. Some interest groups are consumer based. Without being exhaustive, some of the important health-related interest groups are noted next.

Hospitals can join the American Hospital Association (www.aha.org), long-term care organizations can join the American Health Care Association (www.ahca.org) or the American Association of Homes and Services for the Aging, now known as LeadingAge (www.leadingage.org), and health insurers and health plans can join America's Health Insurance Plans (www.ahip.org).

Other interest groups represent individual health practitioners. Physicians can join the American Medical Association (AMA; www.ama-assn.org). African American physicians may choose to join the National Medical Association (www.nmanet.org), and female physicians may choose to join the American Medical Women's Association (www.amwa-doc.org). In addition, physicians have the opportunity to affiliate with groups, usually termed *colleges* or *academies,* where membership is based on medical specialty. Prominent examples are the American College of Surgeons (www.facs.org) and the American Academy of Pediatrics (www.aap.org). Other personal membership groups include the American College of Healthcare Executives (www.ache.org), the American Nurses Association (www.ana.org), and the American Dental Association (www.ada.org), to name a few.

Often, in addition to national interest groups, health services provider organizations and individual practitioners can join state and local groups—usually affiliates or chapters of national groups—that also represent their interests. For example, states have state hospital associations and state medical societies. Many urban centers and densely populated areas even have groups at the regional, county, or city level.

There are numerous other health-related interest groups in addition to those whose members provide health services directly. Examples include the following:

- America's Health Insurance Plans (www.ahip.org)
- Association of American Medical Colleges (www.aamc.org)
- Association of University Programs in Health Administration (www.aupha.org)
- Biotechnology Industry Organization (www.bio.org)
- Blue Cross and Blue Shield Association (www.bcbs.com)
- Pharmaceutical Research and Manufacturers of America (www.phrma.org)

Like groups whose members are health services providers, these groups focus particularly on policies that affect their members directly.

There are also a number of interest groups that serve consumers. Reflecting the populations from which their members are drawn, groups with individual member constituencies are diverse. Some are based in part on a shared characteristic such as race, gender, age, or connection to a specific disease or condition. Examples include the following:

- Alliance for Retired Americans (www.retiredamericans.org)
- American Association of Retired Persons (AARP; www.aarp.org)
- American Heart Association (www.heart.org)
- Consortium for Citizens with Disabilities (www.c-c-d.org)
- Families USA (www.familiesusa.org)
- National Association for the Advancement of Colored People (NAACP; www.naacp.org)
- National Organization for Women (NOW; www.now.org)

Interest groups such as NAACP and NOW serve the health interests of their members as part of agendas focused broadly on racial and gender equality. Although the Fourteenth Amendment to the US Constitution guarantees equal protection under the law, American history clearly shows how difficult this equality has been to achieve. Interest groups such as NAACP and NOW have made equality their central public policy goal at the polls; in the workplace; and in education, housing, health services, and other facets of life in the United States. Income inequality in the United States is the newest of these variables.

The specific health policy interests of groups representing African Americans include adequately addressing this population segment's unique health problems: widespread disparities in health status and access to health services, higher infant mortality, higher exposure to violence among adolescents, higher levels of substance abuse among adults, and, compared to other segments of the population, earlier deaths from cardiovascular disease and other causes. Similarly, groups representing the interests of women seek to address their unique health problems. In particular, they focus on such interests as breast cancer, childbearing, osteoporosis, domestic violence, family health, and funding for biomedical research on women's health problems.

A growing proportion of the American population is older than 65. Older adults have specific health interests related to their stage of life; as people age, they consume relatively more healthcare services, and their healthcare needs differ from those of younger people. They also become more likely to consume long-term care services and community-based services intended to help them cope with limitations in the activities of daily living.

In addition to their health needs, older citizens have a unique health policy history and, therefore, a unique set of expectations and preferences regarding the nation's health policy. The Medicare program, a key feature of this history, includes extensive provisions for health benefits for older citizens. Building on the specific interests of older people and their preferences to preserve and extend their healthcare benefits through public policies, organizations such as AARP and the Alliance for Retired Americans (www.retiredamericans.org) play an important role in addressing the health policy interests of their members.

Other interest groups with individual constituencies reflect member interests based primarily on specific diseases or conditions, such as the American Cancer Society (www.cancer.org) or the Consortium for Citizens with Disabilities (www.c-c-d.org). The American Heart Association (AHA; www.heart.org), for example, has 22.5 million volunteers and supporters pursuing the organization's mission of building healthier lives, free of cardiovascular diseases and stroke. The association pursues its mission through such avenues as direct funding of research, public and professional education programs, and community programs designed to prevent heart disease. It also seeks to serve its members' interests through influencing public policy related to heart disease. As AHA (2014) notes on its web page, its federal policy agenda is organized into the following categories:

- Research, with a focus on stable and predictable funding streams for NIH, AHRQ, and the National Center for Health Statistics
- Prevention, with a focus on measures for improving cardiovascular health such as obesity prevention, tobacco control, and public funding for prevention and air pollution control
- Quality care, including health equity for minorities and women, evidence-based cardiovascular care, stroke prevention and treatment programs, rehabilitation services, and telemedicine
- Access to care, including adequate and affordable healthcare coverage; appropriate systems of emergency care for stroke, ST segment elevation myocardial infarction, and sudden cardiac arrest; cardiopulmonary resuscitation training; and access to automated external defibrillators and cardiovascular surveillance systems
- Stroke, including the creation and enhancement of high-quality stroke systems of care incorporating prevention, community education, notification and response of emergency medical services, acute treatment, and rehabilitation

Tactics of Interest Groups in Agenda Setting

As influential participants in public policymaking, interest groups are integral to the process. They are especially ubiquitous in the health domain. But how do they exert their influence? Interest groups rely heavily on four tactics: lobbying, electioneering, litigation, and, especially recently, shaping public opinion so that it might in turn influence the policymaking process to the groups' advantage (Edwards, Wattenberg, and Lineberry 2012). Each of these tactics is described in the following sections.

Lobbying

This widely used influencing tactic has deep roots in public policymaking in the United States, and it involves large sums of money. Lobbying expenditures on health issues at the federal level were about $480 million in 2013 (Center for Responsive Politics 2014c). In the minds of many people, lobbying conjures a negative image of money exchanging hands for political favors and backroom deals. But ideally it is nothing more than communicating with public policymakers to influence their decisions to be more favorable to, or at least consistent with, the preferences of the lobbyist (Andres 2009; Herrnson, Shaiko, and Wilcox 2005).

Lobbying, the word for these influencing activities, and *lobbyists*, the word for people who do this work, arose in reference to the place where such activities first took place. Before members of Congress had offices or telephones, people who sought to influence their thinking waited for the legislators and talked to them in the lobbies of the buildings they frequented. The original practitioners of this influencing tactic spent so much time in lobbies that they came, naturally enough, to be called lobbyists, and their work, lobbying.

The vast majority of lobbyists operate in an ethical and professional manner, effectively representing the legitimate interests of the groups they serve. However, the few who behave in a heavy-handed, even illegal manner have to some extent tarnished the reputations of all who do this work. Their image is further affected by the fact that their work, properly done, is essentially selfish in nature. Lobbyists seek to persuade others that the position of the interests they represent is the correct one. Lobbyists' whole professional purpose is to persuade others to make decisions that are in the best interests of those who employ or retain them.

Opinions and results of studies on the effectiveness of lobbying are mixed at best (Bergan 2009). Some ambivalence over the role of lobbying derives from the inherent difficulty in isolating its effect from the other influencing tactics discussed later. There is no doubt that lobbying affects the policymaking process, but it seems to work best when applied to policymakers who are already committed, or at least sympathetic, to the lobbyist's position on a public policy issue (Edwards, Wattenberg, and Lineberry 2012). Lobbyists certainly played a prominent role in the enactment of the Medicare Prescription Drug, Improvement, and Modernization Act of 2003 (P.L. 108-173), the ACA, and other health policies (Kersh 2014; Weissert and Weissert 2012). Appendix 14 provides an example of highly focused and cooperative lobbying to improve the Meaningful Use program standards and increase health information technology interoperability. The influence lobbyists exert on policymaking is facilitated by several well-recognized sources (Godwin, Ainsworth, and Godwin 2013; Herrnson, Shaiko, and Wilcox 2005):

- Lobbyists are an important source of information for policymakers. Although most policymakers must be concerned with many policy issues simultaneously, most lobbyists can focus and specialize. They can become expert and can draw on the insight of other experts in the areas they represent.
- Lobbyists can assist policymakers with the development and execution of political strategy. Lobbyists typically are politically savvy and can provide what amounts to free consulting to the policymakers they choose to assist.
- Lobbyists can assist elected policymakers in their reelection efforts. (More is said about this role in the next section on electioneering.) This assistance can take several forms, including campaign contributions, votes, and workers for campaigns.
- Lobbyists can be important sources of innovative ideas for policymakers. Policymakers are judged on the quality of their ideas as well as their abilities to have those ideas translated into effective policies. For most policymakers, few gifts are as valued as a really good idea, especially when they can turn that idea into a bill that bears their name.
- Finally, lobbyists can be friends with policymakers. Lobbyists are often gregarious and interesting people in their own right. They entertain, sometimes lavishly, and they are socially engaging. Many of them have social and educational backgrounds similar to those of policymakers. In fact, many lobbyists have been policymakers earlier in their careers. Friendships between lobbyists and policymakers are neither unusual nor surprising.

Electioneering
Electioneering, or using the resources at their disposal to aid candidates for political office, is a common means through which interest groups seek to influence the policymaking process. Many groups have considerable resources to devote to this tactic. The effectiveness of electioneering in influencing the

policymaking process is based on the simple fact that policymakers who are sympathetic to a group's interests are far more likely to be influenced than are policymakers who are not sympathetic. Thus, interest groups seek to elect and keep in office policymakers whom they view as sympathetic to the interests of the group's members.

Interest groups have, to varying degrees, a set of resources that involve electoral advantages or disadvantages for political candidates. For example, some groups whose members are widely dispersed across congressional districts throughout the country, that can mobilize their members, and whose members have status or wealth can affect election outcomes (Kingdon 2010).

One of the most visible aspects of electioneering is the channeling of money into campaign finances. Exhibit 5.4 shows the extent of this activity in the House and Senate midterm elections in 2012. Health-related interest groups participate heavily in this form of electioneering. Appendix 15 describes the types of groups permitted to be involved in financing political campaigns.

In 1975, Congress created the Federal Election Commission (FEC; www.fec.gov) to administer and enforce the Federal Election Campaign Act—the law that governs the financing of federal elections. The duties of the FEC, which is an independent regulatory agency, are to disclose campaign finance information; enforce the provisions of the law, such as the limits and prohibitions on contributions; and oversee the public funding of presidential elections.

The Center for Responsive Politics, a nonpartisan, not-for-profit research group based in Washington, DC, is a rich source of information on the use of money in politics and its effect on elections and public policymaking. The center's website (www.opensecrets.org) provides extensive, detailed information on the flow of money in the political process.

Although participation in campaign financing is an important source of influence for interest groups, the most influential groups are those who exert their influence through lobbying and electioneering activities. The hospital industry is a notable example. The AHA is a leading campaign contributor through its political action committee. Furthermore, it has many additional resources at its disposal. As Kingdon (2010) points out, every congressional district has hospitals whose trustees are community leaders and whose managers and physicians are typically articulate and respected in their community. These spokespersons can be mobilized to support sympathetic candidates or to contact their representatives directly regarding any policy decision.

As Ornstein and Elder (1978, 74) observed decades ago, "The ability of a group to mobilize its membership strength for political action is a highly valuable resource; a small group that is politically active and cohesive can have more political impact than a large, politically apathetic, and unorganized

EXHIBIT 5.4
Money Raised in the 2012 Election Cycle

Party	No. of Candidates	Total Raised	Total Spent	Total Cash on Hand	Total from PACs	Total from Individuals
House						
All	1,711	$1,111,628,101	$1,066,133,319	$188,367,571	$356,365,626	$630,572,348
Democrats	760	$485,807,408	$475,717,820	$80,237,763	$157,708,117	$284,891,677
Republicans	848	$615,698,976	$580,407,676	$107,994,009	$198,616,347	$344,465,486
Senate						
All	251	$699,077,039	$701,308,507	$40,061,500	$81,151,846	$462,843,233
Democrats	81	$303,637,298	$309,490,575	$18,987,272	$43,814,883	$245,543,444
Republicans	137	$377,246,329	$377,363,376	$16,816,036	$36,473,722	$208,667,036
President						
All	16	$1,368,861,431	$1,365,753,453	$5,537,101	$1,728,562	$988,737,778
Democrats	1	$738,503,770	$737,505,368	$3,301,800	N/A	$549,580,640
Republicans	10	$625,415,939	$623,361,597	$2,075,152	$1,728,562	$435,760,387

Source: Center for Responsive Politics (2014b). Reprinted with permission.

group." The ability to mobilize people and other resources at the grass-roots level helps explain the capabilities of various groups to influence the policymaking process. The most influential health interest groups, including those representing hospitals, physicians, and nurses, have particularly strong grassroots organizations to call into play in their lobbying and electioneering tactics.

Litigation

A third tactic interest groups can use to influence the policymaking process is litigation. Interest groups, acting on behalf of their members, seek to influence the policy agenda and the larger policymaking process through litigation in which they challenge existing policies, seek to stimulate new policies, or try to alter certain aspects of policy implementation. Use of the litigation tactic in state and federal courts is widespread, and interest groups increasingly employ it in their efforts to influence policymaking in the health domain.

Although interest groups are more likely to seek to influence legislative and executive branch decisions, they can and do pursue their policy goals in the courts. This tactic is especially attractive when interest groups do not have the economic resources to mount a large lobbying effort or do not have large and influential memberships. In these circumstances, groups may find the judicial branch a more fertile ground for their efforts. When interest groups turn to the courts, they are likely to use one of two strategies: test cases and *amicus curiae* ("friend of the court") briefs.

Because the judiciary engages in policymaking primarily by rendering decisions in specific cases, interest groups may attempt to ensure that cases that pertain to their interests are brought before the courts, which is known as using the *test-case strategy*. A particular interest group can initiate and sponsor a case, or it can participate in a case initiated by another group that is pertinent to its interests. The latter strategy involves filing *amicus curiae* briefs and is the easiest way for interest groups to become involved in cases. This strategy, which is used in federal and state appellate courts rather than trial courts, permits groups to get their interests before the courts even when they do not control the cases in which they participate by filing the briefs. To file a brief, a private group must obtain permission from the parties to the case or from the court. This requirement does not apply to government interests. In fact, the solicitor general of the United States is especially important in this regard, and in some situations the US Supreme Court invites the solicitor general to present an *amicus* brief.

Friend-of-the-court briefs are often intended not to strengthen the arguments of one of the parties but to assert to the court the filing group's preferences as to how a case should be resolved. *Amicus curiae* briefs are often filed to persuade an appellate court to either grant or deny review of a lower-court decision (US Department of State 2004). For example, in one case a group of commercial insurers and health maintenance organizations in New York City challenged the state of New York's practice of adding a surcharge to certain hospital bills to raise money to help fund health services for indigent people (Green 1995). The US Supreme Court heard this case. Because the outcome was important to their members, a number of health interest groups filed *amicus* briefs in an effort to influence the court's decision. Through such written depositions, groups state their collective position on issues and describe how the decision will affect their members. This practice is widely used by interest groups in health and other domains. It has made the Supreme Court accessible to these groups, who, in expressing their views, have helped determine which cases the Court will hear and how it will rule on them (Collins 2008). This practice is also frequently and effectively used by interest groups in lower courts to help shape the health policy agenda.

The use of litigation is not limited to attempts to shape the policy agenda, however. One particularly effective use of this tactic is seeking clarification from the courts on vague pieces of legislation. This practice provides opportunities for interest groups to exert enormous influence on policymaking overall by influencing the rules, regulations, and administrative practices that guide the implementation of public statutes or laws. We will say more about the role of interest groups in rulemaking in Chapter 8 in the discussion about rulemaking in the overall public policymaking process. For now, recall from Chapter 1 that the rules and regulations established to implement laws and programs are themselves authoritative decisions that fit the definition of public policies.

Shaping Public Opinion

Because policymakers are influenced by the electorate's opinions, many interest groups seek to influence the policymaking process by shaping public opinion (Blendon et al. 2010; Schlesinger 2014). A good example of this influence is seen in some of the activities of the Coalition to Protect America's Health Care. On its Facebook page, the coalition describes itself as "an organization of hospitals, national, state, regional and metropolitan hospital associations . . . united to achieve one goal: to protect high quality patient care by preserving the financial viability of America's hospitals" (Coalition to Protect America's Health Care 2014). It pursues this goal in part by shaping public opinion through ads supporting hospitals.

This tactic, of course, is not new. It was used extensively in the congressional debate over national health reform in the 1990s. Interest groups spent more than $50 million seeking to shape public opinion on the issues involved. For example, many thought the health insurance industry's ubiquitous "Harry and Louise" ads were effective during the debate (Hacker 1997). These ads were not the first use of this public opinion tactic by health-care interest groups, however.

Intense opposition in some quarters to the legislation, especially by the AMA, fueled the congressional debate over the Medicare legislation in the 1960s. The American public had rarely, if ever, been exposed to so feverish a campaign to shape opinions as it experienced in the period leading up to its enactment in 1965.

Among the many activities undertaken in that campaign to influence public opinion (and through it, policymakers), perhaps none is more enter-taining in hindsight—and certainly few better represent the campaign's tone and intensity—than one action taken by the AMA. As part of its campaign to influence public opinion on Medicare, the AMA sent every physician's spouse a recording and advised her (most physicians were men in those days) to host friends and neighbors and play the recording for them. The idea was to encourage these people to write letters to their representatives in Congress in opposition to the legislation. Near the end of the recording, narrated by Ronald Reagan, the following words can be heard (as quoted in Skidmore 1970, 138):

Write those letters now; call your friends and tell them to write them. If you don't, this program, I promise you, will pass just as surely as the sun will come up tomor-row. And behind it will come other federal programs that will invade every area of freedom as we have known it in this country. Until one day . . . [we] will awake to find that we have socialism. And if you don't do this, and I don't do it, one of these days you and I are going to spend our sunset years telling our children and our children's children what it was like in America when men were free.

Attempts to shape public opinion about government's role in health reached their high point in the debate leading up to the 2010 enactment of the ACA. The health sector spent a record $552 million in 2009 seeking to influence the legislation (Center for Responsive Politics 2014a). Some of this money was spent on ads intended to shape public opinion.

Although the effect of the appeals to public opinion made by inter-est groups on policymaking is debatable, the extent and persistence of the practice suggests that interest groups believe that it does make a difference. One factor clearly mitigates the usefulness of this tactic and makes difficult its use by interest groups: the heterogeneity of the American population's perceptions of problems and preferred solutions to them. For example, in the congressional debate over major health reform in the 1990s, the majority viewpoint at the beginning of the debate was that health reform was needed. However, at no time during the debate was a public consensus achieved on the nature of that reform. No feasible alternative for reform ever received majority support in any public opinion poll. During most of the debate, in fact, public opinion was about evenly divided among the possible reform options (Brodie and Blendon 1995). Similarly, public opinion was split during development of the ACA legislation and has continued to be split throughout its implementation (Kaiser Family Foundation 2013). The split was largely partisan in the early debate about reform in 2009, with Democrats (70 percent) supporting reform and Republicans (60 percent) opposing it (Kaiser Family Foundation 2009).

Interest Group Resources and Success in Influencing the Policy Agenda

Using lobbying, electioneering, litigation, and efforts to shape public opinion, interest groups seek to influence the policy agenda and the larger public policymaking process to the strategic advantage of their members. The degree of success they achieve depends on the resources at their disposal. In a classic book on the subject, Ornstein and Elder (1978) categorize the resources of interest groups as follows:

- Physical resources, especially money and the number of members
- Organizational resources, such as the quality of a group's leadership, the degree of unity or cohesion among its members, and the group's ability to mobilize its membership for political purposes
- Political resources, such as expertise in the intricacies of the public policymaking process and a reputation for influencing the process ethically and effectively
- Motivational resources, such as the strength of ideological conviction among the membership
- Intangible resources, such as the overall status or prestige of a group

An especially important physical resource is the size of a group's membership. Large groups, especially when a group can convince policymakers that the group speaks with one united voice representing the preferences of its members, can influence all phases of the policymaking process from agenda setting through modification (Kingdon 2010). Larger groups can obviously have more financial resources, but perhaps even more important, size might provide an advantage simply because the group's membership is spread through every legislative district. However, the costs of organizing a large group can be high, especially if their interests are not extremely concordant and focused.

The mix of physical, organizational, political, motivational, and intangible resources available to an interest group, and how effectively the group uses them, helps determine the group's influence on the policy agenda and other aspects of the policymaking process. A particular group's performance is also affected by its access to resources compared with groups that may be pursuing competing or conflicting policy outcomes (Edwards, Wattenberg, and Lineberry 2012; Feldstein 2006; Kingdon 2010). The policy market- place, as we discussed in Chapter 2, is a place where many people and groups promote their policy preferences.

The Influential Role of Chief Executives in Agenda Setting

Chief executives—presidents, governors, or mayors—also influence the policy agenda, including the agenda for policy in the health domain. Popu- lar chief executives can influence the policy agenda easily (Aberbach and Peterson 2006). Kingdon (2010) attributes the influence of presidents (his point also applies to other chief executives) to certain institutional resources inherent in the executive office. Morone (2014) notes that presidents can energize healthcare policy by setting the agenda and proposing solutions to problems. He also observes that bold federal health policies invariably require presidential leadership.

Political advantages available to chief executives include the ability to present a unified administration position on issues—which contrasts with the legislative branch, where opinions and views tend to be heterogeneous—and the ability to command public attention. Properly managed, the latter ability can stimulate substantial public pressure on legislators. Chief executives can even rival powerful interest groups in their ability to shape public opinion around the public policy agenda.

Chief executives can emphasize problems and preferred solutions in a number of ways, including press conferences, speeches, and addresses. To emphasize problems and preferred solutions may be an especially potent tac- tic in such highly visible contexts as a president's state of the union address or a governor's state of the state address.

Candidates for the presidency are often specific in their campaigns on various health policy issues, sometimes even to the point of endorsing specific legislative proposals. Examples include the emphasis President Kennedy and President Johnson gave to enactment of the Medicare program in their cam- paigns and President Clinton's highly visible commitment to fundamental health reform as a central theme of his 1992 campaign. President Bush made enactment of the Medicare Prescription Drug, Improvement, and Modern- ization Act of 2003 a priority as he entered the campaign for his second term in 2004. In his 2008 campaign, and again in his 2012 reelection campaign,

President Obama made health reform one of the highest priorities for his administration. Implementation of the ACA is one of the highest priorities of his second term.

Another issue-raising mechanism some chief executives favor is the appointment of special commissions or task forces. President Clinton used this tactic in the 1993 appointment of the President's Task Force on Health Care Reform (Johnson and Broder 1996), as did President Obama in the creation of the National Commission on Fiscal Responsibility and Reform in 2010.

Governors can also use commissions and task forces to elevate issues on the policy agenda. For example, Massachusetts made history when that state's Gay and Lesbian Student Rights Law was signed by Governor Weld in 1993. He established the nation's first Governor's Commission on Gay and Lesbian Youth, which helped lead the state legislature to enact the law. This law prohibits discrimination in public schools on the basis of sexual orientation. Gay students are guaranteed redress if they suffer name-calling, threats of violence, and unfair treatment in school. In another example, Governor McAuliffe of Virginia established the Governor's Task Force on Mental Health Services and Crisis Response in 2013 and charged it to seek and recommend solutions to improve the state's mental health crisis services.

Chief executives occupy a position that permits them to influence each phase of the policymaking process. In addition to their issue-raising role in agenda setting, they are well positioned to focus the legislative branch on the development of legislation and to prod legislators to continue their work on favored issues even when other demands compete for their time and attention. In addition, chief executives are central to the implementation of policies by virtue of their position atop the executive (or implementing) branch of government, as we discuss in Chapters 7 and 8, and they play a crucial role in modifying previously established policies, as we discuss in Chapter 9.

The Nature of the Health Policy Agenda

The confluence of problems and potential solutions and the political circumstances that surround them invariably shapes the health policy agenda. This agenda, however, is extraordinarily dynamic, literally changing from day to day. In addition, the nation's health policy agenda coexists with policy agendas in other domains, such as defense, welfare, education, and homeland security. The situation is further complicated by the fact that in a pluralistic society where difficult problems exist and clear-cut solutions are rare, every problem and potential solution has different "sides," each with its supporters and detractors. The number, ratio, and intensity of these supporters and detractors are determined by the effect on them of a problem and its possible solution. One consequence of this phenomenon is severe crowding and confounding of the health policy agenda. This agenda is impossible to describe in its full form at any point in time; it is enormous and in constant flux.

As policymakers seek to accommodate the needs and preferences of different interests in particular problem–potential solution combinations, the inevitable result is a large and diverse set of policies that are riddled with incompatibilities and inconsistencies. The subset of US policies on the production and consumption of tobacco products—a mix that simultaneously facilitates and discourages tobacco use—provides a good example of the coexistence of public policies at cross-purposes.

Another example can be seen in the health policy agenda, and in the eventual pattern of public policies, related to medical technology. Policymakers have sought to spread the benefits of new medical technology and at the same time to protect the public from unsafe technologies and slow the growth in overall health costs through controlling the explosive growth of new technologies. The result is a large group of technology-related policies that seek to foster (e.g., NIH, National Science Foundation, other biomedical funding, tax credits for biomedical research in the private sector), to inhibit (e.g., state-run certificate-of-need programs that restrain the diffusion of technology), and to control (e.g., Food and Drug Administration regulation and product liability laws) the development and use of medical technology in the United States.

Its complexity and inconsistency aside, the most important aspect of the health policy agenda is that when a problem is widely acknowledged, when possible solutions have been identified and refined, and when political circumstances are favorable, a window of opportunity opens, albeit sometimes only briefly. Through this window, problem–potential solution combinations move forward to a new stage: development of legislation (see Exhibit 5.1). As we describe in Chapter 6, through the development of legislation, policymakers seek to convert some of their ideas, hopes, and hypotheses about addressing problems into concrete policies in the form of new public laws or amendments to existing ones.

Summary

The policy formulation phase involves agenda setting and the development of legislation, as Exhibit 5.1 shows. Agenda setting is the central topic of this chapter. We discuss the development of legislation in Chapter 6.

Following Kingdon's (2010) conceptualization, agenda setting in public policymaking is a function of the confluence of three streams of activity:

problems, possible solutions to those problems, and political circumstances. When all three streams flow together in a favorable alignment, a window of opportunity opens (see Exhibit 5.1), allowing a problem–potential solution combination, which might be developed into a new public law or an amendment to an existing one, to advance to the next point in the policymaking process: development of legislation.

Review Questions

1. Discuss the formulation phase of policymaking in general terms.
2. Discuss agenda setting as the confluence of three streams of activities. Include the concept of a window of opportunity for legislation development in your answer.
3. Describe the nature of problems that drive policy formulation.
4. Discuss the role of research and analysis in defining problems and assessing alternatives.
5. Contrast decision making in the public and private sectors as it relates to selecting from among alternative solutions to problems.
6. Discuss the involvement of interest groups in the political circumstances that affect agenda setting. Incorporate the specific ways they influence agenda setting in your response.
7. Discuss the role of chief executives in agenda setting at the federal level.
8. Discuss the nature of the health policy agenda that results from agenda setting at the federal level.

References

Aberbach, J. D., and M. A. Peterson. 2006. *The Executive Branch*. New York: Oxford University Press.

AcademyHealth. 2014. "What Is Health Services Research?" Accessed January 10. http://academyhealth.org/About/content.cfm?ItemNumber=831&navItem Number=514.

American Heart Association (AHA). 2014. "Federal Issues." Accessed January 13. http://www.heart.org/HEARTORG/Advocate/Advocate_UCM_001133 _SubHomePage.jsp.

Andres, G. J. 2009. *Lobbying Reconsidered: Politics Under the Influence*. White Plains, NY: Pearson Longman.

Atkins, D., J. Siegel, and J. Slutsky. 2005. "Making Policy When the Evidence Is in Dispute." *Health Affairs* 24 (1): 102–13.

Bergan, D. E. 2009. "Does Grassroots Lobbying Work?" *American Politics Research* 37 (2): 327–52.

Blendon, R., M. Brodie, D. E. Altman, and J. Benson. 2010. *American Public Opinion and Health Care*. Washington, DC: CQ Press.

Brodie, M., and R. J. Blendon. 1995. "The Public's Contribution to Congressional Gridlock on Health Care Reform." *Journal of Health Politics, Policy and Law* 20 (2): 403–10.

Center for Responsive Politics. 2014a. "Health: Background." Accessed January 19. www.opensecrets.org/industries/background.php?cycle=2014&ind=H.

———. 2014b. "Price of Admission." Accessed November 21. www.opensecrets. org/bigpicture/stats.php.

———. 2014c. "Ranked Sectors." Accessed January 13. www.opensecrets.org /lobby/top.php?indexType=c&showYear=2013.

Coalition to Protect America's Health Care. 2014. Facebook page. Accessed January 9. www.facebook.com/protectcare/info.

Collins, P. M., Jr. 2008. *Friends of the Supreme Court: Interest Groups and Judicial Decision Making*. New York: Oxford University Press.

Edwards, G. C., M. P. Wattenberg, and R. L. Lineberry. 2012. *Government in America: People, Politics, and Policy*, brief eleventh edition. New York: Pearson.

Feldstein, P. J. 2006. *The Politics of Health Legislation: An Economic Perspective*, third edition. Chicago: Health Administration Press.

Forrest, C. B., D. Martin, E. Holve, and A. Millman. 2008. *Health Services Research Doctoral Core Competencies: Final Report*. Accessed January 10, 2014. http://archive.ahrq.gov/funding/hsrcomp08/hsrcomp08.html.

Godwin, R. K., S. Ainsworth, and E. Godwin. 2013. *Lobbying and Policymaking: The Public Pursuit of Private Interests*. Washington, DC: CQ Press.

Green, J. 1995. "High-Court Ruling Protects Hospital-Bill Surcharges." *AHA News* 31 (18): 1.

Hacker, J. S. 2010. "The Road to Somewhere: Why Health Reform Happened; Or Why Political Scientists Who Write About Public Policy Shouldn't Assume They Know How to Shape It." *Perspectives on Politics* 8 (3): 861–76.

———. 1997. *The Road to Nowhere*. Princeton, NJ: Princeton University Press.

Herrnson, P. S., R. G. Shaiko, and C. Wilcox. 2005. *The Interest Group Connection: Electioneering, Lobbying, and Policymaking in Washington*, second edition. Washington, DC: CQ Press.

Johnson, H., and D. S. Broder. 1996. *The System: The American Way of Politics at the Breaking Point*. Boston: Little, Brown.

Kaiser Family Foundation. 2013. "Kaiser Health Tracking Poll: December 2013." Published December 20. www.kff.org/health-reform/poll-finding /kaiser-health-tracking-poll-december-2013.

———. 2009. "Kaiser Health Tracking Poll: July 2009." Published July. www.kaiser familyfoundation.files.wordpress.com/2013/01/7945.pdf.

Kersh, R. 2014. "Ten Myths About Health Lobbyists." In *Health Politics and Policy*, fifth edition, edited by J. A. Morone and D. Ehlke, 236–53. Stamford, CT: Cengage Learning.

Kingdon, J. W. 2010. *Agendas, Alternatives, and Public Policies*, updated second edition. Upper Saddle River, NJ: Pearson Education.

Martin, A. B., M. Hartman, L. Whittle, A. Catlin, and the National Health Expenditure Accounts Team. 2014. "National Health Spending in 2012: Rate of Health Spending Growth Remained Low for the Fourth Consecutive Year." *Health Affairs* 33 (1): 67–77.

Morone, J. A. 2014. "The Presidency." In *Health Politics and Policy*, fifth edition, edited by J. A. Morone and D. Ehlke, 56–75. Stamford, CT: Cengage Learning.

Ornstein, N. J., and S. Elder. 1978. *Interest Groups, Lobbying and Policymaking*. Washington, DC: Congressional Quarterly Press.

Patient-Centered Outcomes Research Institute (PCORI). 2014. "About Us." Published October 6. www.pcori.org/about-us/landing/.

Price, D. 1978. "Policymaking in Congressional Committees: The Impact of 'Environmental' Factors." *American Political Science Review* 72 (2): 548–75.

Redhead, C. S. 2014. *Appropriations and Fund Transfers in the Patient Protection and Affordable Care Act (ACA)*. Congressional Research Service Report R41301. Published October 10. www.fas.org/sgp/crs/misc/R41301.pdf.

Schlesinger, M. 2014. "Public Opinion." In *Health Politics and Policy*, fifth edition, edited by J. A. Morone and D. Ehlke, 214–35. Stamford, CT: Cengage Learning.

Shah, A. 2013. "Global Financial Crisis." Published March 24. www.globalissues.org/article/768/global-financial-crisis.

Skidmore, M. 1970. *Medicare and the American Rhetoric of Reconciliation*. Tuscaloosa, AL: University of Alabama Press.

Steinberg, E. P., and B. R. Luce. 2005. "Evidence Based? Caveat Emptor!" *Health Affairs* 24 (1): 80–92.

US Department of State. 2004. *Outline of U.S. Legal System*. Published December 20. http://iipdigital.usembassy.gov/st/english/publication/2011/07/20110726143910su0.8681996.html#axzz2qr6f1Sx3.

Weissert, C. S., and W. G. Weissert. 2012. *Governing Health: The Politics of Health Policy*, fourth edition. Baltimore, MD: Johns Hopkins University Press.

Yankelovich, D., and W. Friedman. 2010. "How Americans Make Up Their Minds: The Dynamics of the Public's Learning Curve and Its Meaning for American Life." In *Toward Wiser Public Judgment*, edited by D. Yankelovich and W. Friedman, 1–8. Nashville, TN: Vanderbilt University Press.

POLICY FORMULATION: DEVELOPMENT OF LEGISLATION

Learning Objectives

After reading this chapter, you should be able to

- understand the policy formulation phase of policymaking more thoroughly;
- list and describe the steps in the choreography of legislation development;
- discuss the legislative process in state governments;
- discuss the drafting of legislative proposals, including the forms they can take;
- discuss the legislative committee and subcommittee structure of Congress;
- identify and describe the roles of the key congressional committees and subcommittees with health policy jurisdiction; and
- describe the federal and state budget legislative development processes.

As we noted in Chapters 3 and 5, the formulation phase of health policymaking is made up of two distinct and sequential parts: agenda setting and legislation development. Chapter 5 focused on agenda setting; in this chapter we turn our attention to the development of legislation. Policy formulation can be fully appreciated only through an understanding of the combination of activities associated with agenda setting and legislation development.

As with the discussion of agenda setting in Chapter 5, this discussion of legislation development is confined almost exclusively to its occurrence at the federal level of government. However, state and local governments develop their own legislation, and this is generally done using a similar approach. The problems legislation is developed to address differ at each level, as do many of the participants and the specific mechanisms and procedures used in developing legislation.

The result of the entire formulation phase of policymaking is public policy in the form of new public laws or amendments to existing laws.

New health-related laws or amendments originate from the policy agenda. Recall that the health policy agenda is established through the interactions of a diverse array of problems, possible solutions to those problems, and the dynamic political circumstances that relate to the problems and to their potential solutions. Combinations of problems, potential solutions, and political circumstances that achieve priority on the policy agenda move on to the next component of the policy formulation phase: legislation development (see the darkly shaded portion of Exhibit 6.1).

The laws and amendments to existing laws that result from the formulation phase of policymaking are tangible, and purposely so. They can be seen and read in a number of places (see Appendix 5 for example). The US Constitution prohibits the enactment of laws that are not specifically and directly made known to the people who are to be bound by them. In practice, federal laws are published for the citizenry immediately upon enactment. Of course, it is incumbent on persons who might be affected by laws to know of them and to be certain that they understand the effects of those laws. Health professionals should devote time and attention to the potential and real impact of relevant laws and amendments.

At the federal level, enacted laws are first printed in pamphlet form called *slip law*. Later, laws are published in the *US Statutes at Large* and eventually incorporated into the *US Code*. The *Statutes at Large*, published annually, contains the laws enacted during each session of Congress. In effect, it is a compilation of all laws enacted in a particular year. The *US Code* is a complete compilation of all the nation's laws. A new edition of the code is published every six years, with cumulative supplements published annually. Federal public laws can be read at www.congress.gov.

The Choreography of Legislation Development

Development of legislation is the point in policy formulation at which specific legislative proposals, which are characterized in Chapter 5 as hypothetical or unproved potential solutions to the problems they are intended to address, advance through a series of steps that can end in new or amended public laws. These steps, not unlike those of a complicated dance, are specified or choreographed. The steps followed at the federal level are shown schematically in Exhibit 6.2. A variation of these steps was shown earlier in Exhibit 3.2 and briefly introduced and described in Chapter 3. Only when all of the steps are completed does a new public law or, far more typically, an amendment to a previously enacted law result. The steps that make up the development of legislation activity provide the framework for most of the discussion in this chapter.

EXHIBIT 6.1

Policymaking Process: Development of Legislation in the Formulation Phase

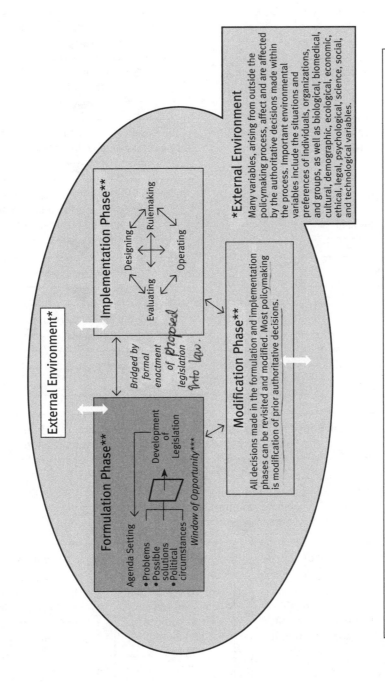

Formulation Phase**

Agenda Setting

Development of Legislation

• Problems
• Possible solutions
• Political circumstances

Window of Opportunity***

Bridged by formal enactment of proposed legislation into law.

Implementation Phase**

Designing ↔ Rulemaking

Evaluating ↔ Operating

External Environment*

Modification Phase**

All decisions made in the formulation and implementation phases can be revisited and modified. Most policymaking is modification of prior authoritative decisions.

*External Environment

Many variables, arising from outside the policymaking process, affect and are affected by the authoritative decisions made within the process. Important environmental variables include the situations and preferences of individuals, organizations, and groups, as well as biological, biomedical, cultural, demographic, ecological, economic, ethical, legal, psychological, science, social, and technological variables.

Policymakers in all three branches of government make policy in the form of position-appropriate, or authoritative, decisions. Their decisions differ in that the **legislative branch is primarily involved in formulation, the **executive branch** is primarily involved in implementation, and both are involved in modification of prior decisions or policies. The **judicial branch** interprets and assesses the legality of decisions made within all three phases of the policymaking process.

***A window of opportunity opens for possible progression of issues through formulation, enactment, implementation, and modification when there is a favorable confluence of problems, possible solutions, and political circumstances.

EXHIBIT 6.2
The Steps in Legislation Development

Bill is originated and drafted.	Bill is originated and drafted.
Representative introduces bill in the House.	Senator introduces bill in the Senate.
Bill is read in the House and assigned to a committee by the speaker.	Bill is read in the Senate and assigned to a committee by the majority leader.
Bill leaves committee, is scheduled for floor consideration and debate, and may be amended.	Bill leaves committee, is scheduled for floor consideration and debate, and may be amended.
House passes bill.	Senate passes bill.
Bill is sent to Senate.	Bill is sent to House.

A conference committee is created to resolve differences if both chambers do not pass an identical bill.

Identical bill is passed by both House and Senate OR one branch agrees to the other branch's version OR bill is amended and both branches vote again and pass amended version.

Bill is presented to the president, who has four options.

Option 1:	*Option 2:*	*Option 3:*	*Option 4:*
President signs bill into law.	During congressional session, bill becomes law after 10 days without presidential signature.	When Congress is not in session, bill does not become law without presidential signature.	President vetoes bill. Two-thirds vote in House and Senate can override veto.

Source: Adapted from Teitelbaum, J. B., and S. E. Wilensky. 2013. *Essentials of Health Policy and Law,* second edition. Burling, MA: Jones and Bartlett Learning. www.jblearning.com. Reprinted with permission.

Legislation development begins with the origination of ideas for legislation and extends through the enactment of some of those ideas into law or the amendment of existing laws. The steps of this process apply equally whether the resulting legislation is a new law or an amendment. Sullivan (2007) provides an extensive description of the steps through which federal legislation is developed. Similarly, most states include descriptions of their legislative processes on their websites. For example, Massachusetts publishes *Lawmaking in Massachusetts* (Galvin 2014). Exhibit 6.3 illustrates the steps in the state of Washington's legislative process, a process typical of the states.

At the federal level, the path through which legislation is developed begins with ideas for proposed legislation or bills in the agenda-setting stage, extends through formal drafting of legislative proposals and then several other steps, and culminates in the enactment of laws derived from some of the proposals. In practice, only a fraction of the legislative proposals that are formally introduced in a Congress—the two annual sessions spanning the terms of office of members of the House of Representatives—are enacted into law. For example, the One Hundred Fourteenth Congress spans the period from January 3, 2015, to January 3, 2017. Proposals that are not enacted by the end of the congressional session in which they were introduced die and must be reintroduced in the next Congress to be considered further.

As the bridge between policy formulation and implementation (shown in Exhibit 6.1), formal enactment of proposed legislation into new or

---

EXHIBIT 6.3
Steps in the Legislative Process in the State of Washington

1. A bill (a proposed law presented to the Legislature for consideration) may be introduced in either the Senate or House of Representatives by a member.
2. It is referred to a committee for a hearing. The committee studies the bill and may hold public hearings on it. It can then pass, reject, or take no action on the bill.
3. The committee report on the passed bill is read in open session of the House or Senate, and the bill is then referred to the Rules Committee.
4. The Rules Committee can either place the bill on the second reading of the calendar for debate before the entire body or take no action.
5. At the second reading, a bill is subject to debate and amendment before being placed on the third reading calendar for final passage.
6. After passing one house, the bill goes through the same procedure in the other house.
7. If amendments are made, the other house must approve the changes.
8. When the bill is accepted in both houses, it is signed by the respective leaders and sent to the governor.
9. The governor signs the bill into law or may veto all or part of it. If the governor fails to act on the bill, it may become law without a signature.

Source: Washington State Legislature (2014).

amended law represents a significant transition between these two phases of the overall public policymaking process. The focus in this chapter is on ways in which public laws are developed and enacted in the policymaking process; their implementation is discussed in Chapters 7 and 8.

As we described in Chapter 5, individuals, health-related organizations, and especially the interest groups to which they belong are instrumental in the agenda setting that precedes legislation development. They also actively participate in the development itself: Once a health policy problem or issue achieves an actionable place on the policy agenda and moves to the next stage of policy formulation—development of legislation—those with concerns and preferences often continue to seek to exert influence.

Individuals and health-related organizations and interest groups can participate directly in originating ideas for legislation, helping with the actual drafting of legislative proposals, and attending the hearings sponsored by legislative committees. When competing bills seek to address a problem, those with interests in the problems align themselves with favored legislative solutions and oppose those they do not favor. The following sections present a detailed discussion of the steps in legislation development at the federal level, although much of this information also applies to legislative processes in the states.

Originating and Drafting Legislative Proposals

The development of legislation begins with the conversion of ideas, hopes, and hypotheses about how problems might be addressed through changes in policy—ideas that emerge from agenda setting—into concrete legislative proposals or bills (see Exhibit 6.2). Actually, proposed legislation can be introduced in one of four forms. Two of the forms, bills and joint resolutions, are used for making laws. The other two forms of proposed legislation, simple resolutions and concurrent resolutions, are used to handle matters of congressional administration or for expressing nonbinding policy views.

Forms of Legislative Proposals

The discussion of originating and drafting legislative proposals presented here focuses on bills because they are the most common way for legislation to emerge. Congress selects between using bills or joint resolutions to introduce legislative proposals using conventions that have developed over time for the subject matter involved. Although bills are much more common than joint resolutions, a good example of a routinely used joint resolution is one to make continuing appropriations beyond the end of a fiscal year when the regular appropriations bills for the next year have not been completed. This joint resolution is called a *continuing resolution* (CR) (Office of the Legislative Counsel, US House of Representatives 2014).

For a bill or a joint resolution to become law, it must pass both the House of Representatives and the Senate and be signed by the president. Even if a bill or joint resolution is passed and presented to the president, it can be vetoed. Such vetoed legislation can become law if Congress overrides the veto by a two-thirds vote. The legislation can also become law if the president takes no action for a period of ten days while Congress is in session. There is no legal difference and little practical difference between a bill and a resolution, and they are not differentiated operationally here.

Simple resolutions (passed in either the House of Representatives or the Senate) and concurrent resolutions (passed in both the House of Representatives and the Senate) are not presented to the president because they do not become law. Exhibit 6.4 summarizes the four forms that legislative proposals can take.

Origins of Ideas for Public Policies

Ideas for public policies originate in many places. They obviously come from members of the House of Representatives and the Senate. In fact, many Congress members are elected, at least in part, on the basis of the legislative ideas they expressed in their campaigns. Promises to introduce certain proposals, made specifically to the constituents candidates seek to represent, are core aspects of the American form of government and frequent sources of eventual legislative proposals. Once in office, legislators may become more aware of and knowledgeable about the need to amend or repeal existing laws or enact new laws as their understanding of the problems and potential solutions that face their constituents or the larger society evolves.

But legislators are not the only source of ideas for laws or amendments. Individual citizens, health-related organizations, and interest groups representing many individuals or organizations may petition the government—a right guaranteed by the First Amendment—and propose ideas for the development of policy in the form of laws or amendments. In effect, such petitions result directly from the participation of individuals, organizations, and groups in agenda setting as described in Chapter 5. Much of the nation's policy originates in this way because certain individuals, organizations, and interest groups have considerable knowledge of the problem–potential solution combinations that affect them or their members.

Individuals, organizations, and groups also participate in the development of legislation. Interest groups tend to be especially influential in legislation development, as they are in agenda setting, because of their pooled resources. Well-staffed interest groups, for example, can draw on the services

EXHIBIT 6.4
Comparison
of Forms of
Legislative
Proposals

Forms of Legislative Proposals	Passage Required by	Presentment to President	Result	Example
Bill	Both House of Representatives and Senate	Yes	Law	H.R. 2568 (111th Congress)
Joint resolution	Both House of Representatives and Senate	Yes	Law	H.J. Res. 52 (a CR from the 110th Congress)
Concurrent resolution	Both House of Representatives and Senate	No	Not law (binding only as to certain matters of congressional administration)	S. Con. Res. 70 (the concurrent resolution on the budget for fiscal year 2009; 110th Congress)
Simple resolution	Either House of Representatives or Senate	No	Not law (binding only as to certain matters of administration of the house that passed it)	H. Res. 88 (a "special rule" governing House debate on a bill; 111th Congress)

Source: Adapted from Office of the Legislative Counsel, US House of Representatives (2014).

of legislative draftspersons to transform ideas and concepts into suitable legislative language.

An increasingly important source of ideas for legislative proposals is "executive communication" from members of the executive branch to members of the legislative branch. Such communications, which also play a role in agenda setting, usually take the form of a letter from a senior member of the executive branch such as a member of the president's cabinet, the head of an independent agency, or even the president. These communications typically include comprehensive drafts of proposed bills. They are sent simultaneously to the speaker of the House of Representatives and the president of the Senate, who can insert them into the legislation development procedures at appropriate places.

The executive branch's role as a source of policy ideas is based in the US Constitution. Although the Constitution establishes a government characterized by the separation of powers, Article II, Section 3, imposes an obligation on the president to report to Congress from time to time on the state of the union and to recommend such policies in the form of laws or amendments as the president considers necessary, useful, or expedient. Many of the executive communications to Congress follow up on ideas first aired in annual presidential State of the Union addresses to Congress.

Executive communications that pertain to proposed legislation are referred by the legislative leaders who receive them to the appropriate legislative committee or committees that have jurisdiction in the relevant areas. The chairperson of an affected committee may introduce the bill either in the form in which it was received or with whatever changes the chairperson considers necessary or desirable. Only members of Congress can actually introduce proposed legislation, no matter who originates the idea or drafts the proposal.

The practice of having committee chairpersons introduce legislative proposals that arise through executive communication is followed even when the majority of the House or Senate and the president are not of the same political party, although there is no constitutional or statutory requirement that a bill be introduced to put the executive branch's recommendations into effect. When the chairperson of the committee with jurisdiction does not introduce a bill that is based on executive communication, the committee or one of its subcommittees considers the proposed legislation to determine whether the bill should be introduced.

The most important regular executive communication is the proposed federal budget the president transmits annually to Congress (Oleszek 2014). Recently prepared budgets and related supporting documents are available from the Office of Management and Budget (OMB; www.whitehouse.gov /omb/budget). More is said about the budget process later in this chapter; here, suffice it to say that the president's budget proposal, together with supportive testimony by officials of the various executive branch departments and agencies, individuals, organizations, and interest groups concerned about the budget—before one of the 12 subcommittees of the appropriations committees of the House and Senate—is the basis of the appropriation bills that these committees eventually draft.

Drafting Legislative Proposals

Drafting legislative proposals is an art in itself, one requiring considerable skill, knowledge, and experience. Any member of the Senate or House of Representatives can draft bills, and these legislators' staffs are usually instrumental in drafting them, often with assistance from the Office of Legislative Counsel in the Senate or House of Representatives.

Information on how the Office of the Legislative Counsel in the House of Representatives supports legislation development is available at www.house.gov/legcoun. Information on how the Senate's Office of the Legislative Counsel supports legislation development is available at www.slc.senate.gov.

Sandra Strokoff (2014), senior counsel in the Office of the Legislative Counsel, US House of Representatives, describes the work of the attorneys who work in the counsel's office as follows:

> Frequently, on the floor of the House of Representatives, one will hear a Member refer to another as the "author" of a bill who has "carefully crafted" the language of the proposed legislation. Statements like these make me smile, because if the Members are the authors, then I and my colleagues in the Office of the Legislative Counsel of the House of Representatives are the ghost writers.
>
> The Office of the Legislative Counsel, created by statute originally in 1918, is currently composed of 30-plus attorneys who generally toil in anonymity, at least as far as those outside the legislative process are concerned. Attorneys are charged with taking the idea of any Member or committee of the House of Representatives requesting the services of the Office and transforming it into legislative language or, as one of my clients used to say, "the magic words." We participate in all stages of the legislative process, be it preparing a bill for introduction, drafting amendments, participating in any conference of the two Houses of Congress to resolve differences between the two versions of the bill, or incorporating changes in the bill at each stage for publication and ultimately for presentation to the president. Frequently, we draft while debate is going on—both during committee consideration and on the House Floor, and may be asked to explain the meaning or effect of legislative language.

When bills are drafted in the executive branch, trained legislative counsels are typically involved. These counsels work in several executive branch departments, and their work includes drafting bills to be forwarded to Congress. Similarly, proposed legislation that arises in the private sector, typically from interest groups, is drafted by people with expertise in this intricate task.

On occasion, legislation drafting is undertaken as a public–private partnership (Hacker 1997, 2010). Such legislation drafting has occurred twice in recent decades in the health policy arena, first in the case of the Clinton administration's attempt at substantial health reform, and again in the more successful Obama administration proposal that eventually was enacted in 2010 as the Affordable Care Act (ACA).

In the first example, in late 1993, after many months of feverish drafting by a team including some of the nation's foremost health policy experts, President Clinton presented his proposal for legislation that would fundamentally reform the American healthcare system. The document, 1,431 pages in length, outlined the drafters' vision of the way health services should be provided and financed in the United States. The proposal was in the form of a comprehensive draft of a bill (to be called the Health Security Act) that could potentially be enacted into law.

However, the proposal faced a long and difficult path from legislation development to possible enactment. Hacker and Skocpol (1997, 315–16) note that "President Clinton sought to enact comprehensive federal rules that would, in theory, simultaneously control medical costs and ensure universal insurance coverage. The bold Health Security initiative was meant to give everyone what they wanted, delicately balancing competing ideas and claimants, deftly maneuvering between major factions in Congress, and helping to revive the political prospects of the Democratic Party in the process."

In the end, the Clinton health reform proposal failed to make it successfully through the remaining steps in legislation development to enactment into law (Johnson and Broder 1996; Skocpol 1996). Peterson (1997, 291) characterized the failure of this proposal as a situation in which "the bold gambit of comprehensive reform had once again succumbed to the power of antagonistic stakeholders, a public paralyzed by the fears of disrupting what it already had, and the challenge of coalition building engendered by the highly decentralized character of American government."

The second example of developing legislation through a public–private partnership led to a more successful outcome. The ACA was enacted into law in 2010. (You may want to review Appendix 1, an overview of the ACA.) There have been difficulties in implementing this law and extraordinary attempts have been made to repeal it (Jost 2014), but this legislation was successfully developed into public law, and a complex law at that.

Technically, in March 2010, the One Hundred Eleventh Congress enacted the ACA (P.L. 111-148). The law was substantially amended by the health provisions in the Health Care and Education Reconciliation Act of 2010 (P.L. 111-152). Several other laws that were subsequently enacted made more targeted changes to specific ACA provisions. The ACA emerged from bills in the House of Representatives and the Senate. In the Senate, two committees—the Committee on Health, Education, Labor and Pensions (HELP) and the Committee on Finance—participated in the drafting. The law was formed in an amazingly convoluted series of negotiations involving numerous members of Congress working through various committees, the administration, congressional and administration staff, external stakeholders such as the pharmaceutical and insurance industries, and the professionals who wrote the actual language of the law. Cannan (2013) wrote an excellent history of the ACA's dynamic path through the legislation development step.

The ACA has multiple goals. Among the most important are to increase access to affordable health insurance for the millions of Americans without coverage and make health insurance more affordable for those already covered. The act makes numerous changes in the way healthcare is financed, organized, and delivered. Among its many provisions, the ACA restructures the private health insurance market, sets minimum standards for health coverage, creates a mandate for most US residents to obtain health insurance coverage, and provides for the establishment of state-based insurance exchanges for the purchase of private health insurance. Certain individuals and families receive federal subsidies to reduce the cost of purchasing coverage through the exchanges. The ACA also expands eligibility for Medicaid; amends the Medicare program in ways that are intended to reduce the growth in Medicare spending; imposes an excise tax on insurance plans found to have high premiums; and makes numerous other changes to the tax code, Medicare, Medicaid, the Children's Health Insurance Program, and many other federal programs. Full implementation of the law involves all the major healthcare stakeholders, including the federal and state governments, as well as employers, insurers, and healthcare providers (Redhead et al. 2012).

Packed into 1,024 pages, the ACA is a product of input from many sources. For example, the individual mandate provision requiring most residents to obtain health insurance, coupled with public subsidies for many, has deep historical roots in previous health reform attempts. The conservative Heritage Foundation proposed an individual mandate as an alternative to single-payer healthcare as far back as 1989 (Avik 2012). In 2006, Massachusetts enacted health reform at the state level that included an individual mandate and an insurance exchange (Wees, Zaslavsky, and Ayanian 2013).

No matter who drafts legislation, however, only members of Congress can officially sponsor a proposal, and the legislative sponsors are ultimately responsible for the language in their bills. Bills commonly have multiple sponsors and many cosponsors. Once ideas for solving problems through policy are drafted in legislative language, they are ready for the next step: introduction for formal consideration by Congress. Although the Health Security proposal the Clinton administration drafted was formally introduced in Congress, it was not enacted into law. The ACA, on the other hand, was formally introduced and moved through the other steps in legislation development to ultimate enactment into law.

Introducing and Referring Proposed Legislation to Committees

Members of the Senate and the House of Representatives who have chosen to sponsor or cosponsor legislation introduce their proposals in the form of bills (see Exhibit 6.2). On occasion, identical bills are introduced in the Senate and House for simultaneous consideration. When bills are introduced in either chamber of Congress, they are assigned a sequential number (e.g., H.R. 1, H.R. 2, H.R. 3, etc.; S. 1, S. 2, S. 3, etc.) based on the order of introduction by the presiding officer, and are referred to the appropriate standing committee or committees for further study and consideration. Exhibit 6.5 illustrates the path of a bill introduced in the House of Representatives through its enactment into public law. (Follow the path from the bottom of the exhibit up.)

Date	Chamber	Actions
01/24/2014		Became P.L. 113-77, Poison Center Network Act of 2014
01/24/2014		Signed by president.
01/15/2014	House	Presented to president.
01/15/2014	Senate	Message on Senate action sent to the House.
01/14/2014	Senate	Passed Senate without amendment by unanimous consent.
01/09/2014	Senate	Received in the Senate.
01/08/2014 – 3:47pm	House	On motion to suspend the rules and pass the bill as amended, agreed to by the Yeas and Nays: (2/3 required): 388–18.
01/08/2014 – 3:39pm	House	Considered as unfinished business.
01/08/2014 – 1:12pm	House	At the conclusion of debate, the Yeas and Nays were demanded and ordered. Pursuant to the provisions of clause 8, rule XX, the chair announced that further proceedings on the motion would be postponed.

EXHIBIT 6.5
Path of a Bill to Public Law: H.R. 3527 to P.L. 113-77, Poison Center Network Act of 2014

(continued)

EXHIBIT 6.5
Path of a Bill
to Public Law:
H.R. 3527 to P.L.
113-77, Poison
Center Network
Act of 2014
(continued)

Date	Chamber	Actions
01/08/2014 – 12:57pm	House	Debate—The House proceeded with forty minutes of debate.
01/08/2014 – 12:57pm	House	Considered under suspension of the rules.
01/08/2014 – 12:57pm	House	Mr. Pitts moved to suspend the rules and pass the bill, as amended.
01/07/2014	House	Reported by the Committee on Energy and Commerce.
12/10/2013	House	Committee Consideration and Mark-Up Session Held.
12/10/2013	House	Forwarded by Subcommittee to Full Committee.
12/10/2013	House	Subcommittee Consideration and Mark-Up Session Held.
11/22/2013	House	Referred to the Subcommittee on Health.
11/18/2013	House	Referred to the House Committee on Energy and Commerce.
11/18/2013	House	Introduced in House.

Source: Poison Center Network Act of 2014, H.R. 3527, 113th Cong. (2014).

Legislative Committees and Subcommittees

The Senate and the House of Representatives are organized into legislative committees and subcommittees. The committee structure of Congress is crucial to the development of legislation. Committee and subcommittee deliberations provide the settings for intensive and thorough consideration of legislative proposals and issues. Exhibit 6.6 shows the current legislative committee structure of the US Congress.

Each standing committee has jurisdiction over a certain area of legislation, and all bills that pertain to a particular area are referred to its committee. Information about the committees is available on their websites, which can be accessed through www.congress.gov. Committees are divided into subcommittees to facilitate work. For example, the Ways and Means Committee of the House of Representatives has six subcommittees: Health, Human Resources, Oversight, Select Revenue Measures, Social Security, and Trade.

House	Senate
Standing Committees	
• Agriculture • Appropriations • Armed Services • Budget • Education and the Workforce • Energy and Commerce • Ethics • Financial Services • Foreign Affairs • Homeland Security • House Administration • Judiciary • Natural Resources • Oversight and Government Reform • Rules • Science, Space, and Technology • Small Business • Transportation and Infrastructure • Veterans' Affairs • Ways and Means	• Agriculture, Nutrition, and Forestry • Appropriations • Armed Services • Banking, Housing, and Urban Affairs • Budget • Commerce, Science, and Transportation • Energy and Natural Resources • Environment and Public Works • Finance • Foreign Relations • Health, Education, Labor, and Pensions • Homeland Security and Governmental Affairs • Judiciary • Rules and Administration • Small Business and Entrepreneurship • Veterans' Affairs
Special and Select Committees	
• Intelligence (Permanent) (Select Committee)	• Aging (Special Committee) • Ethics (Select Committee) • Indian Affairs (Other Committee) • Intelligence (Select Committee)
Joint Committees	
• Joint Economic • Joint Library • Joint Printing • Joint Taxation	

EXHIBIT 6.6
Current Committees of the US Congress

Source: Congress.gov (2014).

Sometimes the content of a bill calls for assignment to more than one committee. In this case, the bill is assigned to multiple committees either jointly or, more commonly, sequentially. For example, the Clinton administration's Health Security plan was introduced simultaneously in the House and the Senate as H.R. 3600 and S. 1757. Because of its scope and complexity, the bill was then referred jointly to ten House committees and two Senate committees for consideration and debate.

Membership on the various congressional committees is divided between the two major political parties. The proportion of members from each party is determined by the majority party. Legislators typically seek membership on committees that have jurisdiction in their particular areas of interest and expertise. The interests of their constituencies typically influence the interests of policymakers. For example, members of the House of Representatives from agricultural districts or financial centers often prefer to join committees that deal with these areas. The same is true of senators in terms of whether they hail from primarily rural or highly urbanized states, from the industrialized Northeast, or from the more agrarian West. The seniority of committee members follows the order of their appointment to the committee.

The majority party in each chamber also controls the appointment of committee and subcommittee chairpersons. These chairpersons exert great power in the development of legislation, because they determine the order and the pace in which the committees or subcommittees they lead consider legislative proposals.

Each committee has a professional staff to assist with administrative details involved in its consideration of bills. Under certain conditions, a standing committee may also appoint consultants on a temporary or intermittent basis to assist the committee in its work. By virtue of expert knowledge, the professional staff members who serve committees and subcommittees are key participants in legislation development.

Committees with Health Policy Jurisdiction

Although no congressional committee is devoted exclusively to the health policy domain, several committees and subcommittees have jurisdiction in health-related legislation development. In recent decades, health has been an especially important and prevalent domain in the federal and state policy agendas. The committees and subcommittees with jurisdiction for health matters have been busy.

At the federal level, there is some overlap in the jurisdictions of committees with health-related legislative responsibilities. Most general health bills are referred to the House Committee on Energy and Commerce and the Senate HELP Committee. However, any bills involving taxes and revenues must be referred to the House Committee on Ways and Means and the Senate Committee on Finance. These two committees have substantial health policy jurisdiction because so much health policy involves taxes as a source of funding. The main health policy interests of these committees are outlined here.

- *Committee on Finance* (www.finance.senate.gov), *with its Subcommittee on Health Care.* This Senate committee has jurisdiction over health programs under the Social Security Act and health programs financed by a specific tax or trust fund. This role gives the committee jurisdiction over matters related to the ACA, Medicare, and Medicaid.

- *Committee on Health, Education, Labor, and Pensions* (www.help .senate.gov), *with its Subcommittees on Children and Families, Employment and Workplace Safety, and Primary Care and Aging.* This Senate committee's jurisdiction encompasses most of the agencies, institutes, and programs of the Department of Health and Human Services (HHS), including the Food and Drug Administration, the Centers for Disease Control and Prevention, the National Institutes of Health, the Administration on Aging, the Substance Abuse and Mental Health Services Administration, and the Agency for Healthcare Research and Quality. The committee also oversees public health and health insurance policy.

- *Committee on Ways and Means* (http://waysandmeans.house.gov) *with its Subcommittee on Health.* This House committee has jurisdiction over bills and matters that pertain to providing payments from any source for healthcare, health delivery systems, or health research. The jurisdiction of the Subcommittee on Health includes bills and matters related to the healthcare programs of the Social Security Act (including Titles XVIII and XIX, which are the Medicare and Medicaid programs) and tax credit and deduction provisions of the Internal Revenue Code dealing with health insurance premiums and healthcare costs.

- *Committee on Energy and Commerce* (http://energycommerce .house.gov) *with its Subcommittees, including those on Health and on Environment and the Economy.* This House committee has jurisdiction over all bills and matters related to public health and quarantine; hospital construction; mental health; biomedical research and development; health information technology, privacy, and cybersecurity; public health insurance (Medicare, Medicaid) and private health insurance; medical malpractice insurance; the regulation of food and drugs; drug abuse; HHS; the Clean Air Act; and environmental protection in general, including the Safe Drinking Water Act.

Legislative Committee and Subcommittee Operations

Depending on whether the chairperson of a committee has assigned a bill to a subcommittee, either the full committee or the subcommittee can, if it chooses, hold hearings on the bill. At these public hearings, members of the executive branch, representatives of health-related organizations and interest groups, and other individuals can present their views and recommendations on the legislation under consideration. For example, from the One Hundred

Tenth Congress, H.R. 1014, a bill to amend the federal Food, Drug, and Cosmetic Act and the Public Health Service Act to improve the prevention, diagnosis, and treatment of heart disease, stroke, and cardiovascular diseases in women, was introduced in the House of Representatives on February 13, 2007. An identical bill, S. 573, was simultaneously introduced in the Senate. The bills followed different courses.

In the House, H.R. 1014 was referred to the House Committee on Energy and Commerce on the day it was introduced, and it was sent to the Subcommittee on Health the following day. Hearings on the bill were held on May 1, 2007. Following further discussion and consideration, the bill, with some modification, passed the House on September 23, 2008. In the Senate, S. 573 was introduced on September 13, 2007. The bill was immediately referred to the Senate HELP Committee, where it received no further action. Appendix 16 provides an example of testimony at a hearing related to H.R. 1014 before the House Subcommittee on Health of the Committee on Energy and Commerce.

Following such hearings, and there may be a number of them for a bill, members of committees or subcommittees "mark up" the bills they are considering. This term refers to going through the original bill line by line and making changes. Sometimes, when similar bills or bills addressing the same issue have been introduced, they are combined in the markup process. In cases of subcommittee involvement, when the subcommittee has completed its markup and voted to approve the bill, it reports out the bill to the full committee with jurisdiction.

When no subcommittee is involved, or when a full committee has reviewed the work of a subcommittee and voted to approve the bill, the full committee reports out the bill for a vote, this time to the floor of the Senate or House. At this point, the administration can formally weigh in with support for or opposition to a bill. This input is issued through a Statement of Administration Policy, examples of which are available at the White House website (www.whitehouse.gov/omb/legislative_sap_default).

If a committee votes to report a bill favorably, a member of the committee staff writes a report in the name of a committee member. This report is an extremely important document. The committee report describes the purposes and scope of the bill and the reasons the committee recommends its approval by the entire Senate or House. As an example, the report for H.R. 1014 can be read at the Congress website (www.congress.gov/bill/110th-congress/house-bill/1014).

Committee reports are useful and informative documents in the legislative history of a public law or amendments to it. These reports are used by courts in considering matters related to particular laws that have been enacted and by executive branch departments and agencies as guidance for implementing enacted laws and amendments. They provide information regarding legislative proposals for those who are interested in the history, purpose, and meaning of enacted legislation.

Generally, a committee report contains an analysis in which the purpose of each section of a bill is described. All changes or amendments to existing law that the bill would require are indicated in the report, and the text of laws the bill would repeal are set out. The report begins by describing and explaining committee amendments to the bill as it was originally referred to the committee. Executive communications pertaining to the bill are usually quoted in full in the report.

House or Senate Floor Action on Proposed Legislation

Following approval of a bill by the full committee with jurisdiction, the bill and its report are discharged from the committee. The House or Senate receives it from the committee and places it on the legislative calendar for floor action (see Exhibit 6.2).

Bills can be further amended in debate on the House or Senate floor. However, because great reliance is placed on the committee process in both chambers of Congress, amendments to bills proposed from the floor require considerable support.

Once a bill passes in either the House or the Senate, it is sent to the other chamber. The step of referral to a committee with jurisdiction, and perhaps then to a subcommittee, is repeated, and another round of hearings, markup, and eventual action may or may not take place. If the bill is again reported out of committee, it goes to the involved chamber's floor for a final vote. If it is passed in the second chamber, any differences in the House and Senate versions of a bill must be resolved before the bill is sent to the White House for action by the president.

Conference Committee Actions on Proposed Legislation

To resolve differences in a bill that both chambers of Congress have passed, a conference committee (see Exhibit 6.2) may be established (US Senate 2014). Conferees are usually the ranking members of the committees that reported out the bill in each chamber. If they can resolve the differences, a conference report is written and both chambers of Congress vote on it. If the conferees cannot reach agreement, or if either chamber does not accept the report, the bill dies. However, if both chambers accept the conference report, the bill is sent to the president for action. The conference committee process is described more fully in Appendix 17.

Presidential Action on Proposed Legislation

The president has several options regarding proposed legislation that has been approved by both the House and the Senate (see Exhibit 6.2). The president can sign the bill, in which case it immediately becomes law. The president can veto the bill, in which case it must be returned to Congress along with an explanation for the rejection. A two-thirds vote in both chambers of Congress can override a presidential veto. The president's third option is neither to veto the bill nor to sign it. In this case, the bill becomes law in ten days, but the president has made a political statement of disfavor regarding the legislation. A fourth option may apply when the president receives proposed legislation near the close of a congressional session; the bill can be pocket vetoed if the president does nothing about it until the Congress is adjourned. In this case, the bill dies.

Legislation Development for the Federal Budget

Because enactment of legislation related to the federal government's annual budget is so crucial to the government's performance and the well-being of the American people, special procedures have been developed to guide this process. The Congressional Budget and Impoundment Control Act of 1974 and the Balanced Budget and Emergency Deficit Control Act of 1985 and their subsequent amendments provide Congress with the process through which it establishes target levels for revenues, expenditures, and the overall deficit for the coming fiscal year. The budget process is designed to coordinate decisions on sources and levels of federal revenues and on the objectives and levels of federal expenditures. Such decisions affect other policy decisions, including those that pertain to health.

A distinctive feature of legislation development for the budget is the president's role. The president is required to submit a budget request to Congress each year to initiate the process. By doing so, the president establishes the starting point and the framework for the annual process of legislation development for the federal budget. Once the president submits a budget request, the legislative process for federal budget making unfolds in distinct stages. First, Congress drafts and approves a budget resolution that provides the framework for overall federal government taxation and spending for various agencies and programs for the upcoming year. Next, the agencies and programs are authorized by way of establishment, extension, or modification. This authorization must take place before any money can be appropriated for a particular agency or program, which is the final stage of federal budget making.

The federal budgeting process is enormously complex. It "entails dozens of subprocesses, countless rules and procedures, the efforts of tens of thousands of staff persons in the executive and legislative branches, millions of work hours each year, and the active participation of the president and congressional leaders, as well as other members of Congress and executive officials" (Heniff, Lynch, and Tollestrup 2012, ii). Several federal agencies play especially important research and oversight roles in the budgeting process. These include the OMB, the Government Accountability Office (GAO), and the Congressional Budget Office (CBO).

Exhibit 6.7 shows the actions and timeline through which the annual federal budget is supposed to be developed. As noted earlier, the schedule begins when the president submits a budget request to Congress. Appendix 18 describes these steps in greater detail.

President's Budget Request

The president's budget, officially referred to as the *Budget of the United States Government* (www.whitehouse.gov/omb/budget), is required by law to be submitted to Congress no later than the first Monday in February (see Step 1 in Exhibit 6.7). The budget request by the president includes

Action Steps	Timeline
1. President submits budget request to Congress.	First Monday in February
2. House and Senate Budget Committees pass budget resolutions.	April 15
3. House and Senate Appropriations Subcommittees mark up appropriations bills.	June 10
4. House and Senate vote on appropriations bills and reconcile differences.	June 30
5. President signs each appropriations bill and the budget becomes law.	October 1
6. Congress passes continuing resolutions until budget is in place	As needed
7. Audit and review of expenditures	Ongoing

EXHIBIT 6.7
Steps in the Federal Budget Process

estimates of spending, revenues, borrowing, and debt. In addition, it includes policy and legislative recommendations and detailed estimates of the financial operations of federal agencies and programs. The president's budget request plays three important roles. First, the budget request tells Congress what the president recommends for overall federal fiscal policy. Second, it lays out the president's priorities for spending on health, defense, education, and so on. Finally, the budget request signals to Congress the spending and tax policy changes the president prefers (Center on Budget and Policy Priorities 2011).

The president's budget is only a request to Congress, which can do with it as it pleases. Even so, the formulation and submission of the budget request is an important tool in the president's direction of the executive branch and of national policy. The president's proposals often influence congressional revenue and spending decisions, though the extent of the influence varies from year to year and depends on such variables as political circumstances and the condition of the economy (Heniff, Lynch, and Tollestrup 2012).

Preparation of the president's budget typically begins at least 9 months before it is submitted to Congress. Therefore, preparation begins about 17 months before the start of the fiscal year to which a budget pertains. The early stages of budget preparation occur in federal agencies, primarily in the OMB.

Congressional Budget Resolution

Upon receiving the president's budget request, Congress begins the months-long process of reviewing the request (Step 2 in Exhibit 6.7). Based on the review process, which may include hearings to question administration officials about the budget request, the House and Senate Budget Committees draft their budget resolutions. These resolutions go to the House and Senate floors, where they can be amended (by a majority vote). A House–Senate conference then resolves any differences, and a reconciled version is voted on in each chamber.

Because the budget resolution is a "concurrent" congressional resolution, it is not signed by the president and is not a law. Budget resolutions are supposed to be passed by April 15, but often are not. Resolutions may not be passed because of disagreements about spending levels and priorities. On occasion, no budget resolution is passed, in which case the previous year's resolution remains in effect. Congress has failed to pass a budget resolution by the April 15 deadline on many occasions. When Congress fails to do so, the House can begin to work on most of the appropriations bills without a budget resolution after one month. The Senate can also do so if a majority vote among members favors proceeding.

Congressional Appropriations Process

Before appropriations can be made to any agency or program, they first must be authorized. Authorization can occur through a law that establishes a program or agency and sets the terms and conditions under which it operates, or by a law that specifically authorizes appropriations for that program or agency. Assuming that authorization has occurred, federal spending for agencies and programs occurs in two main forms: mandatory and discretionary. Primarily, mandatory spending, also known as direct spending, is for entitlement programs such as Medicare, Medicaid, and Social Security. The ACA contains some mandatory programs such as the Prevention and Public Health Fund, for example. Mandatory spending is under the jurisdiction of the legislative committees of the House and Senate. The House Ways and Means Committee and the Senate Finance Committee are most responsible for mandatory spending decisions. Discretionary spending decisions occur in the context of annual appropriations acts. All discretionary spending is under the jurisdiction of the appropriations committees in the House and the Senate (Tollestrup 2012).

The appropriations acts passed by Congress provide federal agencies and programs legal authority to incur obligations. These acts also grant the Treasury Department the authority to make payments for designated purposes (Heniff, Lynch, and Tollestrup 2012). Steps 3 and 4 in Exhibit 6.7 constitute the federal appropriations process. Based on the guidance provided by the budget resolution, the House and Senate Appropriations Committees allocate spending levels to their 12 subcommittees, which then determine funding levels for the agencies and programs under their jurisdiction. The subcommittees include those for Labor, Health and Human Services, Education, and Related Agencies as well as 11 others in each chamber of Congress.

As with delays in Congress failing to pass a budget resolution by the deadline, disagreements over spending levels and priorities also delay the work of the appropriations committees' subcommittees. When some or all of the appropriations subcommittees fail to pass their spending bills, the bills can be grouped into a single appropriations bill, called an omnibus bill, and sent to the floor of the House or Senate for a vote.

President Signs Appropriations Bills

For the federal budget to become law, the president must sign each appropriations bill passed by Congress (Step 5 in Exhibit 6.7). Only then is the budget process complete for the year. Rarely, however, is this work completed by the September 30 deadline so that the budget can become law on October 1. When the budget is not completed on time, Congress may pass a CR so that agencies and programs can receive funds and continue to operate on a temporary basis until the appropriations bills become law (Step 6 in Exhibit 6.7). The alternative to a CR is to shut down the nonessential activities of the federal government. Both CRs and shutdowns are problematic for the agencies and programs operating under the federal budget.

Audit and Review of Expenditures

Even when the federal budget for a given fiscal year is completed and operating, however, the budgeting cycle continues in the form of ongoing oversight by legislative committees, auditing, and review of expenditures. Specifically, GAO serves as an independent, nonpartisan agency that works for Congress. Among its duties are "auditing agency operations to determine whether federal funds are being spent efficiently and effectively; investigating allegations of illegal or improper activities; and reporting on how well government programs and policies are meeting their objectives" (GAO 2014). CBO produces "independent analyses of budgetary and economic issues to support the Congressional Budget process" (CBO 2014). Among its products is a monthly analysis of federal spending and revenue totals for the previous month, current month, and fiscal year to date. OMB works directly for the president and has major responsibility for budget development and execution and oversight of agency and program performance (OMB 2014).

Legislation Development for State Budgets

The states also develop budget legislation, although the process varies considerably from state to state. In all states, however, the budget is among the most—if not *the* most—important mechanisms for establishing policy priorities. Pennsylvania, for example, uses a process that includes the following four key stages (Office of the Budget 2014):

1. *Budget preparation.* The budget is developed and submitted to the General Assembly.
2. *Legislative review and approval.* The budget is reviewed by appropriations committees of the House and the Senate. The General Assembly enacts its decisions about the budget in the form of the General Appropriation Bill and several individual appropriation bills.
3. *Budget execution.* The governor assumes responsibility for implementing the budget, although the various state agencies share this responsibility and the Office of the Budget is heavily involved.
4. *Audit.* There is an ongoing audit of financial performance and monitoring and evaluating performance of the state's various programs.

The activities in each of the four stages in this example of legislation development for state budgets are described more fully in the following section.

Stage 1: Budget Preparation

The preparation stage of the budget process for a fiscal year that begins July 1 in Pennsylvania is initiated nearly 12 months prior to that date. The governor controls the first phase of building the budget. The governor establishes initial direction for the budget in August, and state agencies are guided by these priorities as they develop funding requests. The agency heads seek to balance the wants and needs of their constituencies with the administration's priorities and guidelines on total spending.

The Office of the Budget, whose director reports directly to the governor, exerts considerable influence as the office evaluates the agencies' requests and begins to help them formulate preliminary spending and revenue recommendations. Agency heads meet with the governor to express their views on desired changes to those recommendations. This input influences the governor's final recommendations. The governor's Executive Budget, the result of the preparation stage, is finalized in January and submitted to a joint session of the General Assembly through the governor's budget address in early February.

Stage 2: Legislative Review and Approval

Upon receiving the Executive Budget, the House and Senate Appropriations Committees hold hearings to review agency requests for funds. Cabinet secretaries and others participate in these hearings, which provide legislators with an opportunity to review the specific programmatic, financial, and policy aspects of each agency's programs and requests. At the same time, legislative staff members analyze the details of the proposals. These review activities provide interest groups with their greatest opportunities to influence the outcome in specific areas by interacting with the legislature. The General Assembly makes its decisions on the budget in the form of the General Appropriation Bill and individual appropriation bills.

Pennsylvania's governor has the power of "line-item veto," which means the governor can reduce or eliminate, but not increase, specific items in the budget legislation. Line-item veto power allows the governor to insist on certain items in the budget and exert additional influence over the legislative process before the budget legislation reaches the governor's desk. Pennsylvania's constitution requires a balanced budget, which means the governor must veto spending that exceeds the estimated available revenues.

Stage 3: Budget Execution

The governor's signing of the General Appropriation Bill signals the beginning of the execution stage of the budget cycle. With the signing, the Office

Most states include descriptions of their budget process on state web-sites. For example, California's process can be seen at www.dof.ca.gov/ fisa/bag/process.htm; New York's at www.budget.ny.gov/citizen/pro-cess/process.html; North Carolina's at www.osbm.state.nc.us/files/ pdf_files/2003_budget_manual.pdf; and Texas's at www.senate.state. tx.us/SRC/pdf/Budget_101-2011.pdf.

of the Budget issues detailed "rebudget," or spending plan, instructions. The agencies rebudget the funds appropriated in the legislation. The governor assumes responsibility for implementing the budget, although the various state agencies share this responsibility and the Office of the Budget is highly involved in these activities. The Office of the Budget has the authority to establish the authorized salaried complement for agencies and to request and approve agency spending plans or rebudgets. The executive branch must periodically report the progress of spending to the General Assembly.

Stage 4: Audit

The final stage of the budget cycle for a particular year encompasses an audit and a review of financial and program performance. The Office of the Budget monitors and reviews performance and may conduct program audits or evaluations of selected programs. In addition, the state's auditor general performs a financial post audit. Audits may be administrative reviews or more official performance audits with published results available to other govern-ment officials and the public. Agency officials or the Pennsylvania General Assembly acts on significant audit findings and recommendations.

Pennsylvania's budget process authorizes the Office of the Budget to evaluate the effectiveness and management efficiency of programs supported by any agency under the governor's jurisdiction. The process also requires the secretary of the budget to prepare reports detailing the results of program evaluations for distribution to the governor, the General Assembly, interested agencies, stakeholders and interest groups, and the public. A more complete description of another state's budget process, Michigan in this case, is pre-sented in Appendix 19.

From Formulation to Implementation

When a legislature, whether the US Congress or a state legislature, approves proposed legislation, and the chief executive, whether the president or a governor, signs it, the policymaking process crosses an important threshold. The point at which proposed legislation is formally enacted into law is the point of transition from policy formulation to policy implementation. As shown in Exhibit 6.1, the formal enactment of legislation bridges the formulation and implementation phases of policymaking and triggers the implementation phase. Policy implementation is considered in the next chapter.

Summary

The policy formulation phase of policymaking involves agenda setting and the development of legislation. Agenda setting, which we discussed in Chapter 5, entails the confluence of problems, possible solutions to those problems, and political circumstances that permit certain problem–possible solution combinations to progress to the development of legislation.

Legislation development, the other component of policy formulation and the central topic of this chapter, follows carefully choreographed steps that include the drafting and introduction of legislative proposals, their referral to appropriate committees and subcommittees, House and Senate floor action on proposed legislation, conference committee action when necessary, and presidential action on legislation voted on favorably by the legislature. These steps apply whether the legislation is new or, as is often the case, an amendment of prior legislation.

The tangible final products of legislation development are new public laws, amendments to existing ones, or budgets, in the case of legislation development in the budget process. At the federal level, laws are first printed in pamphlet form called *slip law*. Subsequently, laws are published in the *Statutes at Large* and then incorporated into the *US Code*.

Review Questions

1. Discuss the link between agenda setting and the development of legislation.
2. Describe the steps in legislation development.
3. Discuss the various sources of ideas for legislative proposals.
4. What congressional legislative committees are most important to health policy? Briefly describe their roles.
5. Describe the federal budget process. Include the relationship between the federal budget and health policy in your response.

References

Avik, R. 2012. "The Tortuous History of Conservatives and the Individual Mandate." *Forbes*. Posted February 7. www.forbes.com/sites/theapothecary/2012/02/07/the-tortuous-conservative-history-of-the-individual-mandate/.

Cannan, J. 2013. "A Legislative History of the Affordable Care Act: How Legislative Procedure Shapes Legislative History." *Law Library Journal* 105 (2): 131–73.

Center on Budget and Policy Priorities. 2011. "Introduction to the Federal Budget Process." Accessed March 24, 2014. www.cbpp.org/cms/index.cfm?fa=view&id=155.

Congress.gov. 2014. "Committees of the U.S. Congress." Accessed February 4. www.congress.gov/committees.

Congressional Budget Office (CBO). 2014. "Overview." Accessed March 25. www.cbo.gov/about/overview.

Galvin, W. F. 2014. "Lawmaking in Massachusetts." Accessed January 31. www.sec.state.ma.us/trs/trslaw/lawidx.htm.

Government Accountability Office (GAO). 2014. "About GAO." Accessed March 24. www.gao.gov/about/index.html.

Hacker, J. S. 2010. "The Road to Somewhere: Why Health Reform Happened; Or Why Political Scientists Who Write About Public Policy Shouldn't Assume They Know How to Shape It." *Perspectives on Politics* 8 (3): 861–76.

———. 1997. *The Road to Nowhere*. Princeton, NJ: Princeton University Press.

Hacker, J. S., and T. Skocpol. 1997. "The New Politics of U.S. Health Policy." *Journal of Health Politics, Policy and Law* 22 (2): 315–38.

Heniff, B., Jr., M. S. Lynch, and J. Tollestrup. 2012. "Introduction to the Federal Budget Process." Washington, DC: Congressional Research Service Report 7-5700.

Johnson, H., and D. S. Broder. 1996. *The System: The American Way of Politics at the Breaking Point*. New York: Little, Brown.

Jost, T. S. 2014. "Implementing Health Reform: Four Years Later." *Health Affairs* 33 (1): 7–10.

Office of Management and Budget (OMB). 2014. "The Mission and Structure of the Office of Management and Budget." Accessed March 25. www.whitehouse.gov/omb/organization_mission.

Office of the Budget. 2014. "The Budget Process in Pennsylvania." Accessed February 5. www.budget.state.pa.us/portal/server.pt/community/office_of_the_budget_home/4408.

Office of the Legislative Counsel, US House of Representatives. 2014. "House Office of the Legislative Counsel (HOLC) Guide to Drafting Legislation." Accessed February 3. www.house.gov/legcoun/HOLC/Drafting_Legislation/Drafting_Guide.html.

Oleszek, W. J. 2014. *Congressional Procedures and the Policy Process*, ninth edition. Thousand Oaks, CA: CQ Press.

Peterson, M. A. 1997. "Introduction: Health Care into the Next Century." *Journal of Health Politics, Policy and Law* 22 (2): 291–313.

Redhead, C. S., H. Chaikind, B. Fernandez, and J. Staman. 2012. "ACA: A Brief Overview of the Law, Implementation, and Legal Challenges." Washington, DC: Congressional Research Service Report R41664.

Skocpol, T. 1996. *Boomerang: Clinton's Health Security Effort and the Turn Against Government in U.S. Politics.* New York: Norton.

Strokoff, S. 2014. "How Our Laws Are Made: A Ghost Writer's View." US House of Representatives, Office of the Legislative Counsel. Accessed February 3. www.house.gov/legcoun/HOLC/Before_Drafting/Ghost_Writer.html.

Sullivan, J. V. 2007. *How Our Laws Are Made.* Published July 25. www.gpo.gov /fdsys/pkg/CDOC-110hdoc49/pdf/CDOC-110hdoc49.pdf.

Teitelbaum, J. B., and S. E. Wilensky. 2013. *Essentials of Health Policy and Law*, second edition. Burlington, MA: Jones & Bartlett Learning.

Tollestrup, J. 2012. *The Congressional Appropriations Process: An Introduction.* Washington, DC: Congressional Research Service Report R42388. Accessed February 19, 2014. www.senate.gov/CRSReports/crs-publish.cfm ?pid=%260BL%2BP%3C%3B3%0A.

US Senate. 2014. "Senate Glossary." Accessed March 23. www.senate.gov/reference/glossary_term/conference_committee.htm.

Washington State Legislature. 2014. "How a Bill Becomes a Law." Accessed January 31. www.leg.wa.gov/legislature/Pages/Bill2Law.aspx.

Wees, P., A. M. Zaslavsky, and J. Z. Ayanian. 2013. "Improvements in Health Status After Massachusetts Health Care Reform." *Milbank Quarterly* 91 (4): 663–89.

POLICY IMPLEMENTATION AND IMPLEMENTING ORGANIZATIONS

Learning Objectives

After reading this chapter, you should be able to

- describe the responsibilities of the executive, legislative, and judicial branches of government in policy implementation;
- explain why the Centers for Medicare & Medicaid Services (CMS) is an important policy-implementing organization;
- describe the legislative history of CMS's formation and evolution;
- describe the organizational structure of CMS;
- discuss the functions of CMS;
- discuss the management aspects of policy implementation; and
- discuss the management challenges CMS faces in carrying out its policy implementation responsibilities.

In this chapter, we shift our focus from policy formulation to policy implementation. As outlined in Chapter 3 and described in more detail in Chapters 5 and 6, the policy formulation phase of policymaking is made up of two sets of interrelated activities—agenda setting and legislation development. Sometimes these formulation activities lead to policies in the form of new or amended public laws. Enactment of laws and amendments marks the transition from policy formulation to the policy implementation phase of policymaking, although the boundary between the two phases is porous and two-way, as shown in the center of Exhibit 7.1.

Implementing organizations, primarily the departments and agencies in the executive branches of governments, are established and maintained, and the people within them employed, to carry out the intent of public laws and amendments as enacted by the legislative branch. The relationship between those who formulate policies and those who implement them is symbiotic. Policy formulators must have implementers if their policies are to have effect, and implementers work on implementing formulated policies.

EXHIBIT 7.1
Policymaking Process: Implementation Phase

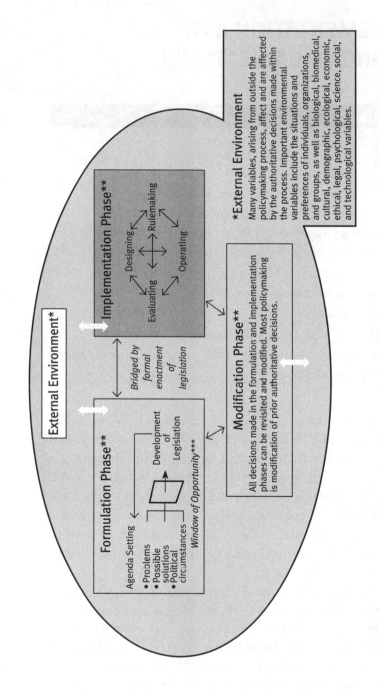

Formulation Phase**

Agenda Setting

Development of Legislation

• Problems
• Possible solutions
• Political circumstances

Window of Opportunity***

Bridged by formal enactment of legislation

Implementation Phase**

Designing ↔ Rulemaking
↕   ↕
Evaluating ↔ Operating

External Environment*

Modification Phase**

All decisions made in the formulation and implementation phases can be revisited and modified. Most policymaking is modification of prior authoritative decisions.

*External Environment

Many variables, arising from outside the policymaking process, affect and are affected by the authoritative decisions made within the process. Important environmental variables include the situations and preferences of individuals, organizations, and groups, as well as biological, biomedical, cultural, demographic, ecological, economic, ethical, legal, psychological, science, social, and technological variables.

Policymakers in all three branches of government make policy in the form of position-appropriate, or authoritative, decisions. Their decisions differ in that the **legislative branch is primarily involved in formulation, the **executive branch** is primarily involved in implementation, and both are involved in modification of prior decisions or policies. The **judicial branch** interprets and assesses the legality of decisions made within all three phases of the policymaking process.

***A window of opportunity opens for possible progression of issues through formulation, enactment, implementation, and modification when there is a favorable confluence of problems, possible solutions, and political circumstances.

As was discussed briefly in Chapter 3, until policies are implemented they are only so much paper and rhetoric. An implemented law or amendment can affect one or more determinants of health by changing the physical or social environment in which people live and work, affecting their behavior and even their biology, and by influencing the availability and accessibility of health services.

The implementation phase of public policymaking involves managing human, financial, and other resources in ways that facilitate achievement of the goals and objectives embodied in enacted legislation. Policy implementation is primarily a management undertaking. That is, policy implementation in its essence is the use of resources to pursue the objectives inherent in public laws and amendments. Implementation is carried out through an interrelated set of activities as shown in the darkly shaded portion of Exhibit 7.1. These activities—designing, rulemaking, operating, and evaluating—may lead to subsequent rounds of these activities. These implementing activities are discussed in more detail in Chapter 8.

Depending on the scope of policies being implemented, the managerial tasks involved can be simple and straightforward, or they can require massive effort. Implementation of the Affordable Care Act (ACA), for example, is proving to be a monumental and challenging management undertaking (Jost 2014).

In this chapter, we focus on the Centers for Medicare & Medicaid Services (CMS; www.cms.gov) as an exemplar of an implementing agency or organization. This provides background and context for the more in-depth discussion of the activities in the implementation phase of policymaking in the next chapter. First, however, we discuss an important feature of public policymaking in the United States: how the three branches of government share responsibility for policy implementation.

Responsibility for Policy Implementation

As noted earlier, in the implementation phase, more responsibility for policymaking shifts from the legislative branch to the executive branch, although implementation is a shared responsibility among the branches of government. While the executive branch bears much of the responsibility for implementation and plays a central role in policy implementation, the legislative branch oversees implementation, and the judicial branch also plays a role, largely refereeing implementation. Each branch's implementation responsibility is described in the following sections, beginning with the executive branch agencies.

Executive Branch Organizations' Implementation Responsibilities

Organizations and agencies such as the Department of Health and Human Services (HHS) and the Department of Justice (DOJ), and subdivisions of those departments; independent federal agencies such as the Environmental Protection Agency (EPA), the Consumer Product Safety Commission, and the Food and Drug Administration (FDA); and many other executive branch organizations exist primarily to implement the laws formulated by the legislative branch.

CMS is one example of an implementing organization. We use it as an exemplar because it is so heavily involved in implementing important health policies such as Medicare, Medicaid, and the ACA. CMS is a federal agency located organizationally within HHS, as shown in Exhibit 7.2. The agency was established specifically to implement the Medicare and Medicaid programs. In addition, CMS now has major responsibilities for implementing the ACA, which requires that CMS coordinate with states to establish health insurance marketplaces, expand Medicaid, and regulate private health insurance plans, among other things. Because CMS is heavily involved in implementing so much of the nation's health policy, we will use it as an exemplar of an implementing organization. First, however, we consider the roles of the legislative and judicial branches in policy implementation.

Legislative Branch Oversight of Implementation

Although organizations in the executive branch bear most of the responsibility for implementing policies, the legislative branch maintains oversight responsibility of the implementation phase. The US Senate's *Glossary* defines *oversight* as "committee review of the activities of a federal agency or program" (US Senate 2014). Legislative branch oversight has a long history, having been mandated by the Legislative Reorganization Act of 1946. Generally, legislative oversight is intended to accomplish the following:

- Ensure that implementing organizations adhere to congressional intent
- Improve the efficiency, effectiveness, and economy of government's operations
- Assess the ability of implementing organizations and individuals to manage and accomplish implementation, including investigation of alleged instances of inadequate management, waste, fraud, dishonesty, or arbitrary action
- Ensure that implementation of policies reflects the public interest

Effective legislative oversight is accomplished through several means. One powerful technique involves the funding appropriations that Congress must make to continue implementation of many of the policies it enacts. Although some health policies, such as the Medicare program, are

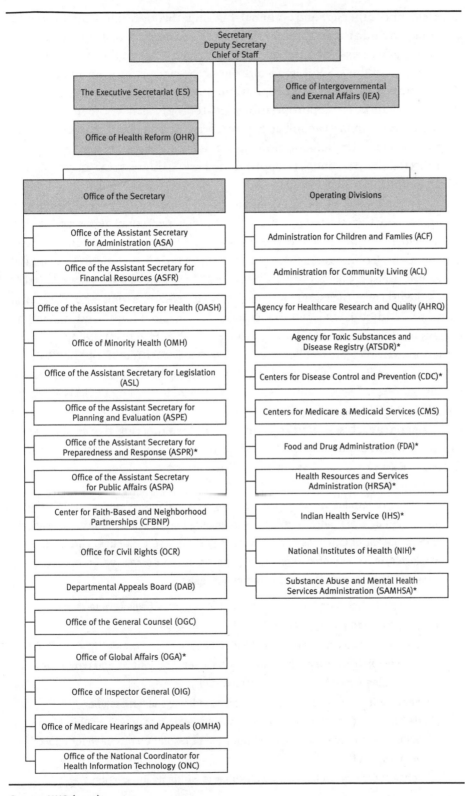

Source: HHS (2014).
*Components of the Public Health Service

EXHIBIT 7.2
Organization Chart of the Department of Health and Human Services (HHS)

entitlements, others require annual funding through appropriations acts. Examples include the research programs of the National Institutes of Health, the health activities of the Department of Veterans Affairs (www.va.gov), and the activities of the US Public Health Service (www.usphs.gov) and the FDA. The House and Senate appropriations committees (www.appropriations .house.gov and www.appropriations.senate.gov) review the performance of these and similar organizations in carrying out their implementation responsibilities. Implementation inadequacies—real or perceived—may be reflected in the budgets appropriated by Congress for implementing organizations.

Other means of oversight include direct contact between members of Congress and their staffs and executive branch personnel who are involved in implementing policies and the use of implementation oversight agencies, including the Congressional Budget Office and the Government Accountability Office (Kaiser, Oleszek, and Tatelman 2011; Nadel 1995; Oleszek 2014).

Legislative oversight responsibility extends beyond the appropriations procedure. Each standing committee of the House and Senate has certain oversight responsibilities. Those for the House standing committees, for example, are spelled out in Clause 2 of Rule X of the Rules of the House of Representatives for the One Hundred Thirteenth Congress, which can be viewed online (www.gpo.gov/fdsys/pkg/HMAN-113/pdf /HMAN-113-houserules.pdf). Rule X requires that early in the first session of a Congress, each standing committee shall, in a meeting that is open to the public and with a quorum present, adopt its oversight plan for that Congress. Clause 2(b)(1) of Rule X states the following:

In order to determine whether laws and programs addressing subjects within the jurisdiction of a committee are being implemented and carried out in accordance with the intent of Congress and whether they should be continued, curtailed, or eliminated, each standing committee (other than the Committee on Appropriations) shall review and study on a continuing basis:

- the application, administration, execution, and effectiveness of laws and programs addressing subjects within its jurisdiction;
- the organization and operation of Federal agencies and entities having responsibilities for the administration and execution of laws and programs addressing subjects within its jurisdiction;
- any conditions or circumstances that may indicate the necessity or desirability of enacting new or additional legislation addressing subjects within its jurisdiction (whether or not a bill or resolution has been introduced with respect thereto); and
- future research and forecasting on subjects within its jurisdiction.

Appendix 20 shows relevant parts of a typical oversight plan, in this instance of a committee with important oversight responsibilities for health policy, the House Committee on Energy and Commerce.

Judicial Branch Involvement in Implementation

Enacted legislation and the rules made to guide its implementation can be challenged in the courts as is discussed in depth in Chapter 4. Administrative law judges in the implementing agencies hear the appeals of people or organizations who are dissatisfied with the way the implementation of a policy affects them. For example, the Office of Administrative Law Judges (www.epa.gov/oalj) is an independent office in the Office of the Administrator of EPA. These judges conduct hearings and render decisions in proceedings between EPA and people, businesses, government entities, and other organizations that are regulated under environmental laws. They also preside over enforcement and permit proceedings under the Administrative Procedure Act, and they conduct other proceedings involving alleged violations of environmental laws, including the following:

- Clean Air Act
- Clean Water Act
- Comprehensive Environmental Response, Compensation, and Liability Act
- Emergency Planning and Community Right-to-Know Act
- Federal Insecticide, Fungicide, and Rodenticide Act
- Marine Protection, Research, and Sanctuaries Act
- Safe Drinking Water Act
- Solid Waste Disposal Act, as amended by the Resource Conservation and Recovery Act
- Toxic Substances Control Act (TSCA)
- Subchapter II of TSCA, known as the Asbestos Hazard Emergency Response Act

Federal administrative law judges are certified by the Office of Personnel Management and ensured decisional independence. Decisions issued by administrative law judges at EPA are subject to review by the Environmental Appeals Board (EAB). The initial decision of these judges—unless a party appeals to EAB, or EAB on its own initiative elects to review the initial decision—becomes EPA's final order.

Although the executive branch bears much of the responsibility for implementation and plays a central role in policy implementation, the other branches of government also play important implementation roles. The legislative branch oversees implementation and the judicial branch referees many aspects of policy implementation. In the next section we turn our attention to CMS, using it as an example of a federal implementing organization. Knowing more about CMS will provide important background for the discussion in Chapter 8 of the activities of implementation.

CMS as an Exemplar Implementing Agency

As shown in Exhibit 7.2, CMS is an operating division within HHS. CMS is the largest purchaser of healthcare in the United States, currently paying for almost one-third of the nation's health expenditures. In FY2015, CMS's budget for benefit outlays and operations is about $1 trillion. The organization provides health benefits to about 123 million Medicare, Medicaid, and Children's Health Insurance Program (CHIP) beneficiaries—more than one in three Americans. With implementation of the ACA, CMS will provide benefits to millions of additional people (HHS 2015). CMS is indeed a large and especially important health policy implementing organization.

Legislative History of CMS

Created in 1977 as the Health Care Financing Administration, the agency brought together, under unified leadership, implementation responsibility and authority for the two largest federal healthcare programs—Medicare and Medicaid. This agency has changed over time, including changing its name to CMS in 2001. The brief story of CMS's growth and evolution described here is drawn from the agency's budget justification document for FY2015, especially the Executive Summary (HHS 2015). The evolutionary pattern of CMS's development has been one in which new legislation keeps significantly expanding the organization's implementation responsibilities.

CHIP was added to its responsibilities in 1997. In 2003, the Medicare Prescription Drug, Improvement, and Modernization Act added a prescription drug benefit, creating substantial new implementation responsibilities. In 2005, the Deficit Reduction Act created a Medicaid Integrity Program to address fraud and abuse in the Medicaid program. The Tax Relief and Health Care Act of 2006 established a physician quality reporting program and quality improvement initiatives and increased CMS's program integrity efforts. The Medicare Improvements for Patients and Providers Act of 2008 extended and expanded the physician quality reporting program and established an electronic prescribing incentive program. It also established value-based purchasing for end-stage renal disease services. The Children's Health Insurance Program Reauthorization Act of 2009 improved outreach, enrollment, and access to benefits within the Medicaid and CHIP programs, and mandated development of child health quality measures and reporting for children enrolled in Medicaid and CHIP. The American Recovery and Reinvestment Act of 2009 provided investments for technological advances, including health information technology and the use of electronic health records, along with prevention and wellness activities.

The 2010 ACA contained numerous provisions affecting CMS's traditional role in Medicare, Medicaid, and CHIP, including a major expansion of the Medicaid program; a two-year extension of CHIP; the establishment of a new Federal Coordinated Health Care Office in CMS to improve care for beneficiaries who are eligible for both Medicare and Medicaid; the gradual elimination of the Medicare prescription drug coverage gap; payment reform; quality improvement incentives; and the creation of a CMS Innovation Center to explore different care delivery and payment models in Medicare, Medicaid, and CHIP.

In 2011, CMS became responsible for the implementation of the ACA's consumer protections and private health insurance provisions, including new coverage options for previously uninsured Americans with preexisting conditions; reimbursement for employers to help pay part of the cost of providing health benefits for early retirees, their spouses, and their dependents; new requirements regarding the market conduct of private healthcare insurers; and new consumer outreach and education efforts to help consumers assess their options and determine their eligibility for public health programs. In 2014, CMS worked with states to create new health insurance marketplaces.

Organizational Structure and Functions of CMS

Exhibit 7.3 is an organization chart of CMS. The agency is organized into centers, each responsible for key functions as described in the following sections. The descriptions provided here are adapted and abstracted from CMS's website (CMS 2014).

Center for Medicare

The Center for Medicare serves the following functions:

- Serves as CMS's focal point for the formulation, coordination, integration, implementation, and evaluation of national Medicare program policies and operations
- Identifies and proposes modifications to Medicare programs and policies to reflect changes or trends in the healthcare industry, program objectives, and the needs of Medicare beneficiaries
- Coordinates with the Office of Legislation on the development and advancement of new legislative initiatives and improvements

EXHIBIT 7.3

Organization Chart of the Centers for Medicare & Medicaid Services

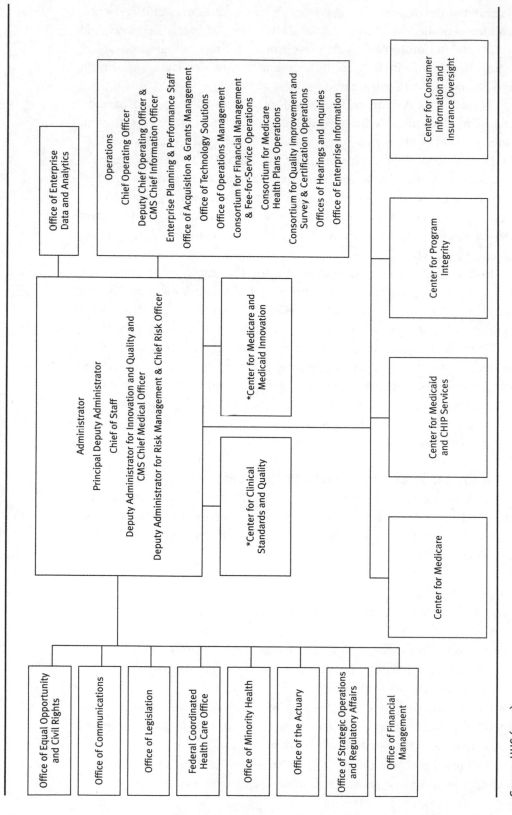

Source: HHS (2014).

*Reports to Deputy Administrator for Innovation and Quality

- Serves as CMS's lead for management, oversight, budget, and performance issues relating to Medicare Advantage and prescription drug plans, and Medicare fee-for-service providers and contractors
- Oversees all CMS interactions and collaboration with key stakeholders relating to Medicare (i.e., plans, providers, other government entities, advocacy groups, Consortia) and communication and dissemination of policies, guidance, and materials to the same to understand their perspectives and to drive best practices in the healthcare industry
- Develops and implements a comprehensive strategic plan, objectives, and measures to carry out CMS's Medicare program mission and goals and position the organization to meet future challenges with the Medicare program and its beneficiaries
- Coordinates with the Center for Program Integrity on the identification of program vulnerabilities and implementation of strategies to eliminate fraud, waste, and abuse

Center for Medicaid and CHIP Services

The Center for Medicaid and CHIP Services serves the following functions:

- Serves as CMS's focal point for the formulation, coordination, integration, implementation, and evaluation of all national program policies and operations relating to Medicaid and CHIP
- In partnership with states, evaluates the success of state agencies in carrying out their responsibilities for effective state program administration and beneficiary protection, and, as necessary, assists states in correcting problems and improving the quality of their operations
- Identifies and proposes modifications to Medicaid and CHIP program measures, regulations, laws, and policies to reflect changes or trends in the healthcare industry, program objectives, and the needs of Medicaid beneficiaries
- Collaborates with the Office of Legislation on the development and advancement of new legislative initiatives and improvements
- Serves as CMS's lead for management, oversight, budget, and performance issues relating to Medicaid, CHIP, and the related interactions with the states
- Coordinates with the Center for Program Integrity on the identification of program vulnerabilities and implementation of strategies to eliminate fraud, waste, and abuse
- In conjunction with the Office of Public Engagement, oversees all CMS interactions and collaboration relating to Medicaid and

CHIP with beneficiaries, states and territories, and key stakeholders (e.g., health facilities and other healthcare providers, other federal government entities, local governments) and communication and dissemination of policies, guidance, and materials to the same to understand their perspectives, support their efforts, and drive best practices for beneficiaries, in states and throughout the healthcare industry

- Develops and implements a comprehensive strategic plan, objectives, and measures to carry out CMS's Medicaid and CHIP mission and goals and position the organization to meet future challenges with the Medicaid and CHIP programs

Center for Consumer Information and Insurance Oversight

The Center for Consumer Information and Insurance Oversight serves the following functions:

- Provides national leadership in setting and enforcing standards for health insurance that promote fair and reasonable practices to ensure affordable, quality healthcare coverage is available to all Americans
- Provides consumers with comprehensive information on insurance coverage options currently available so they may make informed choices on the best health insurance for themselves and their families and issues consumer assistance grants to states
- Implements, monitors compliance with, and enforces the new rules governing the insurance market such as the prohibition on rescissions and on preexisting condition exclusions for children
- Conducts external appeals for states that do not have that authority
- Implements, monitors compliance with, and enforces the new rules regarding medical loss ratio standards and the insurance premium rate review process, and issues premium rate review grants to states
- Administers the Pre-Existing Condition Insurance Plan program and associated grant funding to states, the Early Retiree Reinsurance Program, and the Consumer Operated and Oriented Plan program
- Collects, compiles, and maintains comparative pricing data for an Internet portal providing information on insurance options and provides assistance to enable consumers to obtain maximum benefit from the new health insurance system
- Collects, compiles, and maintains comparative pricing data for the department's website, provides assistance to enable consumers to

understand the new health insurance laws and regulations, and establishes and issues consumer assistance grants to states

- Develops and implements policies and rules governing state-based exchanges, establishes and issues exchange planning and establishment to states, oversees the operations of state-based exchanges, and administers exchanges in states that elect not to establish their own

Center for Medicare and Medicaid Innovation

The Center for Medicare and Medicaid Innovation serves the following functions:

- Identifies, validates, and disseminates information about new care models and payment approaches to serve Medicare and Medicaid beneficiaries seeking to enhance the quality of health and healthcare and reducing cost through improvement
- Consults with representatives of relevant federal agencies, and clinical and analytical experts with expertise in medicine and healthcare management, including providers, payers, states, businesses, and community agencies, to develop new and effective models of care
- Creates and tests new models in clinical care, integrated care, and community health, and disseminates information on these models through CMS, HHS, states, local organizations, and industry channels
- Performs rapid cycle evaluation of innovation and demonstration activities to determine effectiveness and feasibility for broader dissemination, scale, and sustainability
- Works closely with other CMS components and regional offices to study healthcare industry trends and data to design, implement, and evaluate innovative payment and service delivery models, and to disseminate information about effective models
- Creates and tests innovative payment and service delivery models, building collaborative learning networks to facilitate the collection and analysis of innovation, as well as the implementation of effective practices, and developing necessary technology to support this activity
- Creates and tests innovative payment and service delivery models, developing fellows with expertise in innovation, demonstration, and diffusion to help support the introduction of effective practices across the nation
- Carries out core business functions (e.g., budget, facilities, HR, communications)

Center for Clinical Standards and Quality

The Center for Clinical Standards and Quality serves the following functions:

- Serves as the focal point for all quality, clinical, and medical science issues; survey and certification; and policies for CMS's programs
- Provides leadership and coordination for the development and implementation of a cohesive, CMS-wide approach to measuring and promoting quality and leads CMS's priority-setting process for clinical quality improvement
- Coordinates quality-related activities with outside organizations; monitors quality of Medicare, Medicaid, and the Clinical Laboratory and Improvement Amendments (CLIA)
- Evaluates the success of interventions
- Identifies and develops best practices and techniques in quality improvement; implementation of these techniques will be overseen by appropriate components
- Develops and collaborates on demonstration projects to test and promote quality measurement and improvement
- Develops, tests, evaluates, adopts, and supports performance measurement systems (i.e., quality measures) to evaluate care provided to CMS beneficiaries except for demonstration projects residing in other components
- Ensures that CMS's quality-related activities (survey and certification, technical assistance, beneficiary information, payment policies, and provider/plan incentives) are fully and effectively integrated
- Carries out the Health Care Quality Improvement Program for the Medicare, Medicaid, and CLIA programs
- Oversees the planning, policy, coordination, and implementation of the survey, certification, and enforcement programs for all Medicare and Medicaid providers and suppliers, and for laboratories under the auspices of CLIA
- Serves as CMS's lead for management, oversight, budget, and performance issues relating to the survey and certification program and the related interactions with the states
- Leads in the specification and operational refinement of an integrated CMS quality information system, which includes tools for measuring the coordination of care between healthcare settings; and analyzes data supplied by that system to identify opportunities to improve care and assess success of improvement interventions

- Develops requirements of participation for providers and plans in the Medicare, Medicaid, and CLIA programs; revises these requirements based on statutory change and input from other components
- Operates the Quality Improvement Organization and End-Stage Renal Disease Network program in conjunction with regional offices, providing policies and procedures, contract design, program coordination, and leadership in selected projects
- Identifies, prioritizes, and develops content for clinical and health-related aspects of CMS's Consumer Information Strategy; collaborates with other components to develop comparative provider and plan performance information for consumer choices
- Prepares the scientific, clinical, and procedural basis for coverage of new and established technologies and services and provides coverage recommendations to the CMS administrator
- Coordinates activities of CMS's Technology Advisory Committee and maintains liaison with other departmental components regarding the safety and effectiveness of technologies and services
- Prepares the scientific and clinical basis for and recommends approaches to quality-related medical review activities of carriers and payment policies

Center for Program Integrity

The Center for Program Integrity serves the following functions:

- Serves as CMS's focal point for all national and statewide Medicare and Medicaid programs and CHIP integrity fraud and abuse issues
- Promotes the integrity of the Medicare and Medicaid programs and CHIP through provider/contractor audits and policy reviews, identification and monitoring of program vulnerabilities, and providing of support and assistance to states
- Recommends modifications to programs and operations as necessary and works with CMS centers, offices, and the chief operating officer (COO) to effect changes as appropriate
- Collaborates with the Office of Legislation on the development and advancement of new legislative initiatives and improvements to deter, reduce, and eliminate fraud, waste, and abuse
- Oversees all CMS interactions and collaboration with key stakeholders relating to program integrity (i.e., DOJ, HHS Office of Inspector General, state law enforcement agencies, other federal entities, CMS components) to detect, deter, monitor, and combat fraud and abuse,

as well as to take action against those who commit or participate in fraudulent or other unlawful activities

- In collaboration with other CMS centers, offices, and the COO, develops and implements a comprehensive strategic plan, objectives, and measures to carry out CMS's Medicare, Medicaid, and CHIP program integrity mission and goals and to ensure program vulnerabilities are identified and resolved

Policy Implementation as Policymaking, but with a Management Aspect

Although implementation of policies is different from their formulation by legislative bodies of governments, authoritative decisions are also made during implementation. In other words, policy is being made in the formulation and implementation phases of the process shown in Exhibit 7.1. As we will see later in Chapter 9, policymaking (or authoritative decision making) continues in the modification phase.

In the implementation phase of policymaking, in addition to the fact that policy is being made as authoritative decisions are made about implementing policies, there is also an important management aspect to activities in this phase. Actually, there are two important management aspects. Implementing organizations must manage the implementation of policies, and to do so is these organizations' reason for being. In addition to managing policy implementation, the managers of these organizations must also oversee their own organizations.

Effective management of entities such as CMS, or any of the large number of implementing organizations in the executive branch, requires managers to do essentially what managers of all kinds of organizations do. Management of organizations and units of organizations can be defined generically as a "process, composed of interrelated social and technical functions and activities, occurring in a formal organizational setting for the purpose of helping establish objectives and accomplishing the predetermined objectives through the use of human and other resources" (Longest and Darr 2014). Effective managers of policy-implementing organizations do this kind of management. For example, in managing CMS as an organization, its leaders must

- analyze variables in CMS's external environment, assessing their importance and relevance, and responding to them appropriately;
- determine CMS's mission and objectives;

- assemble the resources necessary to achieve the mission and objectives;
- determine the processes necessary to accomplish the mission and objectives and ensure that the processes are carried out effectively and efficiently; and
- lead others in contributing to the accomplishment of CMS's mission and objectives.

However, beyond the traditional management responsibilities involved in running a large and complex organization, CMS's leaders must also manage the implementation of the policies established through policy formulation for which CMS bears implementation responsibility. We consider this latter form of management here. Information on the more traditional form of managing in formal organizational settings can be found in the general management literature, which is abundant. See, for example, Daft (2014).

Challenges of Managing Policy Implementation

Information about the nature and extent of the challenges CMS faces in managing implementation can be found in an annual summary of the top ten management challenges facing HHS, prepared by HHS's Office of Inspector General (OIG; www.oig.hhs.gov/reports-and-publications/top-challenges). Although the summary pertains to all of HHS, seven of the top ten challenges are faced by CMS in its implementing activities. The OIG's list of challenges for HHS in 2013 was as follows (OIG 2013):

1. Overseeing the health insurance marketplaces
2. Transitioning to value-based payments for healthcare
3. Ensuring appropriate use of prescription drugs in Medicare and Medicaid
4. Protecting the integrity of an expanding Medicaid program
5. Fighting fraud and waste in Medicare Parts A and B
6. Preventing improper payments and fraud in Medicare Advantage
7. Ensuring quality of care in nursing facilities and home- and community-based settings
8. Effectively using data and technology to protect program integrity
9. Protecting HHS grants and contract funds from fraud, waste, and abuse
10. Ensuring the safety of food, drugs, and medical devices

To provide an example of the nature of these challenges, the OIG's statement on the first challenge, overseeing the health insurance marketplaces, is reproduced in the following box.

Management Challenge 1: Overseeing the Health Insurance Marketplaces

Why This Is a Challenge

The Health Insurance Marketplaces (Marketplaces), also known as the Health Insurance Exchanges, add a substantial new dimension to the Department's program landscape.

The Marketplaces include State, Federal, and Partnership Marketplaces, each of which must implement and successfully operate a complex set of program requirements. Individuals use the Marketplaces to get information about their health insurance options, be assessed for eligibility (for, among other things, qualified health plans, premium tax credits, and cost sharing reductions), and enroll in the health plan of their choice. Sufficient enrollment, including enrollment of relatively healthy individuals, is essential for producing a stable and effective insurance market.

The Department faces significant challenges in several key areas, including eligibility systems, payment accuracy, contractor oversight, and data security and consumer protection. Coordination among Federal and State agencies, private insurers, and contractors is necessary to achieve program objectives and poses an additional challenge to the Department.

Eligibility Systems. The Federally Facilitated Marketplace (FFM) operates via the Department's healthcare.gov website. Healthcare.gov also serves as a gateway for consumers to reach State-run Marketplaces. The Department has acknowledged that it faces significant, well-publicized challenges in ensuring that healthcare.gov operates successfully. These reported challenges include hardware and software issues. The Department must ensure that healthcare.gov verifies consumers' personal information; accurately determines eligibility for Marketplace insurance, tax credits, and cost-sharing subsidies; operates effectively and easily for consumers; and transmits complete, accurate, and timely information to insurers regarding enrollees. The Marketplaces must also successfully facilitate Medicaid enrollment for those who qualify (see Challenge 4, protecting the integrity of an expanding Medicaid program).

CMS operates and oversees the Data Services Hub (Hub), which allows for exchange of data between the Marketplaces and Government databases to verify applicant eligibility, in coordination with partners

(continued)

at the Social Security Administration, Internal Revenue Service (IRS), Department of Homeland Security, Department of Justice (DOJ), and the States.

The Department must also be attentive to State Marketplace operations to ensure States' compliance with requirements, including requirements for making eligibility determinations and for transmitting accurate and timely data used for purposes of Federal payments, such as determinations related to subsidies.

Contractor Oversight. Contractors have played, and will continue to play, a vital role in building, maintaining, and fixing the systems that underpin the FFM. Early reports reflected that these systems, as constructed, did not function as they were intended. The Department must ensure, to the greatest extent possible, that the Government obtains specified products and services from its various contractors on time and within budget. The Department faces a challenge to ensure proper management of, and payment under, the various contracts entered into for implementation and operation of the FFM, including the Hub. This challenge is heightened by, among other things, the large number of contracts and the need to coordinate work across multiple contractors. For general information on challenges associated with contract administration, see Management Challenge 9.

Payment Accuracy. Ensuring accurate payments related to the Marketplaces also poses a substantial management challenge. The Department needs to implement financial management and payment systems to ensure accurate and timely payments to insurers of advance premium tax credits, cost-sharing subsidies, and premium stabilization payments. These payments involve complex calculations and offsets, adjustments, and reconciliations, which pose challenges for making accurate payments. Monitoring and accounting for these payments can also be challenging. In addition, some payments will rely on information obtained from private insurers. The Centers for Medicare & Medicaid Services (CMS) will need to work closely with insurers to ensure that information is timely, complete, and accurate. Given the amount of Federal funds involved, the Department should undertake a thorough risk assessment and, where appropriate, develop error rates to measure the integrity of program payments.

Security. Effective operation of the Marketplaces requires rapid, accurate, and secure integration of data from numerous Federal and State sources and individuals who use the Marketplaces. It requires

(continued)

means for real-time communication among many Federal and State systems on a large scale. Because these systems handle consumers' sensitive personal information, security of data and systems is paramount. Where the Department offers consumers alternate pathways for enrollment that do not require consumers to use healthcare.gov, such as submitting paper applications or using a call center, the Department also must ensure that those pathways incorporate effective security and eligibility safeguards and work well for consumers and insurers.

Another key responsibility is educating consumers about the Marketplaces and how to use them. Educating consumers about protecting themselves from fraud schemes, such as identity theft, is important since criminals often take advantage of new programs. Potential fraud schemes include identity thieves posing as legitimate assisters offering to help individuals purchase insurance in exchange for money or personal identifying information; imposters misleading Medicare beneficiaries into falsely believing they need to purchase new insurance; and sham websites that appear to be legitimate. The Department must also ensure that navigators, agents and brokers, and other assisters are qualified and properly trained to help consumers and provide reliable information.

Progress in Addressing the Challenge

On December 1, 2013, the Administration reported significant improvement in the operations of healthcare.gov. The report identified improvement on several system performance metrics, including response time, error rate, system stability, and number of concurrent users.

With respect to the Hub, CMS obtained its necessary security authorization on September 6, 2013. OIG had reviewed CMS's implementation of security controls for the Hub from March through June 2013. CMS has reported that all key steps that remained at the time of our review have since been completed.

CMS has issued regulations and guidance regarding numerous aspects of the Marketplaces and the related subsidies and premium stabilization programs. This includes a final rule on program integrity provisions for the Marketplaces and related programs intended to safeguard Federal funds and protect consumers. In addition to these regulations, CMS reports providing technical assistance and other support to States regarding Marketplace implementation.

(continued)

The Department and Office of Inspector General (OIG) are working closely with Government partners, including the Federal Trade Commission (FTC), DOJ, and State Attorneys General, among others, to prevent and respond to consumer fraud in connection with the Marketplaces. OIG and the Department have conducted consumer education and outreach on how to protect oneself against fraud and identity theft. The FTC and States have primary jurisdiction for responding to consumer fraud allegations, and OIG has updated the OIG fraud hotline to seamlessly route consumer fraud complaints to the FTC, as well as routing consumer inquiries about the Marketplaces to CMS.

What Needs To Be Done

The Department must continue to upgrade and improve healthcare.gov, including both the front-facing consumer functions, as well as the back-end administrative and financial management functions. The Department also must ensure that alternate pathways for enrollment operate with integrity and that consumers' personal information is secure. The Department must ensure that issuers and consumers receive accurate enrollment and subsidy information and that systems for paying insurers operate with sound safeguards and internal controls. States and consumers must receive accurate information about potential Medicaid enrollment. Vigilant monitoring and testing of the Marketplaces and rapid mitigation of identified vulnerabilities are essential.

The Department must address challenges in the short run to facilitate the ongoing open enrollment for 2014, when most people will be required to have health insurance. In addition, where the Department uses temporary mechanisms for the current enrollment period, the Department must develop permanent solutions that ensure the smooth and successful operation of the Marketplaces for special enrollment periods, the 2015 open enrollment period that is scheduled to start on November 15, 2014, and beyond. Moreover, the Department must address full implementation of the online SHOP Exchange.

The Department must also complete its development and implementation of financial management and payment systems and ensure that payments to insurers, which are scheduled to begin in January 2014, are accurate. While in the near-term the Department faces immediate challenges related to healthcare.gov operations, eligibility verification, payment accuracy, contracting, and security of data, the

(continued)

Department will face continuing challenges as the program evolves over time. The Department will need to adjust its management and oversight approaches accordingly to ensure that problems are prioritized and addressed. As with other new programs, the Department must monitor for known fraud, waste, and abuse risks and detect emerging new risks to protect the Federal investment in health care reform. If fraud schemes are identified, the Department must respond quickly and effectively.

Further, the Department must continue to coordinate closely with States and with other Federal agencies to monitor the operations and security of the Marketplaces and to implement the subsidies and other programs that begin on January 1, 2014. OIG will monitor the implementation and operations of the Marketplaces and plans to conduct oversight work initially focused on core risk areas, such as eligibility systems, payment accuracy, IT security, and contracting. In particular, OIG will conduct an audit of safeguards to prevent the submission of fraudulent or inaccurate information pursuant to the mandate at Public Law 113-46, Section 1001(c) (an Act making continuing appropriations for the fiscal year ending September 30, 2014). OIG is coordinating closely with its oversight partners at GAO, other IGs (such as the Treasury IG for Tax Administration), and State auditors to develop complementary work and maximize the Government's limited oversight resources.

Source: OIG (2013).

As we have seen in this chapter, CMS is an important example of a health policy implementing organization. It is large and complex, with substantial and diverse policy implementation responsibilities. We turn our attention to what CMS does in carrying out its implementation activities of designing, rulemaking, operating, and evaluating in the next chapter.

Summary

The implementation phase of public policymaking involves managing human, financial, and other resources in ways that facilitate achievement of the objectives embodied in enacted legislation. In this sense, policy implementation is primarily a management undertaking. The essence of policy implementation is described as the use of resources to pursue the objectives inherent in legislatively enacted policies.

Implementing organizations, primarily the departments and agencies in the executive branches of governments, are established and maintained and the people within them employed to carry out the intent of public policies enacted by legislative branches. The relationship between those who formulate policies and those who implement them is symbiotic. CMS is described as an exemplar implementing organization in the federal government.

Implementation is carried out through an interrelated set of activities as shown in Exhibit 7.1. These activities are designing, rulemaking, operating, and evaluating, which may lead to subsequent rounds of these activities. These implementing activities are discussed in more detail in Chapter 8.

Review Questions

1. Describe in general terms the implementation phase of public policymaking.
2. Who is responsible for policy implementation?
3. Discuss legislative oversight of policy implementation.
4. What are some of the key points in the legislative history of the establishment and evolution of CMS?
5. Describe the key functions of CMS's Center for Medicare.
6. Discuss the challenges CMS faces in managing the health insurance marketplaces.

References

Centers for Medicare & Medicaid Services (CMS). 2014. "CMS Leadership." Published February 6. www.cms.gov/About-CMS/Agency-Information/CMS Leadership/index.html.

Daft, R. L. 2014. *Management*, eleventh edition. Mason, OH: South-Western Cengage Learning.

Jost, T. S. 2014. "Implementing Health Reform: Four Years Later." *Health Affairs* 33 (1): 7–10.

Kaiser, F. M., W. J. Oleszek, and T. B. Tatelman. 2011. *Congressional Oversight Manual*. Washington, DC: Congressional Research Service.

Longest, B. B., Jr., and K. Darr. 2014. *Managing Health Services Organizations and Systems*, sixth edition. Baltimore, MD: Health Professions Press.

Nadel, M. 1995. "Congressional Oversight of Health Policy." In *Intensive Care: How Congress Shapes Health Policy*, edited by T. E. Mann and N. J. Ornstein,

127–42. Washington, DC: American Enterprise Institute and the Brookings Institution.

Office of Inspector General (OIG). 2013. "2013 Top Management & Performance Challenges." Accessed February 20, 2014. http://oig.hhs.gov/reports-and-publications/top-challenges/2013/.

Oleszek, W. J. 2014. *Congressional Procedures and the Policy Process*, ninth edition. Thousand Oaks, CA: CQ Press.

US Department of Health and Human Services (HHS). 2015. "Centers for Medicare and Medicaid Services, Justification of Estimates for Appropriations Committees, FY 2015." Accessed January 7. http://cms.hhs.gov/About-CMS/Agency-Information/PerformanceBudget/Downloads/FY2015-CJ-Final.pdf.

———. 2014. "CMS Organizational Chart." Accessed January 7, 2015. www.cms.gov/About-CMS/Agency-Information/CMSLeadership/Downloads/CMS_Organizational_Chart.pdf.

US Senate. 2014. *Senate Glossary*. Accessed February 20. www.senate.gov/pagelayout/reference/b_three_sections_with_teasers/glossary.htm.

POLICY IMPLEMENTATION ACTIVITIES: DESIGNING, RULEMAKING, OPERATING, AND EVALUATING

Learning Objectives

After reading this chapter, you should be able to

- discuss the set of activities that implementing organizations engage in as they implement policies,
- describe the designing activity in policy implementation,
- describe the rulemaking activity in policy implementation,
- describe the operating activity in policy implementation,
- describe the evaluating activity in policy implementation,
- outline the federal rulemaking process,
- discuss the role of interest groups in rulemaking, and
- list and discuss three key variables in policy operation.

As outlined in Chapter 3, when policy formulation leads to policies in the form of new or amended public laws, they must be implemented if they are to have any effect. As noted earlier, without implementation, policies are only so much paper and rhetoric. As we discussed in Chapter 7, implementing organizations, primarily the departments and agencies in the executive branches of governments, are established and maintained and the people within them employed to carry out the intent of public laws as enacted by the legislative branch. Implementing organizations use a set of activities through which policies are implemented. These relationships and activities are shown in the darkly shaded portion of Exhibit 8.1.

In the previous chapter, we also described in considerable detail the structure and functions of the Centers for Medicare & Medicaid Services (CMS), an important exemplar of an implementing organization. In this chapter we are now ready to consider in more detail the activities that implementing organizations, such as CMS, engage in as they go about implementing policies. As was discussed in Chapter 7, the implementation

EXHIBIT 8.1
Policymaking Process: Implementation Activities

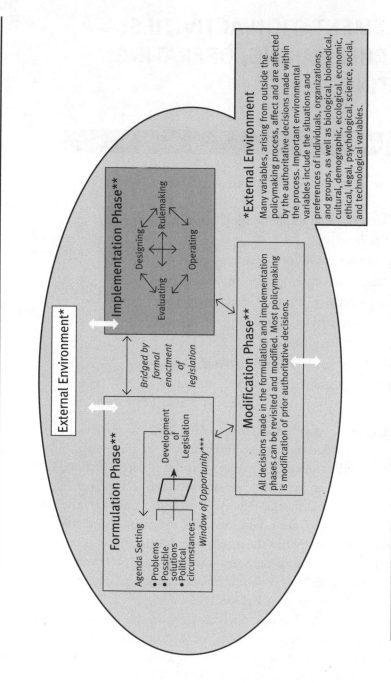

phase of public policymaking involves managing human, financial, and other resources in ways that facilitate achievement of the objectives embodied in enacted legislation. Implementation is carried out through an interrelated set of activities as shown in Exhibit 8.1, during the implementation phase. These activities—designing, rulemaking, operating, and evaluating—are the essence of what implementing organizations do as they implement policies and are the focus of this chapter. As implementing organizations go about their work of implementing policies formulated in the legislative phase, participants in the organizations make additional decisions that are also policies. People in implementing organizations both implement policies and make other policies.

Depending on the objectives, complexity, and associated resources of policies being implemented, their implementation can be relatively straightforward, or it can be difficult. As we have noted before, implementation of the Affordable Care Act (ACA), for example, is proving to be difficult (Jost 2014).

In this chapter, we consider what the people who lead implementing organizations actually do in carrying out their policy implementation responsibilities, keeping in mind that as they are implementing policies they are making additional authoritative decisions, which means that they are implementing policies and policymaking at the same time. In answering the question of what is done in policy implementation, this chapter is organized around the four activities of implementing: designing, rulemaking, operating, and evaluating. Each of these core activities is discussed in the following sections.

Designing

This activity involves efforts to establish the agenda of an implementing organization, plan how to address the agenda, and organize to carry out the plans. Sometimes this is rather straightforward and largely determined by what continuing, new, or revised policies an organization is responsible for implementing. Normally, a policy-implementing organization's work agenda might be rather static year-to-year. Some changes occur routinely, but periodically substantial change in the agenda might occur. The additional implementing responsibilities given to CMS by the ACA are a good example of this phenomenon. In effect, the ACA created major additions to CMS's implementation responsibilities. These are summarized in the following excerpt from the organization's strategy regarding ACA-driven changes in CMS's implementation responsibilities (CMS 2013a):

CMS' role in the larger health care arena has been further expanded beyond our traditional role of administering the Medicare, Medicaid and CHIP Programs. Designed to expand access to affordable health care and make the U.S. health care system more outcome-driven and cost-effective, the ACA requires that CMS coordinate with states to set up Health Insurance Marketplaces, expand Medicaid, and regulate private health insurance plans. The ACA greatly expanded the Agency's role and responsibilities by effectively tasking CMS to lead the charge to provide high quality care and better health at lower costs through improvement to health care for all Americans. This expansion not only involves growth in CMS' traditional base but also includes a greater emphasis on its continuing efforts in program integrity, health care innovation and health disparities reduction, as well as the establishment of Affordable Insurance Marketplaces.

Faced with these added implementation responsibilities, CMS had to plan how it would carry them out and organize itself to meet the responsibilities. Designing in policy-implementing organizations is a constant challenge. In these volatile environments, managers cannot simply design the organization once and then turn their attention elsewhere. Instead, this task is ongoing and involves continuing redesign. Some of the circumstances under which managers of implementing organizations must redesign include the following:

- A significant change occurs in an implementing organization's external environment. This change could be a new or amended public law for the organization to implement or a change in the rules that affect the operationalization of public laws. Environmental changes might also include a major reduction in the organization's budget or a reorganization initiative undertaken in the executive branch.
- An organization adopts new technologies for carrying out its work or is given new implementation responsibilities. A redesign may be required to channel necessary resources into the new activities. Conversely, when old technologies are abandoned or when previous responsibilities are shifted elsewhere, new structural arrangements may be necessary.
- An organization experiences a change in management personnel. Leadership changes are routine in the executive branch organizations that carry out policy implementation. People move in and out of public service. Administrations change. Changes at or near the top level of organizations stimulate redesign. New leadership provides an opportunity to rethink the way the organization is designed and how it conducts its work. New managers typically view their organization's design from a fresh perspective and may want to have its design reflect their own ideas and preferences.

- Often, in government as in the private sector, large-scale design changes that involve substantial reorganization or restructuring occur in the context of larger change programs.
- Routinely, significant changes in implementation responsibilities trigger changes in an agency's organizational structure. For example, the new responsibilities given CMS under the ACA for market reforms and consumer protections in the private health insurance market caused it to establish the Center for Consumer Information and Insurance Oversight (see Exhibit 7.3). The ACA also specified that CMS would house the Center for Medicare and Medicaid Innovation (CMI) and will help coordinate agencywide efforts to promote experimentation and innovation in payment and delivery models, reduce disparities in healthcare outcomes, promote primary care, and improve patient protections.

Designing and redesigning activities of CMS in response to the ACA provide a useful example of this important activity of the implementation phase of policymaking. As we discussed in Chapter 3, designing—involving establishment of the working agenda of an implementing organization and developing plans for how the work will be accomplished, organizing the agency to perform the work, directing the staff of the agency in doing the work, and controlling results—is the essence of management. You may wish to review Exhibit 3.2 for a depiction of how these functions of managing are integrated. You may also recall from Chapter 3 that we defined *management* as "the process, composed of interrelated social and technical functions and activities, occurring within a formal organizational setting for the purpose of helping establish objectives and accomplishing the predetermined objectives through the use of human and other resources" (Longest and Darr 2014, 255).

Rulemaking

Rules are an extraordinarily important aspect of policy implementation, and rulemaking is a core activity in implementation. Rulemaking is an implementation activity with a long history. The Administrative Procedure Act of 1946 defines a *rule* as "the whole or part of an agency statement of general or particular applicability and future effect designed to implement, interpret, or prescribe law or policy." Enacted laws are seldom explicit enough to guide their implementation completely. Rather, they tend to be vague, leaving it to the implementing organizations to specify, publish, and circulate the rules or regulations (remember, these terms have the same meaning in the policy context) that will guide the law's actual operation. For this reason, *rulemaking*, the process through which federal agencies develop, amend, or repeal rules, is an early and vital step in the policy implementation phase.

Exhibit 8.2 is an outline of the process most federal agencies are required to follow in writing or revising a rule. Federal agencies issue approximately 3,000 final rules annually on topics ranging from the timing of bridge openings on some of the nation's rivers to the permissible levels of arsenic and other contaminants in drinking water.

Diver (1989, 199) suggests that rulemaking is "the climactic act of the policy making process." As we will discuss in Chapter 9, this description might be better applied to the modification of previously made policies. Nevertheless, as Kerwin and Furlong (2010) note, the rulemaking process is central to the implementation of public policy in the United States.

As shown at the top of Exhibit 8.2, the federal rulemaking process begins when Congress takes an action (usually the enactment of a new or amended law) that either requires or authorizes an implementing organization in the executive branch to write and issue rules. Much rulemaking is driven by the formulation phase where new laws or amendments to existing ones typically require rules to guide implementation. However, the process is not exclusively determined by legislative action. An implementing agency can decide to undertake rulemaking for a number of other reasons, including (Office of the Federal Register 2014)

- new technologies or new data on existing issues;
- concerns arising from accidents or various problems affecting society;
- recommendations from congressional committees or federal advisory committees;
- petitions from interest groups, corporations, and members of the public;
- lawsuits filed by interest groups, corporations, states, and members of the public;
- presidential directives;
- requests from the Office of Management and Budget or other agencies; and
- studies and recommendations of agency staff.

An example of one of these other factors triggering rulemaking can be seen in the work of the National Advisory Committee on Occupational Safety and Health, which was established under the Occupational Safety and Health Act to advise the secretaries of labor and health and human services on occupational safety and health programs and policies. Members of the

EXHIBIT 8.2

Federal Rulemaking Process

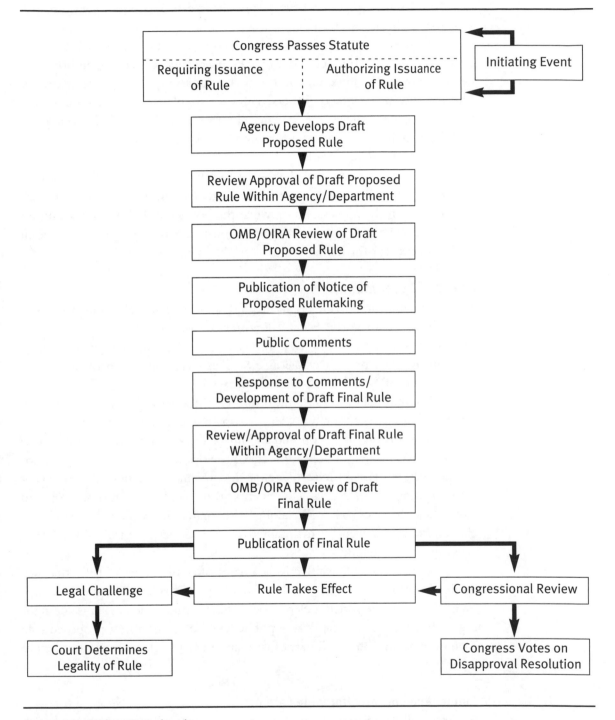

Source: Adapted from Carey (2013).

12-person advisory committee are chosen on the basis of their knowledge and experience in occupational safety and health. Information about the membership and operation of this committee can be seen at www.osha.gov /dop/nacosh/nacosh.html.

No matter what triggers the rulemaking, any rules formally established by executive departments and agencies have legal effect. As authoritative decisions made in government for the purpose of guiding the decisions, actions, and behaviors of others, rules or regulations are, by definition, policies. These policies are codified in the *Code of Federal Regulations (CFR)*, which can be read at www.gpo.gov/fdsys/browse/collectionCfr .action?collectionCode=CFR.

The delegation of rulemaking authority to implementing agencies is an essential feature of rulemaking, although Congress does not relinquish involvement in the process. As shown at the bottom of Exhibit 8.2, Congress and the courts can determine that a rule must be returned to an earlier point in the process for further action or even that a rule be vacated.

Rules of Rulemaking

The promulgation of rules is itself guided by certain rules and protocols, primarily set forth in the Federal Register Act of 1935 and the Administrative Procedure Act of 1946. Key among these is the requirement that implementing agencies publish *proposed* rules. This step is shown in Exhibit 8.2 as "Publication of Notice of Proposed Rulemaking."

The purpose of publishing proposed rules is to give those with interests in the issue an opportunity to participate in the rulemaking prior to the adoption of a *final* rule. Proposed and final rules are published in the *Federal Register (FR)*, a daily publication that provides a uniform system for publishing presidential and federal agency documents. It includes the following major sections: Presidential Documents, Rules and Regulations, Proposed Rules, and Notices. The *FR*, along with many other federal documents, can be read at a website maintained by the Government Printing Office (www.gpo.gov/fdsys).

A proposed rule is effectively a *draft* of a rule or set of rules that will guide the implementation of a law while the final rules are under development. Rules can be added, deleted, or modified; thus, rulemaking is an ongoing component in the life of any public law. Publication of a proposed rule is an open invitation for all parties with an interest in the rule to react before it becomes final.

Rulemaking for the Affordable Care Act

An especially important contemporary example of rulemaking in health policy is the rulemaking to implement the ACA. For example, on June

19, 2013, the Department of Health and Human Services (HHS) issued a
Notice of Proposed Rulemaking related to implementing the ACA, including provisions regarding health insurance marketplaces. This proposed rule
was unusually long, running 63 pages in the *FR*. It can be read in its entirety
at www.gpo.gov/fdsys/pkg/FR-2013-06-19/pdf/2013-14540.pdf. Its key
provisions include the following:

- Oversight of state-operated premium stabilization programs
- Program integrity for advance payments of the premium tax credit and
  cost-sharing reductions
- Program integrity of state marketplaces
- Oversight of Qualified Health Plan issuers in federally facilitated
  marketplaces
- Flexibility for states
- Consumer protections for enrollment assistance
- Establishment of standards for HHS-approved enrollee satisfaction
  survey vendors

Changes to proposed rules often result from the interactions between
implementing officials and those the rules will affect directly. In fact, these
interactions, triggered by the publication of a proposed rule, are among the
most active points of involvement in the policymaking process for individuals, health-related organizations, and interest groups with a stake in how a
particular public law is implemented. The role of interest groups is especially
potent at this point in the process, as the next section will demonstrate.

Appendix 6 contains examples of a proposed rule and a final rule—in
this instance, the rules to implement the Medicare Prescription Drug Benefit
enacted as Title I of the Medicare Prescription Drug, Improvement, and
Modernization Act (MMA) of 2003 (P.L. 108-173). As these examples show,
proposed rules begin with a heading that includes the name of the issuing
agency, the *CFR* title and part(s) that are affected, a brief description of the
specific subject of the document, and, in some cases, an agency docket number identifying the document in the agency's internal filing system. A regulation identifier number may also be included. Instructions for filing comments and the date by which comments must be filed are provided as well.
It has been demonstrated that early commenters can influence the content
of emerging rules and may even thwart unwanted regulations (Naughton et
al. 2009).

The Proposed Rules section of the *FR* also contains documents
related to previously published proposed rules, extending comment periods,
announcing public hearings, making available supplemental information,
withdrawing proposed rules, or correcting previously published proposed

rules. This section also includes advance notices of proposed rulemaking. An advance notice describes a problem or situation and the agency's anticipated regulatory action and seeks public response concerning the necessity of regulation and the adequacy of the agency's anticipated regulatory action.

The Role of Interest Groups in Rulemaking

Implementation of any complex health-related law involves interaction between implementing organizations and affected interest groups (Doonan 2013). For example, some of the rules proposed in implementing the 1974 National Health Planning and Resources Development Act (P.L. 93-641) sought to reduce obstetrical capacity in the nation's hospitals. A 1977 proposal, for example, called for hospitals to perform at least 500 deliveries annually, or close their obstetrical units. Notice of this proposed rule elicited immediate objections, especially from hospitals in rural areas where compliance would be difficult, if not impossible. The implementing organization (the Department of Health, Education, and Welfare, now HHS) received more than 55,000 written reactions to the proposed rule, almost all of them negative (Zwick 1978). As a result, the final rule was far less restrictive and did not specify a required number of deliveries to keep rural obstetrics units open.

Every policy affects one or more interest groups. Because rules established to implement health-related public laws often target members of interest groups, these groups routinely seek to influence rulemaking. Regulatory policies are implemented to prescribe and control the actions, behaviors, and decisions of certain individuals or organizations. Allocative policies provide income, services, or other benefits to certain individuals or organizations at the expense of others. Interest groups that represent the individuals and organizations directly affected by such policies are actively interested in all aspects of policymaking, including rulemaking. As the discussion in Chapter 2 of interest groups in policy markets shows, these groups tend to be well organized and aggressive in pursuit of their preferences, seeking to influence the formulation and implementation of policies that affect them.

Lobbying and other forms of influence become especially intense when some interest groups strongly support the formulation of a particular law or the manner in which it is to be implemented, and other groups oppose it. Policymakers almost always face this dilemma in the formulation and implementation of policies. As we noted in Chapter 2, legislators in such situations will seek to maximize their net political support through their decisions and actions. Those responsible for the management of implementing agencies and organizations are likely to do the same. The result is that rulemaking is often influenced by interest group preferences, with the more politically powerful groups exerting the greatest influence.

The potential for conflicting interests among groups concerned with health policy can be seen in Exhibit 8.3. Although some similarities exist among the preferences of the various categories, there are also important differences. Policymakers can anticipate that these individuals and organizations, largely working through their interest groups, will seek to ensure that any policies that are enacted reflect their preferences and that their preferences influence the subsequent implementation of such policies.

Health policy is replete with examples of the influence of interest groups on rulemaking. One such example can be seen in the rulemaking that stemmed from enactment of the Medicare program. In part to improve its chances for passage, the Medicare legislation (P.L. 89-97) was written so that the Social Security Administration (www.ssa.gov; the original implementing agency, later replaced by the Health Care Financing Administration, which

---

EXHIBIT 8.3
Typical Policy
Preferences
of Selected
Health-Related
Individuals and
Organizations

Federal Government
- Deficit reduction/increased surpluses
- Control over growth of Medicare and Medicaid expenditures
- Fewer uninsured citizens
- Slower growth in healthcare costs

Employers
- Slower growth in healthcare costs
- Simplified benefit administration
- Elimination of cost-shifting
- No mandates

Insurers
- Administrative simplification
- Elimination of cost-shifting
- Slower growth in healthcare costs
- No mandates

Individual Practitioners
- Income maintenance/growth
- Professional autonomy
- Malpractice reform

Suppliers
- Continued demand
- Sustained profitability
- Favorable tax treatment

State Government
- Medicaid funding relief
- More Medicaid flexibility
- Fewer uninsured citizens
- More federal funds and slower growth in healthcare costs

Consumers
- Insurance availability
- Access to care (with choices)
- Lower deductibles and copayments

Technology Producers
- Continued demand
- Sustained research funding
- Favorable tax treatment

Provider Organizations
- Improved financial condition
- Administrative simplification
- Less uncompensated care

Professional Schools
- Continued demand
- Student subsidies

became CMS) would reimburse hospitals and physicians in their customary manner. Reimbursement meant that they would be paid on a fee-for-service (FFS) basis, with the fees established by the providers. Each time providers gave services to Medicare program beneficiaries, they were paid their "usual and customary" fees for doing so.

However, unlike the physicians and hospitals, some prepaid providers, such as health maintenance organizations, had a different method for charging for their services. Their approach was to charge an annual fee per patient no matter how many times the patient might see a physician or use a hospital. In this situation, hospitals and FFS physicians had obviously preferred to have the Social Security Administration reimburse them according to their customary payment pattern. But they could also see an advantage in making the competing prepaid organizations subject to the FFS payment rules. Their preferences, which they vigorously made known to the Social Security Administration through the powerful American Medical Association and to a lesser extent through the American Hospital Association, forced the prepaid organizations to operate under FFS payment rules until the rules were finally changed in 1985 (Feldstein 2006).

The MMA was signed into law in December 2003. Title I of the MMA established Part D of Medicare to provide an outpatient prescription drug benefit beginning in 2006. On August 3, 2004, CMS published a proposed rule in *FR* to implement this benefit. Comments about the proposed rule were due by October 4, 2004. More than 7,000 comments were received, including many from health-related interest groups. The comments helped shape the final rule, which was published on January 28, 2005. (See Appendix 6.)

Other Interactions Between Rulemakers and Those Affected by the Rules

In certain instances, especially when rule development is anticipated to be unusually difficult, when such development seems likely to attract severe disagreement and conflict, or when continual revision is expected, special provisions may be made. For example, after passage of the Health Maintenance Organization Act (P.L. 93-222) in 1973, HHS organized a series of task forces, with some members drawn from outside the implementing organization, to help develop the proposed rules for implementing the law. This strategy produced rules that were more acceptable to those who would be affected by them.

Another strategy used to support rulemaking is the creation of advisory commissions. For example, following enactment of the 1983 Amendments to the Social Security Act (P.L. 98-21), which established the prospective payment system for Medicare reimbursement, Congress established the Prospective Payment Assessment Commission (ProPAC) to provide nonbinding advice to the Health Care Financing Administration (now CMS) in implementing the reimbursement system. A second commission, the Physician Payment Review Commission (PPRC), was established later to advise Congress and CMS regarding payment for physicians' services under the Medicare program. The Balanced Budget Act of 1997 (P.L. 105-33) replaced both commissions with a new commission—the Medicare Payment Advisory Commission (MedPAC; www.medpac.gov)—which incorporates and expands the roles of ProPAC and PPRC. Appendix 21 briefly describes MedPAC's role.

After laws have been enacted by legislatures and implementing agencies have designed plans and structures to implement them, and after initial rules necessary for implementing them have been promulgated, the implementation phase enters an operational stage (see Exhibit 8.1).

Operating

At the point of operating policies, those who implement policies are required to follow the rules promulgated to guide that implementation according to the mandates inherent in the laws. Ideally, this is exactly what happens. However, implementation does not always go smoothly. Some individuals with implementing responsibilities may disagree with the purposes of the enacted laws and may seek to stall, alter, or even subvert the laws in their implementation phases. The power of those with implementation responsibilities to affect the final outcomes and consequences of policies should not be underestimated. It is a power equivalent to that of executives in private-sector organizations with operational responsibilities for the achievement of organizational missions and objectives.

If a policy in the form of a public law is intended to protect people from exposure to toxic substances in their environments, for example, its operation entails the activities involved in actually providing such protection. Operational activities in this situation might include measuring and assessing dangers from substances in the environment or imposing fines as a means to prevent or restrict environmental pollution.

CMS's FY2014 budget request sought the funding needed to administer and oversee CMS's traditional programs—including Medicare, Medicaid, and the Children's Health Insurance Program (CHIP)—as well as the health insurance marketplaces and new private health insurance provisions and consumer protections enacted by the ACA (CMS 2013a). In essence, these are the main operating activities of CMS. To provide a fuller example of the nature of an implementing organization's operation of a policy, we will use CMS's operation of Medicare Parts A and B as a more detailed sample of this activity.

The description of the operation of Medicare Parts A and B provided in the following box is abstracted from CMS's FY2014 Justification of Estimates for Appropriations Committees. Remember that Medicare has four parts. Part A is hospital insurance and Part B is supplemental medical insurance. Part C, also known as Medicare Advantage, offers comprehensive Parts A and B benefits in a managed care setting through private healthcare companies. Medicare Part D provides voluntary prescription drug coverage. This description of policy operation is limited to Parts A and B.

Operation of Medicare Parts A and B

Working with its Medicare contractors, CMS's operation of Medicare Parts A and B includes processing claims, enrolling providers in the Medicare program, handling provider reimbursement services, processing appeals, responding to provider inquiries, educating providers about the program, and administering the participating physician/supplier program (PARDOC). These operating activities are described in more detail below.

Bills/Claims Payments

The Medicare contractors are responsible for processing and paying Part A bills and Part B claims correctly and timely. Currently, almost all providers submit their claims in electronic format—99.8 percent for Part A and over 97.5 percent for Part B.

Provider Enrollment

CMS and its Medicare contractors are responsible for both enrolling providers and suppliers into the Medicare program and ensuring that they continue to meet the requirements for their provider or supplier type. The enrollment process includes a number of verification processes to ensure that Medicare is only paying qualified providers and suppliers. In addition, the Medicare program requires that all new enrollees or those making a change in enrollment obtain Medicare payments by electronic funds transfer.

(continued)

Provider Reimbursement Services

Medicare Part A providers are required to file a cost report on an annual basis. In addition to determining the payment amount for items paid on cost, the cost report is used to finalize prospective payment system (PPS) add-on payments such as graduate medical education (GME), indirect medical education (IME), disproportionate share hospital (DSH), and bad debt payments. The contractors' provider reimbursement area performs several activities, most requiring substantial manual effort, including

- conducting rate reviews to establish and adjust interim reimbursement rates for add-on payments;

- performing quarterly reviews when the provider has elected to be paid on a biweekly basis, in lieu of actual claims payments;

- conducting reviews of payments to all hospice providers to determine if the hospice exceeded the aggregate or inpatient cap;

- maintaining files of provider-specific data (such as the disproportionate share hospital [DSH] adjustment) to calculate the provider's claims payment;

- maintaining systems such as the provider statistical and reimbursement system (PS&R) which contains all of the claims information needed to settle cost reports; and the system for tracking audit and reimbursement (STAR) which tracks the cost report through final settlement;

- making determinations regarding a hospital's provider-based status, which affects the amount of reimbursement the hospital is entitled to receive;

- reporting and collecting provider overpayments; and

- identifying delinquent debt and referring debts to Treasury for collection.

Medicare Appeals

The statutorily mandated Medicare appeals process affords beneficiaries, providers, and suppliers the opportunity to dispute an adverse contractor determination, including coverage and payment decisions. There are five levels in the Medicare Parts A and B appeals process starting with the Medicare Administrative Contractor (MAC) and ending with judicial review in federal district court. In FY2014, CMS anticipates the MACs will process 3.8 million redeterminations.

(continued)

Provider Inquiries

CMS coordinates communication between Medicare contractors and providers to ensure consistent responses. To accomplish this, CMS requires the Medicare contractors to maintain a Provider Contact Center (PCC) that can respond to telephone and written (letters, e-mail, fax) inquiries. The primary goal of the PCC is to deliver timely, accurate, accessible, and consistent information to providers in a courteous and professional manner. These practices are designed to help providers understand the Medicare program and, ultimately, bill for their services correctly.

CMS estimates receiving 34.2 million telephone inquiries in FY2014. CMS has made a number of efforts that contribute to decreased volume in FFS provider calls to MACs' toll-free lines. These efforts include

- major improvements in education beginning in 2005, including major new lines of educational products associated with FFS Medicare;
- improved CMS and MAC websites that host Medicare information;
- improved outreach to FFS providers through national and local provider association partners, expanded MAC provider electronic mailing lists and expanded CMS provider electronic e-mail lists;
- increased number of MAC provider Internet portals for claims-related transaction information; and
- improved training of MAC call center customer service representatives.

Participating Physician/Supplier Program (PARDOC)

This program helps reduce the impact of rising healthcare costs on beneficiaries by increasing the number of enrolled physicians and suppliers who "participate" in Medicare. Participating providers agree to accept Medicare-allowed payments as payment in full for their services. The MACs conduct an annual enrollment process and also monitor limiting charge compliance to ensure that beneficiaries are not being charged more than Medicare allows. Every year, the MACs are instructed to furnish participation enrollment materials to providers. The open enrollment period runs from November 15 through December 31 of each year.

(continued)

CMS has made more information available at www.medicare.gov about physicians participating in Medicare. The National Participating Physician Directory includes the providers' medical school and year of graduation, any board certification in a specialty, gender, hospitals at which they have admitting privileges, and any foreign language capabilities.

Provider Outreach and Education

The goal of Provider Outreach and Education is to reduce the Medicare error rate by helping providers manage Medicare-related matters on a daily basis and properly bill the Medicare program. The Medicare contractors are required to educate providers and their staffs about the fundamentals of the program, policies and procedures, new initiatives, and significant changes including any of the more than 500 change requests that CMS issues each year. They also identify potential issues through analyses of provider inquiries, claim submission errors, medical review data, Comprehensive Error Rate Testing (CERT) data, and the Recovery Audit Program data.

CMS encourages its contractors to be innovative in their outreach approach and to use a variety of strategies and methods for disseminating information including using print, Internet, telephone, CD-ROM, educational messages on the general inquiries line, face-to-face instruction, and presentations in classrooms and other settings.

Enterprise Data Centers

The Enterprise Data Centers (EDCs) are the foundation that supports all CMS production data center operations. Traditionally, the Medicare contractors either operated their own data centers or contracted out these services. As part of CMS's contracting reform initiative, CMS reduced the number of data centers from more than one dozen separate small centers to three large EDCs. CMS manages these contracts and has achieved administrative efficiencies from this consolidation. It will also deliver greater performance, security, reliability, and operational control. In addition, the new EDC infrastructure gives CMS flexibility in meeting current and future data-processing challenges. This flexibility is critical as the FFS claims workloads continue to grow and Medicare claims-processing applications require a more stable environment.

Source: CMS (2013b, 31–34).

Key Variables in Operating Policies

The success of any policy's operation depends on many variables, including (1) how the policy is designed or constructed, (2) certain characteristics of the organization(s) charged with implementation, and (3) the capabilities of the implementing organizations' managers. Each of these variables is examined in the sections that follow.

The Effect of a Policy's Design or Construction on Operation

As with any writing intended to influence the actions, behaviors, or decisions of others (e.g., legal contracts, procedure manuals), the language and construction of a policy—especially in the form of a public law—are crucial to the course and success of its operation. The way laws are written affects how they are subsequently implemented. The effect can be seen throughout implementation. For example, the ACA assigned new responsibilities to CMS and was explicit in directing CMS to engage in certain implementation activities. The design or construction of a policy includes its objectives, the hypotheses or causal relationships embedded in it, and the degree of flexibility allowed those responsible for implementation. As with laws, the design of other forms of policies heavily influences their implementation. Appendix 22 is an example of an executive order issued by a president. The example gives specific guidance as to who is authorized to do what in implementing the order.

Objectives of the Policy

Well-written laws always include clearly articulated objectives, although these are only one element of a good policy. When those who are responsible for implementation know what a law is really intended to accomplish—what its objectives are—they can more easily operate the programs and procedures embedded in it. For example, the Older Americans Act, Section 101 (P.L. 89-73) contained the following ambitious set of objectives:

> The Congress hereby finds and declares that, in keeping with the traditional American concept of the inherent dignity of the individual in our democratic society, the older people of our Nation are entitled to, and it is the joint and several duty and responsibility of the governments of the U.S., of the several States and their political subdivisions, and of Indian tribes to assist our older people to secure equal opportunity to the full and free enjoyment of the following objectives:
>
> 1. An adequate income in retirement in accordance with the American standard of living.
> 2. The best possible physical and mental health which science can make available and without regard to economic status.
> 3. Obtaining and maintaining suitable housing, independently selected, designed, and located with reference to special needs and available at costs which older citizens can afford.

4. Full restorative services for those who require institutional care and a comprehensive array of community-based, long-term care services adequate to appropriately sustain older people in their communities and in their homes, including support to family members and other persons providing voluntary care to older individuals needing long-term care services.

5. Opportunity for employment with no discriminatory personnel practices because of age.

6. Retirement in health, honor, dignity—after years of contribution to the economy.

7. Participating in and contributing to meaningful activity within the widest range of civic, cultural, educational, and training and recreational opportunities.

8. Efficient community services, including access to low-cost transportation, which provide a choice in supported living arrangements and social assistance in a coordinated manner and which are readily available when needed, with emphasis on maintaining a continuum of care for vulnerable older individuals.

9. Immediate benefit from proven research knowledge which can sustain and improve health and happiness.

10. Freedom, independence, and the free exercise of individual initiative in planning and managing their own lives, full participation in the planning and operation of community-based services and programs provided for their benefit, and protection against abuse, neglect, and exploitation.

When the objectives of a policy are unclear, multiple, or conflicting, successful operation is difficult, if not impossible. A clear example of the problem of multiple, conflicting objectives can be seen in the National Health Planning and Resources Development Act of 1974 (P.L. 93-641). Congress hoped this massive policy would fulfill many of the goals it had previously attempted to attain through a wide variety of more focused policies. As outlined in Section 1513 of P.L. 93-641, its multiple objectives included

- improving the health of people;
- increasing the accessibility (including overcoming geographic, architectural, and transportation barriers), acceptability, continuity, and quality of health services; and
- restraining increases in the cost of providing health services.

As Morone (1990, 272) notes regarding P.L. 93-641, "the legislation proposed every health system desideratum its authors could imagine." These inherently contradictory objectives eventually doomed the policy; Congress repealed it in 1986.

Multiple objectives embedded in a single policy can make implementation extremely difficult, especially if the objectives conflict or are not mutually supportive. In one study, managers with implementation responsibility for Medicare report that they are often torn by the competing demands imposed by the multiple objectives established for the program (Gluck and Sorian 2004). This study notes that these managers are simultaneously required under Medicare to

- serve Medicare beneficiaries' healthcare needs;
- protect the financial integrity of the program and preserve the solvency of the Medicare trust funds;
- make sure payments to providers are adequate to ensure their participation in the program;
- ensure the quality of services provided to program beneficiaries;
- guard against fraud and abuse in the program's operation;
- work with numerous private contractors, ensuring their quality and keeping them satisfied with the relationship; and
- work with states, respond to congressional oversight, and serve the political and policy priorities of the executive branch.

For example, "Medicare managers must ensure adequate participation in Medicare by healthcare providers, but also see to it that providers meet performance and quality standards" (Gluck and Sorian 2004, 65).

Hypothesis of the Policy Vague or conflicting objectives are not the only problem that can hinder a policy's operation. The procedural paradigm set forth in a public law can also be flawed. Embedded in every policy, even if only implicitly, is a theory, or hypothesis, about the effect of operating the policy: If someone does *a*, then *b* will result. Only in a perfect world, of course, would policymakers always base laws on entirely plausible hypotheses. However, a policy's underlying hypothesis will affect its implementation.

If the hypothesis underpinning a policy is wrong, its operation will not solve the problem the policy is intended to address. It will not matter that its objectives are appropriate, or even that they are noble. In formulating the National Health Planning and Resources Development Act (P.L. 93-641), for example, Congress combined an oddly matched pair of strategies: voluntary, community-based planning on the one hand and heavy-handed regulation, at least of capital expansion in the health sector, on the other. To no one's surprise (at least in hindsight), the combination did not work well. The core hypothesis of the policy was seriously flawed.

In contrast, when the Older Americans Act (OAA) was introduced in 1965, it had a clear underlying hypothesis. The OAA was intended to provide resources necessary for public and private social service providers to meet the social service needs of the nation's elderly population. The original act received wide bipartisan support and has endured, with amendments, to the present day. The hypothesis of OAA was simple and correct: Establish mechanisms to provide needed services to elderly individuals, and the services will be provided and consumed.

Another aspect of policy construction that can significantly affect implementation is the nature and extent of any decisions left to the implementing organizations. These decisions may be necessitated by directive language in a law, by what a law does not say, or by confusing or vague language in a law. Although some flexibility in developing policy implementation rules can be advantageous, vague directives can create problems for those with implementation responsibilities.

Degree of Flexibility in Operating the Policy

The Occupational Safety and Health Act of 1970 (P.L. 91-596), for example, contained vague directives and phrases that created significant problems for its implementers. Section 2 of the law stressed the importance of fostering healthful working conditions "insofar as possible" rather than specifying objectives or targets for achieving reductions in occupational injuries or diseases. In Section 6, the statute authorized the secretary of labor, in implementing the law, to issue standards dealing with toxic substances in the workplace "to the extent feasible." Considerable time and energy were expended in deciding if this phrase meant that implementers could take the economic costs of their actions to employers into account in establishing standards dealing with workplace toxic substances. In these instances, effective implementation was impeded by the policy's vague and imprecise language.

Language that is too restrictive can also impede the implementation of a policy. In contrast with the imprecise language in the Occupational Safety and Health Act, Congress wrote into the law a precise and extremely restrictive range of fines that could be assessed against firms that violated standards. For less serious violations, the fine would be $1,000. For serious, willful violations, the fine could be up to $10,000. Most analysts considered the limits of these fines far too low to be effective deterrents, especially for large, profitable enterprises. In this instance, effective operation of the law was impeded by specific language.

The Older Americans Act Amendments of 2006 (P.L. 109-365), which reauthorized OAA, provided extensive implementation guidance. However, considerable flexibility was left to the implementing organization, the Administration on Aging (AoA). Much of the language in the law, while providing detailed information about what was to be accomplished in implementation, left to the AoA's managers a great deal of flexibility as to how to accomplish these responsibilities. For example, the 2006 policy added provisions on elder justice, which was defined in the law as the "effort to prevent, detect, treat, intervene in, and respond to elder abuse, neglect, and exploitation and to protect elders with diminished capacity while maximizing their autonomy." The law, which provided guidance for addressing elder justice in Section 201,

> authorizes the Assistant Secretary for Aging to designate within the Administration on Aging responsibility for elder abuse prevention and services. Assigns to the Assistant Secretary the duty of developing objectives, priorities, policy, and a plan for: (1) facilitating the implementation of an elder justice system in the U.S.; (2) supporting states' efforts in carrying out elder justice programs; (3) establishing federal guidelines and disseminating best practices for uniform data collection and reporting by states; (4) collecting and disseminating data relating to the abuse, neglect, and exploitation of older individuals (abuse); (5) establishing an information clearinghouse; (6) researching such abuse; (7) providing technical assistance to states and other entities; (8) conducting a study concerning the degree of abuse; and (9) promoting collaborative efforts and diminishing duplicative efforts in elder justice programs in all levels of government.

This wording gave the AoA explicit direction for what was to be done, leaving the organization's managers to decide how it was to be done, for the most part. This flexibility facilitated the operation of these provisions.

Congress has tended in recent decades to enact longer and more detailed laws to enhance their implementation. For example, the MMA (2003) is 416 pages long. The PDF version of the ACA (http://house docs.house.gov/energycommerce/ppacacon.pdf) is 974 pages long, and the pages of rules and other guidance to help shape implementation are adding up quickly.

Characteristics of Implementing Organizations

The essence of the implementation phase of policymaking is that one or more organizations or agencies operate enacted legislation, ideally in a manner that realizes the intent behind the legislation. As we noted earlier, the bulk of implementation responsibilities rest with executive branch organizations. For example, CMS is primarily responsible for implementing Medicare, the FDA is primarily responsible for implementing many of the nation's food and drug policies, state insurance departments are responsible for implementing the states' policies regarding health insurance, and so on.

A good fit between an implementing organization and the objectives of the policies it implements is an important determinant of operational success. Fit is determined by whether (1) the organization is sympathetic to a policy's objectives and (2) the organization has the necessary resources—authority, money, personnel, status or prestige, information and expertise, technology, and physical facilities and equipment—to implement a policy effectively.

Whether a policy-implementing organization is sympathetic to the objectives of a policy depends on the attitudes and perspectives of its senior leaders and managers. They are the people who ensure that the necessary support for implementation is garnered. In the case of CMS, for example, attitudes and commitments critical to the organization's success in carrying out its implementation responsibilities include those of the administrator, principal deputy administrator, and chief operating officer of the agency, and the managers of CMS's centers (you may wish to review Exhibit 7.3).

If an implementing organization's leaders are not sympathetic to the policies they are responsible for implementing, they are unlikely to protect those policies from unwarranted amendments or intrusions by nonsupporters. Legislators who are hostile to a policy and those who seek to influence those legislators pose a particular threat. Strong allies in the legislative branch and among interest groups can assist with this protective task, but much of the responsibility rests with the leaders of the implementing organization.

The connection between any organization's resources and its capacity to fulfill its purposes is straightforward. CMS's budget and staff must be adequate matches for the implementation challenges facing the organization. Another factor in the fit between an implementing organization and the policies it is supposed to implement is technology. Implementing organizations rely on a variety of methods and technologies to implement policies. Just as policies differ in substantial ways (recall the distinction made in Chapter 1 between allocative and regulatory policies), the technologies needed to implement them also differ (Dye 2012).

Regulatory policies require implementation technologies that prescribe and control the behaviors of whoever is being regulated. Such technologies include capacity for rule promulgation, investigatory capacity, and ability to impose sanctions. Allocative policies, on the other hand, require technologies through which implementing organizations deliver income, goods, or services. Such technologies include targeting recipients or beneficiaries, determining eligibility for benefits, and managing the supply and quality of goods or services provided through the policy. For instance, the Occupational Safety and Health Administration relies heavily on regulatory technologies as it seeks to protect workers from hazards in the workplace. In contrast, CMS relies heavily, although not exclusively, on allocative technologies in the operation of Medicare, Medicaid (including the ACA-based Medicaid expansion), and CHIP. In fulfilling some of its implementation responsibilities under the ACA, CMS relies increasingly on regulatory technologies.

Only when the leaders of an implementing organization are fully sympathetic to a policy's objectives, and have adequate operational resources, including the appropriate technologies to get the job done, can they effectively carry out their implementation duties. Even then, however, other factors affect the degree of success achieved, including the contributions of the organization's managers.

The Capabilities of Managers

Managers make a difference in implementation (Trattner and McGinnis 2004). Their performance directly affects organizational performance (White and Newcomer 2005). They often face substantial managerial challenges. Appendix 23 illustrates one of the challenges facing managers in implementing organizations, the nature of the workplace culture.

Management is essential in any purposeful organization. Someone must determine, initiate, integrate, and oversee the work of others. Senior-level managers in implementing organizations are responsible for

- molding internal and external agreement on the organization's purposes and priorities;
- building support for the organization's purposes and priorities among internal and external stakeholders, especially among administrative branch superiors, legislators with oversight responsibility for the organization, and relevant interest groups;
- striking a workable balance among the economic and professional interests of the organization's members, the demands and preferences of its external stakeholders, and the public interest the organization is required to serve; and
- negotiating and maintaining effective relationships with people and organizations, regulated by or otherwise affected by the implementing organization, who supply resources to the implementing organization or with whom the implementing organization must work closely in carrying out its policy implementation responsibilities.

Effective implementing organizations need managers who can develop and instill a common vision of what the organization is to accomplish and how it is to be accomplished and to stimulate determined and widespread adherence to that vision. They must focus on decisions and activities that affect the entire organization, including those intended to ensure its survival and overall well-being. They must establish missions and objectives; inculcate appropriate values in the individuals who make up the organization; manage the organizational culture; build intraorganizational and interorganizational coalitions; and interpret and respond to challenges and opportunities presented by the external environment (Longest and Darr 2014).

As in any organization, the managers of implementing agencies and organizations can benefit from knowing the histories and experiences of their organization. For example, managerial performance generally improves where

- long-standing shared values and commonly accepted principles and norms help shape the organization's mission and operating practices and resolve conflicts among competing views;
- a history of success in implementing policies helps legitimize the organization's claims for support from internal and external stakeholders; and
- a history of effective relationships with oversight actors and relevant interest groups and the availability of adequate financial resources provide a sense of organizational pride, stability, self-determination, and autonomy.

Basic management skills—especially in communication, conflict resolution, and motivation—also facilitate management effectiveness. Managers who can effectively communicate their views and preferences have a distinct advantage in guiding the behaviors of their followers. Similarly, successful managers are able to minimize conflict, mobilize widespread commitment to their preferences regarding the organization, and motivate stakeholders to help realize these preferences.

Appendix 24 illustrates the magnitude of the challenges facing managers in implementing organizations, in this case some of the state experiences with implementing features of the ACA. Meeting such challenges will depend on how well the agency's managers perform the management functions shown in Exhibit 3.2. Success also depends on managers' possession of specific competencies, perhaps none more important than competency in collaboration.

The ability of managers of implementing organizations to collaborate and partner with other entities is increasingly important to successful implementation. This ability includes the skills to create and maintain multiparty organizational arrangements; to negotiate complex agreements, perhaps even contracts, that sustain these arrangements; and to produce mutually beneficial outcomes through such arrangements.

The ability to develop shared cultures, or at least to minimize the differences that exist in the cultures of collaborating entities, is crucial to establishing and maintaining effective intergovernmental, interorganizational, or interagency collaborations. In this context, culture is the pattern of shared values and beliefs ingrained in an organization or agency over time that influences the behaviors and decisions of the people in it. Collaborating organizations and agencies frequently have different cultures, which complicates relationships between or among them.

When more than one level of government, organization, or agency is involved in the implementation of a policy, as is frequently the case, the capability of the implementing organizations to collaborate in a coordinated manner is important to success. Laws often require an implementing agency to coordinate or collaborate with other agencies. For example, the Older Americans Amendments of 2006 required the assistant secretary for aging to "coordinate with other federal agencies responsible for formulating and implementing programs, benefits, and services related to providing long-term care" and to "facilitate, in coordination with the administrator of CMS and other federal entities, the provision of long-term care in home and community-based settings." This legislation also required the secretary of HHS to "establish an Interagency Coordinating Committee on Aging that meets at least once a year," and further required this committee to "establish a system to improve coordination of federal agencies."

Rarely does a single organization implement a health policy, and never when the scope of the policy is large. The responsibility for implementing the Medicaid program, for example, does not rest entirely with a single organization. It involves CMS working with the Medicaid agencies in each state and with such private-sector organizations as hospitals, nursing homes, and health plans. Successful implementation of the Medicaid program depends heavily on interactions among these and other organizations.

Even more likely to call collaborative capabilities into play are situations in which several implementing organizations are required to coordinate and integrate their implementation responsibilities for a variety of policies intended to address a particular problem. A chief executive (president or governor) often issues an executive order directing two or more agencies to collaborate or to establish a mechanism to facilitate collaboration. For example, President Obama issued Executive Order #13544 to establish the National Prevention, Health Promotion, and Public Health Council in 2010. Establishment of the council was called for in the ACA. This executive order can be read at www.whitehouse.gov/the-press-office /executive-order-establishing-national-prevention-health-promotion-and-public-health. Among the purposes of the council stated in the executive order is to "provide coordination and leadership at the Federal level, and among all executive departments and agencies, with respect to prevention, wellness, and health promotion practices, the public health system, and integrative health care in the United States."

Information about the council, now called the National Prevention Council, is available at www.surgeongeneral.gov/initiatives/prevention /index.html. The council produced the *National Prevention Strategy* (National Prevention Council 2011) and, subsequently, the *National*

Prevention Council Action Plan (National Prevention Council 2012), which outlines a strategy for implementing the plan. The council is chaired by the surgeon general, and its members include leaders from 20 federal departments, agencies, and offices:

- Secretary, Department of Health and Human Services
- Secretary, Department of Agriculture
- Secretary, Department of Education
- Chairperson, Federal Trade Commission
- Secretary, Department of Transportation
- Secretary, Department of Labor
- Secretary, Department of Homeland Security
- Administrator, Environmental Protection Agency
- Director, Office of National Drug Control Policy
- Director, Domestic Policy Council
- Assistant Secretary—Indian Affairs, Department of the Interior
- Attorney General, Department of Justice
- CEO, Corporation for National and Community Service
- Secretary, Department of Defense
- Secretary, Department of Veterans Affairs
- Secretary, Department of Housing and Urban Development
- Director, Office of Management and Budget
- Secretary, Department of the Interior
- Administrator, General Services Administration
- Director, Office of Personnel Management

Evaluating

The fourth core activity in implementing policy is evaluating (see Exhibit 8.1). This activity brings the other elements of implementation full circle and can lead to new rounds of designing, rulemaking, and operating. Evaluating is a critical activity in effectively implementing policy.

At its most basic level, *evaluating* something means determining "its merit, worth, value, or significance" (Patton 2012, 2). When managers of implementing organizations evaluate a policy, or some component part of it, they are interested in determining its value among other things. However, these determinations are made by seeking answers to more practical questions. Examples of these questions include: Is the policy being effectively implemented? How effective is the policy, or some component of it? Were the policy's objectives achieved or were the objectives of some component of the policy achieved? What are the strengths and weaknesses of the policy or component part? To what extent do the benefits of the policy or component part justify its costs? Does the policy or a component part of it deserve continued funding? Increased funding? There are many ways that these and other, similar questions can be answered.

Policy evaluation can be defined as systematically collecting, analyzing, and using information to answer basic questions about a policy, and ensuring that those answers are supported by evidence. As we discussed earlier, policies typically have hypotheses, or theories, embedded in them. The hypothesis is simply a plausible model of how the policy is intended to work. Of course, there are policies for which no one has bothered to use a theory as a basis for the policy. When a policy hypothesis is present, even if only implicitly, the underlying theory can be expressed as follows: If inputs or resources a, b, and c are assembled and processed by doing m, n, and o with them, then the results will be x, y, and z. The important point here is that using their underlying hypotheses as guidelines, policies can be described in terms of the interrelationships among the inputs/resources available for them, what is done with the resources, and the results achieved.

Types of Evaluations

Numerous types of evaluations exist. Among the most widely used types are process and outcome evaluations, formative and summative evaluations, and cost–benefit and cost-effectiveness evaluations. Each of these types of evaluations has specific characteristics, as follows (Office of Planning, Research and Evaluation 2010):

- Process evaluation examines the extent to which a policy or component part of it is operating as intended by assessing ongoing operations. A process evaluation involves collecting data that describes operations in detail, including such variables as the types and levels of services being provided, the location of service delivery, sociodemographic characteristics of those being served; and the linkages with collaborating agencies.
- Outcome evaluation is designed to assess the extent to which a policy or a component of it results in outcomes in terms of specific variables or data elements. These results are expected to be caused by a policy and tested by comparison to actual results. This type of evaluation is also known as impact evaluation.
- Formative evaluation is a type of process evaluation of new or amended policy or component of it that focuses on collecting data on operations so that needed changes or modifications can be made to a policy

or component in its early stages. Formative evaluations are used to provide feedback to managers about what aspects of a policy are working and those that need to be changed.

- Summative evaluation is a type of outcome evaluation that assesses the results or outcomes of a policy or component. This type of evaluation is concerned with the overall effectiveness of a policy. Summative evaluations can occur at the conclusion of a policy or as a major modification is occurring. This timing has its uses, but evaluations that occur while a policy is operating can result in a steady stream of improvements for a policy or component and are of greatest benefit in guiding implementation of policies.

- Cost–benefit evaluation involves comparing the relative costs of operating a policy or component (expenses, staff salaries, etc.) to the benefits (gains to individuals or society) the policy generates. For example, a policy guiding an intervention to reduce cigarette smoking would focus on the difference between the dollars expended for converting smokers into nonsmokers with the dollar savings from reduced medical care for smoking-related disease, days lost from work, and the like.

- Cost-effectiveness evaluation involves comparing the relative costs of operating a policy or component with the extent to which the policy or component met its objectives. For example, evaluating a policy to guide an intervention to reduce cigarette smoking on a cost-effectiveness basis would estimate the dollars that had to be expended to convert each smoker into a nonsmoker.

Timing of Evaluations

Another way to consider policy evaluation is in terms of when in the life of a policy the evaluation occurs. This continuum can be organized as ex-ante policy evaluation, policy maintenance, policy monitoring, and ex-post policy evaluation (Patton, Sawicki, and Clark 2012):

- *Ex-ante policy evaluation*, also called *anticipatory or prospective evaluation*, mainly influences agenda setting, whether in the original formulation of a policy or in its subsequent modification.

- *Policy monitoring evaluation* is typically undertaken to help ensure that policies are implemented as their formulators designed them and intended them to be implemented. It is relatively straightforward and part of the exercise of legislative oversight and managerial control in implementation. As such, monitoring can play a powerful role in identifying when and how to change a policy, either by reformulating it or by making changes in its implementation, both in rules and in operations. Such monitoring frequently provides valuable information for subsequent ex-post analysis.

- *Ex-post policy evaluation*, also called *retrospective evaluation*, is a way to determine the real value of a policy. This determination depends on an assessment of the degree to which a policy's objectives are achieved through its implementation.

Support for Policy Evaluation and Policy Analysis

The legislative and executive branches of the federal government are involved in policy evaluation and other forms of analysis because they are interested in the performance of the policies they enact and implement. Key federal policy analytical organizations are briefly described in the following sections. The first two agencies are executive branch organizations and the next three are legislative branch agencies. The analytical work done by all five agencies supports policy formulation and implementation.

Agency for Healthcare Research and Quality

The Agency for Healthcare Research and Quality (AHRQ; www.ahrq.gov) was originally established in 1989 as the Agency for Health Care Policy and Research. It was reauthorized with a name change to Agency for Healthcare Research and Quality in 1999. AHRQ's mission is to "produce evidence to make health care safer, higher quality, more accessible, equitable, and affordable, and to work with HHS and other partners to make sure that the evidence is understood and used" (AHRQ 2014).

AHRQ has a staff of about 300 people, with an annual budget exceeding $400 million. Approximately 80 percent of the agency's budget is used to support grants and contracts intended to improve healthcare. AHRQ's current priority areas of focus are to

- improve healthcare quality by accelerating implementation of patient-centered outcomes research;
- make healthcare safer;
- increase accessibility by evaluating ACA coverage expansions; and
- improve healthcare affordability, efficiency, and cost transparency.

The agency's duties to evaluate ACA coverage expansions provide a good example of the role of evaluation in policy implementation. AHRQ, in collaboration with the Office of the Assistant Secretary for Planning and Evaluation and CMS, will evaluate the effects of the Medicaid and Marketplace coverage expansions under provisions in the ACA. In conducting the evaluations, AHRQ will focus on developing evidence that will support the secretary of HHS and Congress in making better-informed decisions about the implementation of the ACA. The evaluations will be designed to determine the effects of the coverage expansions on access, disparities reduction, use and expenditures, outcomes, financial security, and employer offers and coverage take-up.

Center for Medicare and Medicaid Innovation

CMI (www.innovation.cms.gov) was established by the ACA to test "innovative payment and service delivery models to reduce program expenditures . . . while preserving or enhancing the quality of care" for those individuals who receive Medicare, Medicaid, or CHIP benefits.

In establishing the center, Congress provided the secretary of HHS with the authority to expand the scope and duration of a model being tested through rulemaking, including the option of testing on a nationwide basis. For the secretary to exercise this authority, a model must either reduce spending without reducing the quality of care, or improve the quality of care without increasing spending, and must not deny or limit the coverage or provision of any benefits. These determinations are made based on evaluations performed by CMS and certified by CMS's chief actuary.

The Innovation Center is currently focused on the following priorities:

- testing new payment and service delivery models,
- evaluating results and advancing best practices, and
- engaging a broad range of stakeholders to develop additional models for testing.

The Innovation Center has divided its models into seven categories as follows (CMS 2014):

Accountable Care

Accountable Care Organizations and similar care models are designed to incentivize health care providers to become accountable for a patient population and to invest in infrastructure and redesigned care processes that provide for coordinated care, high quality and efficient service delivery.

Bundled Payments for Care Improvement

Medicare currently makes separate payments to various providers for the services they furnish to the same beneficiary for a single illness or course of treatment (an episode of care). Offering these providers a single, bundled payment for an episode of care makes them jointly accountable for the patient's care. It also allows providers to achieve savings based on effectively managing resources as they provide treatment to the beneficiary throughout the episode.

Primary Care Transformation

Primary care providers are a key point of contact for patients' health care needs. Strengthening and increasing access to primary care is critical to promoting health and reducing overall health care costs. Advanced primary care practices—also called "medical homes"—utilize a team-based approach, while emphasizing prevention, health information technology, care coordination, and shared decision making among patients and their providers.

Initiatives Focused on the Medicaid and CHIP Population

Medicaid and the Children's Health Insurance Program (CHIP) are administered by the states but are jointly funded by the federal government and states. Initiatives in this category are administered by the participating states.

Initiatives Focused on the Medicare-Medicaid Enrollees

The Medicare and Medicaid programs were designed with distinct purposes. Individuals enrolled in both Medicare and Medicaid (the "dual eligibles") account for a disproportionate share of the programs' expenditures. A fully integrated, person-centered system of care that ensures that all their needs are met could better serve this population in a high quality, cost effective manner.

Initiatives to Speed the Adoption of Best Practices

Recent studies indicate that it takes nearly 17 years on average before best practices—backed by research—are incorporated into widespread clinical practice—and even then the application of the knowledge is very uneven. The Innovation Center is partnering with a broad range of health care providers, federal agencies, professional societies and other experts and stakeholders to test new models for disseminating evidence-based best practices and significantly increasing the speed of adoption.

Initiatives to Accelerate the Development and Testing of New Payment and Service Delivery Models

Many innovations necessary to improve the health care system will come from local communities and health care leaders from across the entire country. By partnering with these local and regional stakeholders, CMS can help accelerate the testing of models today that may be the next breakthrough tomorrow.

Appendix 25 is a fact sheet describing some of CMS's initiatives intended to reform healthcare delivery in the United States.

Government Accountability Office

The Government Accountability Office (GAO; www.gao.gov) is the investigative arm of Congress. It is often called the "congressional watchdog" because it investigates how the federal government spends taxpayer dollars. The agency advises Congress and the heads of executive branch agencies on making government more efficient, effective, ethical, equitable, and responsive. The stated mission of GAO is to "support the Congress in meeting its constitutional responsibilities and to help improve the performance and ensure the accountability of the federal government for the benefit of the American people" (GAO 2014). The agency seeks to provide Congress with timely information that is objective, fact-based, nonpartisan, nonideological, fair, and balanced.

In carrying out its mission, GAO audits and analyzes a host of programs and activities that arise from the implementation of federal policies. Organizationally, GAO is under the direction of the comptroller general of the United States, who is appointed by the president, with the advice and consent of the Senate, to a 15-year term. This organizational structure gives GAO a level of independence and continuity of leadership that is rare in government. The Budget and Accounting Act of 1921 established the organization for the limited purpose of independently auditing federal agencies. Over the years, however, Congress has expanded GAO's audit authority, added extensive new responsibilities and duties, and strengthened the organization's ability to perform its work independently.

GAO does its work largely at the request of congressional committees or subcommittees or by mandate of public laws or committee reports. In fact, GAO is required to perform work requested by committee chairpersons and assigns equal status to requests from ranking minority members of congressional committees. When possible, GAO also responds to requests for analyses and audits from individual members of Congress. The agency supports congressional oversight by (GAO 2014)

- auditing agency operations to determine whether federal funds are being spent efficiently and effectively,
- investigating allegations of illegal and improper activities,
- reporting on how well government programs and policies are meeting their objectives,
- performing policy analyses and outlining options for congressional consideration, and
- issuing legal decisions and opinions such as bid protest rulings and reports on agency rules.

Appendix 26 is a summary of GAO-provided testimony to the House of Representatives' Committee on Homeland Security, Subcommittee on Cybersecurity, Infrastructure Protection, and Security Technologies, on the Department of Homeland Security's efforts to identify, prioritize, assess, and inspect potentially dangerous chemical facilities. This testimony and the analyses on which it is based provide an example of the agency's work.

Because GAO conducts a wide range of analyses, its staff is drawn from a variety of disciplines, including accounting, law, public and business administration, economics, and the social and physical sciences. The work is organized so each staff member concentrates on a specific subject area, facilitating the development of expertise and in-depth knowledge. When an analytical assignment requires specialized experience not available inside GAO, outside experts assist the permanent staff.

Congressional Budget Office

The Congressional Budget Office (CBO; www.cbo.gov) was created by the Congressional Budget and Impoundment Control Act of 1974. The agency's mission is to provide Congress with the objective, timely, and nonpartisan analyses needed for economic and budget decisions and with the information and estimates required for the congressional budget process. Compared with the missions of Congress's other support agencies—the Congressional Research Service (CRS) and the GAO—CBO's mission is narrow and focused. Even so, because the federal budget covers a wide array of activities, the agency is involved in wide-ranging health policy activity.

The Budget Act requires CBO to produce a cost estimate for every bill "reported out" (approved) by a congressional committee. CBO's cost estimates show how the legislation would affect spending or revenues over the subsequent five years or more. They also provide information about the proposal and explain how CBO prepared the estimate.

Appendix 27 is an example of CBO's work, in this case its estimate of the effect on the federal deficit of increasing taxes on alcoholic beverages. On occasion, CBO's estimates become extremely complicated, as they did in projecting the costs of adding a prescription drug benefit to the Medicare program or to the cost projections for the ACA.

CBO's primary responsibility is to assist the congressional budget committees with the matters under their jurisdiction—principally the congressional budget resolution and its enforcement. To help the budget committees enforce the budget resolution, CBO provides estimates of the budgetary costs of legislation approved by the various congressional committees and tracks the progress of spending and revenue legislation.

Overall, CBO's services can be grouped into four categories: helping Congress formulate budget plans, helping it stay within the scope of these plans, helping it assess the impact of federal mandates, and helping it consider the impact of policies on the federal budget. In the last role, for example, the analyses examine current and proposed policies, sometimes suggesting alternative approaches and projecting how the alternatives would affect current programs, the federal budget, and the economy. In line with its nonpartisan mandate, CBO does not offer specific policy recommendations.

Congressional Research Service

CRS (www.loc.gov/crsinfo/about/) is another analytical resource available to members of Congress. Established in 1914 through legislation creating a separate department within the Library of Congress called the Legislative Reference Service, the agency was established to provide Congress with information and analysis that would allow it to make more informed decisions. The Legislative Reorganization Act of 1970 renamed the agency the Congressional Research Service and significantly expanded its responsibilities. Today, the agency's mission is to serve "the Congress throughout the legislative process by providing comprehensive and reliable legislative research and analysis that are timely, objective, authoritative, and confidential, thereby contributing to an informed national legislature" (CRS 2012).

As a legislative branch organization, CRS serves as a shared staff to congressional committees and members, assisting at every stage of the legislative process—from the early considerations in agenda setting that precede bill drafting, through committee hearings and floor debate, to the oversight and modification of enacted laws and various agency activities. CRS operates in many ways as an extension of, or supplement to, the members' own office staff.

The agency's staff includes more than 400 policy analysts, attorneys, information professionals, and experts in a variety of disciplines: law, economics, foreign affairs, defense and homeland security, public administration, education, healthcare, immigration, energy, environmental protection, science, and technology.

CRS is organized into five interdisciplinary research divisions, which are clustered around American law; domestic social policy; foreign affairs, defense, and trade; government and finance; and resources, science, and industry. A knowledge services group serves the five divisions. Within each division, CRS analysts and specialists are organized into smaller sections that focus on specific areas of public policy such as education, labor, taxes, and health.

CRS provides its services in many forms, including (CRS 2013)

- reports on major policy issues;
- tailored confidential memoranda, briefings, and consultations;
- seminars, workshops, and expert congressional testimony; and
- responses to individual inquiries.

By concluding our discussion of the policy implementation phase of policymaking (Chapter 7 and this chapter), we are ready to move on to the third phase in the policymaking process, modification. As we will see in Chapter 9, a modification phase of policymaking is necessary because perfection is not achievable in either policy formulation or implementation.

Summary

The implementation phase of public policymaking involves managing human, financial, and other resources in ways that facilitate achievement of the objectives embodied in enacted legislation. Implementing organizations, primarily the departments and agencies in the executive branches of governments, are established and maintained and the people within them employed to carry out the intent of public laws and amendments to them as enacted by the legislative branch.

Implementation is carried out through the interrelated set of activities shown in the implementation phase in Exhibit 8.1. These activities are designing, rulemaking, operating, and evaluating, which may lead to subsequent rounds of these activities.

Designing involves establishing the agenda of an implementing organization, planning how to address the agenda, and organizing to carry out the plans. Sometimes this process is straightforward, but at other times designing can be difficult. Designing the implementation of the ACA, for example, remains a challenge for CMS.

Rulemaking is an especially important and necessary part of policymaking because enacted laws are seldom explicit enough concerning the steps necessary to guide their implementation adequately. Implementing organizations routinely promulgate rules to guide the operation of enacted laws. The drafting and issuing of rules are themselves guided by certain rules and established procedures that ensure that those affected by a policy will have ample opportunity to participate in the rulemaking associated with its implementation. Interest groups may be heavily involved in rulemaking because they frequently express their preferences regarding rules.

Operating policies puts them into effect. If an objective of a policy is to expand Medicaid enrollment, for example, its operation means adding new enrollees. Operation requires that those who implement policies follow the rules promulgated to guide that implementation according to the mandates inherent in the laws.

Finally, evaluating, the fourth core activity in implementing policy, brings the other elements of implementation full circle and can lead to new rounds of designing, rulemaking, and operating. Policy evaluation is defined as systematically collecting, analyzing, and using information to answer basic questions about a policy. When managers of implementing organizations evaluate a policy, or some component part of it, they are interested in determining answers to such questions as: Was the policy effectively implemented? How effective is the policy or component? Were the policy's or component's objectives achieved? What are the strengths and weaknesses of the policy or component part? To what extent do the benefits of the policy or component part justify its costs? Does the policy or component deserve continued funding? Increased funding? There are many ways that these and other, similar questions can be answered because there are several types of evaluations. In addition, implementing organizations can turn to several organizations to assist with evaluations, including AHRQ, CMI, GAO, CBO, and CRS.

Review Questions

1. Describe the designing activity in policy implementation.
2. Describe the federal rulemaking process.
3. Describe the operating activity in policy implementation.
4. Describe the evaluating activity in policy implementation.
5. List and briefly describe five organizations that support policy evaluating activity.
6. Discuss rulemaking. Include the role of interest groups in rulemaking in your response.

References

Agency for Healthcare Research and Quality (AHRQ). 2014. "About Us." Accessed February 13. www.ahrq.gov/about/index.html.

Carey, M. P. 2013. *The Federal Rulemaking Process: An Overview*. Congressional Research Service Report RL32240. Published June 17. www.fas.org/sgp/crs/misc/RL32240.pdf.

Centers for Medicare & Medicaid Services (CMS). 2014. "Innovation Models." Accessed February 13. www.innovation.cms.gov/initiatives/index.html#views=models.

———. 2013a. "CMS Strategy: The Road Forward, 2013–2017." Published March. www.cms.gov/About-CMS/Agency-Information/CMS-Strategy/Downloads/CMS-Strategy.pdf.

———. 2013b. "Justification of Estimates for Appropriations Committees, FY 2014." Accessed February 11, 2014. www.cms.gov/About-CMS/Agency-Information/PerformanceBudget/Downloads/FY2014-CJ-Final.pdf.

Congressional Research Service (CRS). 2013. "About CRS." Library of Congress. Updated May 1. www.loc.gov/crsinfo/about.

———. 2012. "History and Mission." Library of Congress. Updated November 15. www.loc.gov/crsinfo/about/history.html.

Diver, C. 1989. "Regulatory Precision." In *Making Regulatory Policy*, edited by K. Hawkins and J. Thomas, 199–232. Pittsburgh, PA: University of Pittsburgh Press.

Doonan, M. T. 2013. *American Federalism in Practice: The Formulation and Implementation of Contemporary Health Policy*. Washington, DC: Brookings Institution Press.

Dye, T. R. 2012. *Understanding Public Policy*, fourteenth edition. Upper Saddle River, NJ: Pearson Education.

Feldstein, P. J. 2006. *The Politics of Health Legislation: An Economic Perspective*, third edition. Chicago: Health Administration Press.

Gluck, M. E., and R. Sorian. 2004. *Administrative Challenges in Managing the Medicare Program*. American Association of Retired Persons Report #2004-15. Washington, DC: American Association of Retired Persons.

Government Accountability Office (GAO). 2014. "About GAO." Accessed February 21. http://gao.gov/about/index.html.

Jost, T. S. 2014. "Implementing Health Reform: Four Years Later." *Health Affairs* 33 (1): 7–10.

Kerwin, C. M., and S. R. Furlong. 2010. *Rulemaking: How Government Agencies Write Law and Make Policy*, fourth edition. Washington, DC: CQ Press.

Longest, B. B., Jr., and K. Darr. 2014. *Managing Health Services Organizations and Systems*, sixth edition. Baltimore, MD: Health Professions Press.

Morone, J. A. 1990. *The Democratic Wish: Popular Participation and the Limits of American Government*. New York: Basic Books.

National Prevention Council. 2012. *National Prevention Council Action Plan: Implementing the National Prevention Strategy*. Published June. www.surgeongeneral.gov/initiatives/prevention/2012-npc-action-plan.pdf.

———. 2011. *National Prevention Strategy*. Published June. www.surgeongeneral.gov/initiatives/prevention/strategy/report.pdf.

Naughton, K., C. Schmid, S. W. Yackee, and X. Zhan. 2009. "Understanding Commenter Influence During Agency Rule Development." *Journal of Policy Analysis and Management* 28 (2): 258–77.

Office of Planning, Research and Evaluation. 2010. *The Program Manager's Guide to Evaluation*, second edition. Washington, DC: US Department of Health and Human Services (HHS), Administration for Children and Families, Office of Planning, Research and Evaluation.

Office of the Federal Register. 2014. "A Guide to the Rulemaking Process." Accessed February 9. www.federalregister.gov/uploads/2011/01/the_rulemaking_process.pdf.

Patton, C. V., D. S. Sawicki, and J. J. Clark. 2012. *Basic Methods of Policy Analysis and Planning*, third edition. Upper Saddle River, NJ: Pearson Education.

Patton, M. Q. 2012. *Essentials of Utilization-Focused Evaluation*. Thousand Oaks, CA: Sage.

Trattner, J. H., and P. McGinnis. 2004. *The 2004 Prune Book: Top Management Challenges for Presidential Appointees*. Washington, DC: Brookings Institution Press and the Council for Excellence in Government.

White, B., and K. E. Newcomer (eds.). 2005. *Getting Results: A Guide for Federal Leaders and Managers*. Vienna, VA: Management Concepts.

Zwick, D. I. 1978. "Initial Development of Guidelines for Health Planning." *Public Health Reports* 93 (5): 407–20.

POLICY MODIFICATION

Learning Objectives

After reading this chapter, you should be able to

- discuss how the policy modification phase brings the policymaking process full circle;
- distinguish between policy modification and policy initiation;
- define *incrementalism* and explain the preference for it in policymaking;
- describe the role each branch of government plays in policy modification;
- explain how modification occurs in policy formulation, including in agenda setting and legislation development;
- explain how modification occurs in the designing, rulemaking, operating, and evaluating activities of policy implementation; and
- explain how modification occurs through the cycle of rulemaking and operating.

Policymaking is not a perfect process. Mistakes of omission and commission are routinely made in the formulation and implementation phases. The policymaking process model used throughout this book is brought full circle by the third phase of the process, modification. This phase is necessary because perfection eludes policymakers in the formulation and implementation phases. Even policy decisions that are correct when they are made must adjust to accommodate changing circumstances.

In a hypothetical policymaking process without a modification phase, policies would be formulated in their original version and then implemented, and that would be the end of the process—except, of course, for the policies' consequences. In practice, however, policymaking does not work this way. The consequences of policies—including consequences for those who formulate and implement the policies and for the individuals, organizations, and interest groups outside the process but affected by policies—cause people to seek modification. They do so throughout the life of the policy.

At a minimum, individuals, organizations, or interest groups who benefit from a particular policy may seek modifications that increase or maintain these benefits over time. Similarly, those who are negatively affected by a policy will seek to modify it to minimize the negative consequences. In addition, when the policymakers who formulate and implement a public policy observe it in operation, they will evaluate it against their objectives for that policy. When preferences and reality do not match, efforts to modify the policy typically ensue. Some policymakers do not have to see any evidence of performance to want to modify a policy. They opposed its enactment and pursue modification thereafter. The clearest example of such opposition and pursuit of modification in health policy in recent decades is the continuing battle over the Affordable Care Act (ACA). Beginning with the law's enactment, its repeal or modification has been high on the Republican agenda. Between 2011 and early 2015 there were 56 attempts to repeal or modify the ACA in the Republican-controlled House of Representatives (Pear 2015). These efforts were aimed at complete repeal, with or without replacement, or at specific provisions of the ACA, including health insurance marketplaces, the individual mandate, taxes on medical device companies, and many others.

Almost every policy has a history. In the case of public laws, an initial version is formulated which then evolves as it is implemented, either through amendments to the original legislation or through new or revised rules and changes in operation. Some policies eventually die—they are repealed by the legislative branch—but most have long and dynamic lives during which they are continually modified in various ways. This chapter addresses the policy modification phase of public policymaking.

Careful consideration of the modification phase of policymaking as shown in the darkly shaded portion of Exhibit 9.1 is fundamental to understanding the process as a continual cycle of interrelated activities. Negative consequences of an existing policy will trigger modification efforts by those affected. Changes in the external environment, such as economic conditions, demographic shifts, or scientific or technological advances, can stimulate modifications in policy. If the consequences of an existing policy are positive for individuals, organizations, or groups, they may seek modifications that give them more benefits or protect existing ones. In addition to efforts to modify policy by those whom it affects, those who formulate and implement policies may seek modifications based on the performance and consequences of existing policies. Although such people—and many of those affected by the policies—typically prefer incremental policy changes, which we discuss further later in this chapter, pressure for policy modification is relentless.

As this chapter describes, pressure to modify is exerted at many points in the policymaking process. Authoritative decisions made anywhere in the process are always subject to review and revision. Policy modifications—large and small—emphasize that the separate components of the policymaking

EXHIBIT 9.1

Policymaking Process: Modification Phase

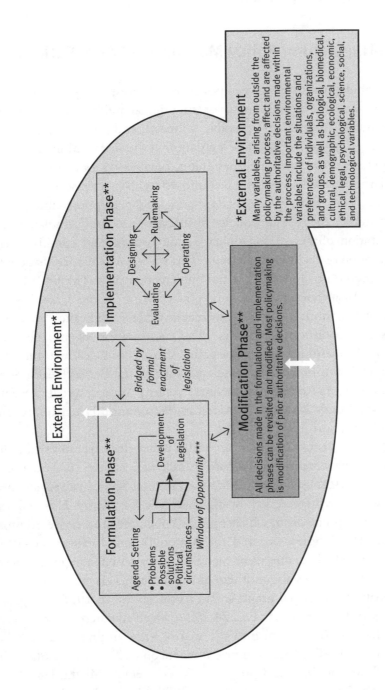

Policymakers in all three branches of government make policy in the form of position-appropriate, or authoritative, decisions. Their decisions differ in that the **legislative branch is primarily involved in formulation, the **executive branch** is primarily involved in implementation, and both are involved in modification of prior decisions or policies. The **judicial branch** interprets and assesses the legality of decisions made within all three phases of the policymaking process.

***A window of opportunity opens for possible progression of issues through formulation, enactment, implementation, and modification when there is a favorable confluence of problems, possible solutions, and political circumstances.

process are, in reality, highly interactive and interdependent. We begin our consideration of modification by drawing a distinction between policy initiation and policy modification.

Distinguishing Policy Modification from Policy Initiation

We can differentiate between policy modification and policy initiation. Policy initiation—the establishment of an original public law—results when the confluence of problems, possible solutions, and political circumstances leads to the initial development of legislation in the formulation phase and then to implementation, including designing, rulemaking, operating, and evaluating activities needed to put the law into effect. By contrast, policy modification results when the performance, impact, and perceptions about performance and impact of existing policies feeds back into the formulation and implementation phases of the policymaking process and stimulates changes in legislation or its implementation. This is shown as the feedback arrows from modification to formulation and implementation in Exhibit 9.1.

An important fact about policymaking in the United States is that policy initiation is a rare occurrence, while modification of existing policies is a common occurrence. The modification phenomenon, especially through amendments to prior policy, can be seen clearly in the ACA, which amended a number of existing laws such as the Public Health Services Act; Employment Retirement Income Security Act; Internal Revenue Code; Social Security Act; and the Medicare Prescription Drug, Improvement, and Modernization Act.

The history of American health policy demonstrates that policymakers can, and on occasion do, initiate entirely new policies. For example, in 1798 Congress established the US Marine Hospital Service to provide medical care for seamen who were sick or disabled. The US Marine Hospital Service was the initial policy from which the US Public Health Service eventually grew. In 1921, Congress enacted the Maternity and Infancy Act (P.L. 67-97), through which grants were made to states to encourage the development of health services for mothers and children. This new policy became the prototype for federal grants in aid to the states. In 1935, Congress enacted the Social Security Act (P.L. 74-271), which initiated the major entrance of the federal government into the area of social insurance. This policy, which has been modified many times, now encompasses, among other things, the Medicare and Medicaid programs. The Veterans' Mental Health and Other Health Care Improvements Act of 2008 (P.L. 110-387) and the American Recovery and Reinvestment Act of 2009 (P.L. 111-5), which also contains extensive health policy provisions, are more recent examples of new policies.

As these examples illustrate, some health or health-related policies are indeed formulated and implemented without being related to prior policies. The vast majority of contemporary health policies, however, spring from existing policies. In other words, most health policies are the result of modifying prior policies, which is why understanding the modification phase is so important.

A review of health policies, such as those presented in the Briefly Annotated Chronological List of Selected US Federal Laws Pertaining to Health shown in Appendix 4, readily illustrates just how many contemporary health policies are amendments to previously enacted public laws or the result of changes—often, a string of changes—in the rules and practices that determine how laws are implemented. In fact, no policy is permanent. Modification of prior policies—whether in the form of decisions representing public laws, implementation rules or regulations, rulings of a court, or operational practices—pervades the entire policymaking process. Perhaps the clearest possible example of policy modification in practice can be found in the long line of policy modifications to Medicare policy over the years since its enactment, a pattern described in the next section.

Medicare: A Long History of Policy Modification in Practice

The role of policy modification can be seen vividly in the legislative history of Medicare. Much of this history is chronicled in Appendix 4. Many examples of how the modification phase plays out are embedded in the history of Medicare-related legislation. A review of this history begins with the enactment of the 1935 Social Security Act (P.L. 74-271); from that point forward, however, the establishment and continuation of the Medicare program is largely a matter of modifying previous policies.

The Medicare program emerged on the nation's policy agenda in large part through the operation of the Social Security program over a span of three decades, from the mid-1930s to the mid-1960s. President Franklin D. Roosevelt formed the Committee on Economic Security in 1934 and charged its members to develop a program that could ensure the "economic security" of the nation's citizens. The committee considered the inclusion of health insurance in the Social Security program from the outset. In fact, sentiment for its inclusion was strong among members of the committee (Oberlander 2003; Starr 2013). But in the end, they decided against recommending the inclusion of health insurance because of the tremendous political burdens associated with such a proposal. The American Medical Association (AMA) in particular strongly opposed the concept.

As stated in the original legislation, the objective of the Social Security Act of 1935 was

> to provide for the general welfare by establishing a system of federal old age benefits, and by enabling the several States to make more adequate provision for aged persons, blind persons, dependent and crippled children, maternal and child welfare, public health, and the administration of their unemployment compensation laws.

Although health insurance was not included among the program's original provisions, its addition was considered from time to time in the ensuing years. President Truman considered national health insurance a key part of his legislative agenda. But AMA's continued powerful opposition and the Truman administration's need to divert its attention to Korea in 1950 meant that the president was unable to stimulate the development and enactment of any sort of universal health insurance policy. Faced with dim political prospects for universal health insurance, proponents turned to a much more limited idea—hospital insurance for the aged.

Following a number of modest proposals for such insurance, none of which could muster the necessary political support for enactment, two powerful members of Congress, Senator Robert Kerr and Representative Wilbur Mills, were able to pass a bill that provided federal support for state programs in welfare medicine. The Amendments to the Social Security Act of 1960 (P.L. 86-778) provided health benefits to the aged poor. Not until the Democratic margin in Congress was significantly increased in President Johnson's landslide election in 1964 did a more expansive initiative have much chance of passage.

With Medicare's prospects significantly improved by the 1964 election, it reached a high priority among President Johnson's Great Society programs and was enacted as part of the Social Security Amendments of 1965 (P.L. 89-97). Medicare emerged on the nation's policy agenda through a series of attempts to modify the original Social Security Act by expanding the benefits provided to include health insurance. Although these attempts at modifying the original Social Security Act failed more often than not, they set the stage for the eventual modification that resulted in the Medicare program.

Following the enactment of the original legislation that established the Medicare program, the chronology of related legislation shows a remarkable pattern of evolutionary, incremental modification of a single, although massive, public policy. In a progression of modifications that continues today, among other changes, Medicare benefits have been added and deleted, who is covered by the program has been adjusted, premiums and copayment provisions have been changed, reimbursement rates and payment mechanisms for service providers have shifted, and features to ensure quality and medical necessity of services have been added, changed, and deleted. A history of these changes written by staff members of the Social Security Administration (2014) is lengthy and informative. A brief sample of the pattern of changes is provided in the accompanying box to illustrate how dynamic the modification of Medicare policy has been and to serve as an example of the critical role modification plays in the overall policymaking process. This sample is limited to changes in policy pertaining to payment to providers. It excludes the numerous changes as to whom Medicare covers, the benefits offered by Medicare, the premiums paid by beneficiaries, and other aspects of Medicare policy. Even with this limitation, however, this chronology reflects significant legislative change over time, a pattern likely to continue as long as this complex and expensive program exists. Indeed, considering its current financial challenges, Medicare faces one of the most volatile periods in its history, and many more modifications are likely in the coming years. In regard to the sample of payment to provider policy changes, remember that Medicare pays providers under provisions of Part A (inpatient hospital, home health, skilled nursing facility, and hospice), Part B (physician, outpatient hospital, and other services), Part C (the Medicare Advantage program), and Part D (prescription drugs).

A Brief History of Medicare Payments to Providers

Before 1983, Part A payments to providers were made on a reasonable cost basis. Medicare payments for most inpatient hospital services are now made under a reimbursement mechanism known as the prospective payment system (PPS). Under the PPS for acute inpatient hospitals, each stay is categorized into a diagnosis-related group (DRG). Each DRG has a specific predetermined amount associated with it, which serves as the basis for payment. A number of adjustments are applied to the DRG's specific predetermined amount to calculate the payment for each stay. In some cases the payment the hospital receives is less than the hospital's actual cost for providing Part A–covered inpatient hospital services for the stay; in other cases it is more. The hospital absorbs the loss or makes a profit. Certain payment adjustments exist for extraordinarily costly inpatient hospital stays and other situations. Payments for skilled nursing care, home health care, inpatient rehabilitation hospital care, long-term care hospitals, inpatient psychiatric hospitals, and hospice are made under separate prospective payment systems.

(continued)

For non-physician Part B services, home health care is reimbursed under the same prospective payment system as Part A, most hospital outpatient services are reimbursed on a separate prospective payment system, and most payments for clinical laboratory and ambulance services are based on fee schedules. A fee schedule is a comprehensive listing of maximum fees used to pay providers. Most durable medical equipment has also been paid on a fee schedule in recent years but is paid based on a competitive bidding process in some areas beginning January 1, 2011. This competitive bidding process will be expanded to all areas within the next several years.

In general, the prospective payment systems and fee schedules used for Part A and non-physician Part B services are increased each year either by indices related to the "market basket" of goods and services that the provider must purchase or by indices related to the Consumer Price Index (CPI). These indices vary by type of provider. The Affordable Care Act mandates reductions in most of these payment updates. In most cases, the payment updates are reduced by stipulated amounts for 2010–2019 and are further and permanently reduced by growth in economy-wide productivity. Starting dates and amounts of reductions vary by provider. It is likely that the lower payment increases will not be viable in the long range. The best available evidence indicates that most healthcare providers cannot improve their productivity to this degree because of the labor-intensive nature of most of these services.

For Part B, before 1992, physicians were paid on the basis of reasonable charge. This amount was initially defined as the lowest of (1) the physician's actual charge, (2) the physician's customary charge, or (3) the prevailing charge for similar services in that locality. Since January 1992, allowed charges have been defined as the lesser of (1) the submitted charges or (2) the amount determined by a fee schedule based on a relative value scale. In practice, most allowed charges are based on the fee schedule, which is supposed to be updated each year by a Sustainable Growth Rate (SGR) system prescribed in the law. However, over the past 10 years, the SGR system would have required significant fee reductions for physicians, and Congress has passed a series of bills to override the reductions.

If a doctor or supplier agrees to accept the Medicare-approved rate as payment in full ("takes assignment"), then payments provided must be considered as payments in full for that service. The provider

(continued)

may not request any added payments (beyond the initial annual deductible and coinsurance) from the beneficiary or insurer. If the provider does not take assignment, the beneficiary will be charged for the excess (which may be paid by Medigap insurance). Limits now exist on the excess that doctors or suppliers can charge. Physicians are "participating physicians" if they agree before the beginning of the year to accept assignment for all Medicare services they furnish during the year. Since beneficiaries in the original Medicare fee-for-service program may select their doctors, they can choose participating physicians.

Medicare Advantage plans and their precursors have generally been paid on a capitation basis, meaning that a fixed, predetermined amount per month per member is nature of services used by the members. The specific mechanisms to determine the payment amounts have changed over the years. In 2006, Medicare began paying capitated payment rates to plans based on a competitive bidding process.

For Part D, each month for each plan member, Medicare pays stand-alone Prescription Drug Plans (PDPs) and the prescription drug portions of Medicare Advantage plans their risk-adjusted bid, minus the enrollee premium. Plans also receive payments representing premiums and cost-sharing amounts for certain low-income beneficiaries for whom these items are reduced or waived. Under the reinsurance provision, plans receive payments for 80 percent of costs in the catastrophic coverage category.

To help them gain experience with the Medicare population, Part D plans are protected by a system of "risk corridors" that allow Medicare to assist with unexpected costs and share in unexpected savings. The risk corridors became less protective after 2007.

Under Part D, Medicare provides certain subsidies to employer and union PDPs that continue to offer coverage to Medicare retirees and meet specific criteria in doing so. These retiree drug subsidy (RDS) payments became taxable under the Affordable Care Act beginning in 2013.

Source: Social Security Administration (2014, 44–45).

Modification is a ubiquitous component of the overall policymaking process, as the chronology of modifications to the Medicare provider payment policy just outlined clearly illustrates. This chronology provides a good example of the role of modification in policymaking. In Medicare and in many other areas of health policy as well, the likelihood that prior decisions will be revisited and changed is a readily recognizable feature of public policymaking in the United States. The propensity for modification makes policymaking distinctly cyclical and dynamic.

Another important feature of the modification phenomenon is a strong preference by many involved in or affected by policymaking for changes to be relatively small and slow moving. This feature is termed *incrementalism* and is discussed in the next section.

Incrementalism in Policymaking

Not only are most public policies modifications of previously established policies, but also, historically, most modifications reflect only modest changes (Anderson 2014). The combination of a process that is characterized by continual modification with the fact that these changes tend to be modest led long ago to the apt characterization of US public policymaking as a process of incrementalism (Lindblom 1969).

Of course, some policy modifications are large scale, but these are exceptions to the general trend. The enactment of Medicare was certainly a large modification of the earlier Social Security Act. The ACA contains numerous major modifications to prior health policy. However, the pattern of incrementalism is likely to continue (Gruber 2008).

The affinity for modest, incremental policy change is not restricted to the health arena. The operation of the nation's overall political, social, and economic systems reflects preferences for modest rather than sweeping change. As we noted in Chapter 2, members of the US power elite have a strong preference for incremental changes in public policies. They believe that incrementalism—building on existing policies via modification in small, incremental steps—allows the economic and social systems to adjust without being unduly threatened by change. Incremental policymaking limits economic dislocation or disruption and causes minimal alteration in the social system's status quo.

These strong preferences for stability ran headlong into the worldwide financial crisis that began in late 2008. The preferences didn't disappear, but they were at least temporarily supplanted by the urgent need to stabilize the economy, in part through certain health reforms that may result in additional large-scale policy modifications. However, when the economy eventually stabilizes, the historical preference for incrementalism in policymaking likely will reemerge.

The Basis of the Preference for Incrementalism
In policymaking that is characterized by incrementalism, significant departures from the existing patterns of policies occur only rarely. Most of the

time, the effects and consequences of policies play out slowly and predictably. This pace supports the idea that policymakers in all three branches of government; leaders in health-related organizations and interest groups; and many individuals who benefit from such policies as the Medicare and Medicaid programs, funding for biomedical research, or the subsidies to help people purchase health insurance coverage provided by the ACA typically have a strong preference for incrementalism in health policymaking.

The results and consequences of incremental decisions are more predictable and stable than are those of decisions not made incrementally. Unless a person—whether a policymaker or someone affected by policies—is unhappy with a situation and wishes an immediate and drastic change, the preference for incrementalism will almost always prevail.

Incrementalism in policymaking increases the likelihood of reaching compromises among the diverse interests in the policy marketplace. The potential for compromise is an important feature of an effective and smoothly running policymaking process. Words like *incrementalism* and *compromise* used in the context of public policymaking may bring to mind compromised principles, inappropriate influence peddling, and corrupt deals made behind closed doors. However, "in a democracy compromise is not merely unavoidable; it is a source of creative invention, sometimes generating solutions that unexpectedly combine seemingly opposed ideas" (Starr and Zelman 1993, 8).

The health policy domain is replete with incrementally developed policies. For instance, the history of the National Institutes of Health (NIH) reflects incremental policymaking over almost 130 years. Ranging from 1887, when the federal government's expenditures on biomedical research totaled about $300, and through the 1930s, when a small federal laboratory conducting biomedical research was initiated, NIH has experienced extensive elaboration (the addition of new institutes as biomedical science evolved), growth (its annual budget was more than $31 billion in 2015), and shifts in the emphases of its research agenda (cancer, AIDS, women's health, health disparities, schizophrenia, and pediatric diseases). Every step in NIH's continuing and incremental evolution has been guided by specific policy changes, each an incremental modification intending carefully measured adjustments in NIH's actions, decisions, and behaviors.

Consistent with our earlier discussion that crises (war, collapse of major financial institutions, major economic instability) can alter the incremental nature of most policymaking, the American Recovery and Reinvestment Act of 2009 (P.L. 111-5) included provisions for a onetime infusion of $10 billion into the NIH budget ($8.5 billion for research grants and $1.5 billion for upgrading and renovating university laboratories and science infrastructure). A budgetary increase of this magnitude is certainly not consistent with NIH's history of incremental increases, but this modification resulted from an unprecedented—or nearly so—financial crisis. The general preference for incremental policy changes didn't disappear, but it was suppressed in favor of infusing new money into the NIH budget to stimulate economic activity in the nation. As the economy stabilizes, the historical preference for incrementalism in policymaking, including in the pattern of growth in the NIH budget, is reasserting itself.

Mechanics of the Modification Phase

The policymaking process provides abundant opportunities for the experiences with and opinions about public laws to influence future iterations of formulation and to change some of the decisions and activities that guide their implementation as well. Two important facts overarch the mechanics of policy modification.

The most basic fact about the mechanics of modification is that participants in all three branches of government play active roles in policy modification. Everyone who can make the authoritative decisions that comprise public policy can also participate in modifying prior decisions.

The second vital mechanistic fact about policy modification, as illustrated by the feedback arrows in Exhibit 9.1, is that policies can be modified at multiple points in the policymaking process: in the agenda-setting and legislation development stages that occur in the formulation phase and in the designing, rulemaking, operating, and evaluating activities that occur in the implementation phase. These two important aspects of policy modification are discussed in the following sections, beginning with how participants in each branch of government are involved in policy modification.

Participants in All Three Branches of Government Play Roles in Modification

Participants from each branch of government are involved in policy modification, although their roles differ. Legislators have significant responsibilities to make and decide when to modify laws. They also oversee implementation of enacted laws and can direct changes in the implementation phase. Legislators stimulate modification during policy formulation and implementation. Chief executives (presidents, governors, or mayors, depending on the level of government) and their top appointees monitor implementation and can point out when adjustments and modifications are needed. Courts can also determine when modifications are needed, such as when the results of one policy infringe on or conflict with the desired results of other policies. The roles of each branch are described more fully in the next sections.

Legislative Branch

In the case of Congress, and with parallels in state legislatures, the core activity is making and amending laws. In addition, through committees and subcommittees, legislative bodies have specific oversight responsibilities in the implementation phase. The purpose of oversight in a legislative context is to assess and evaluate the execution and effectiveness of laws administered by the executive branch, which includes determining if there are areas in which new legislation or amendment of existing legislation is needed. The legislative branch is aided in its evaluation and assessment of policy performance by agencies such as the Government Accountability Office, the Congressional Budget Office, and the Congressional Research Service, as was discussed at length in Chapter 8.

While any congressional committee with jurisdiction can hold oversight hearings, the House and Senate appropriations committees (www.appropriations.house.gov and www.appropriations.senate.gov, respectively) have especially important oversight responsibilities in their annual reviews of the budgets of implementing organizations and agencies. Legislators seeking to influence implementation decisions routinely use the budget review mechanism.

The first or clarifying indications that existing legislation needs to be amended or that new legislation may be needed in a particular area often emerge from oversight hearings. For example, Appendix 28 contains the opening statement of the chair of the House of Representatives Subcommittee on Oversight and Investigation of the Committee on Energy and Commerce delivered at the beginning of a hearing titled "Where Have All the Patients Gone? Examining the Psychiatric Bed Shortage." As the statement suggests, a panel with diverse experience in services for individuals who are seriously mentally ill will offer perspective "on the far-reaching implications of the current psychiatric bed shortage" and "some creative approaches to address it."

In addition to the highly formalized aspects of making and modifying policy through legislation and oversight, members of the legislative branch have other ways of modifying policy. For example, responding to the fact that in early 2014 a number of children in California were afflicted with a polio-like disease causing paralysis in their limbs, Senator Boxer of California sent the following letter (www.boxer.senate.gov/press/release/boxer-urges-cdc-to-investigate-rare-polio-like-disease-afflicting-california-children/) to the director of the Centers for Disease Control and Prevention:

February 27, 2014
Thomas Frieden, MD, MPH
Director U.S. Centers for Disease Control and Prevention
1600 Clifton Road
Atlanta, GA 30333
Dear Director Frieden:

I was alarmed to learn that at least 20 children in California over the last 18 months have suffered from a rare polio-like disease that causes paralysis to one or more arms or legs.

I have enclosed articles by the *San Francisco Chronicle* and the *Associated Press* on this topic. We need answers to what is causing this devastating disease in children.

I request that the CDC undertake a geographic analysis of where these cases are occurring in California.

I am also asking the CDC to answer the following questions:

• What is the CDC doing to identify the cause of this disease?
• Could a virus, such as an enterovirus, be a cause of the disease?
• Could environmental factors and exposures be involved?
• Have you instituted national reporting of acute paralytic diseases? If not, why not?

These questions must be answered because it is deeply disturbing to read reports of otherwise healthy children experiencing sudden paralysis.

The CDC has a robust history of investigating and ultimately solving the mysteries of infectious disease. Families in California and across the nation benefit from all of the work that you do. Thank you for your commitment to health, and I ask you to respond in an urgent fashion so that our country can learn what the CDC is doing to find answers to this troubling disease that is affecting California's children.

Sincerely,
Barbara Boxer
United States Senator

This letter falls outside the normal channels of policymaking, but Senator Boxer will be responded to by Dr. Frieden and modification of existing policy by changes in legislation or implementation may follow depending on the facts of the situation. The point is that policy modification may well be triggered by such communication between participants in the legislative and executive branches. Indeed, participants in the legislative branch have several avenues through which to modify existing policy.

Executive Branch

Chief executives (presidents, governors, or mayors) exert oversight and management of the implementation phase of policymaking. They can also be influential in setting the policy agenda, which often includes modification through amendments to existing laws. Their influence provides them with unique opportunities to initiate policy modification. Chief executives are supported in oversight activity by staff in the executive office and the appointees in various departments and agencies who are responsible to the chief executive. As was discussed in Chapter 8, the Agency for Healthcare Research and Quality and the much newer Center for Medicare and Medicaid Innovation (CMI) play important roles is helping guide policy modification. In particular, the federal Office of Management and Budget, which was also described in Chapter 8, plays a powerful role in policy modification through its management of many aspects of policy implementation carried out in the executive branch.

One powerful mechanism for modifying policy available to the executive branch is through the issuance of executive orders. These are directives issued by presidents and governors, which have the force and effect of law. For example, President Obama issued Executive Order #13649 (www.gpo .gov/fdsys/pkg/FR-2013-07-18/pdf/2013-17478.pdf) as a means of directing specific actions in response to scientific advances in the treatment of human immunodeficiency virus (HIV). The order read in part as follows:

EXECUTIVE ORDER

July 15, 2013

ACCELERATING IMPROVEMENTS IN HIV PREVENTION AND CARE IN THE UNITED STATES THROUGH THE HIV CARE CONTINUUM INITIATIVE

By the authority vested in me as President by the Constitution and the laws of the United States of America, and in order to further strengthen the capacity of the Federal Government to effectively respond to the ongoing domestic HIV epidemic, it is hereby ordered as follows:

Section 1. Policy.

Addressing the domestic HIV epidemic is a priority of my Administration. In 2010, the White House released the first comprehensive National HIV/AIDS Strategy (Strategy), setting quantitative goals for reducing new HIV infections, improving health outcomes for people living with HIV, and reducing HIV-related health disparities.

***

Since the publication of the Strategy, data released by the Centers for Disease Control and Prevention show that there are significant gaps along the HIV care continuum—the sequential stages of care from being diagnosed to receiving optimal treatment. Nearly one-fifth of the estimated 1.1 million people living with HIV in the United States are undiagnosed; one-third are not linked to medical care; nearly two-thirds are not engaged in ongoing care; and only one-quarter have the virus effectively controlled, which is necessary to maintain long-term health and reduce risk of transmission to others.

In light of these data, we must further clarify and focus our national efforts to prevent and treat HIV infection. It is the policy of my Administration that agencies implementing the Strategy prioritize addressing the continuum of HIV care, including by accelerating efforts to increase HIV testing, services, and treatment along the continuum. This acceleration will enable us to meet the goals of the Strategy and move closer to an AIDS-free generation.

Section 2. Establishment of the HIV Care Continuum Initiative.

There is established the HIV Care Continuum Initiative (Initiative), to be overseen by the Director of the Office of National AIDS Policy. The Initiative will mobilize and coordinate Federal efforts in response to recent advances regarding how to prevent and treat HIV infection. The Initiative will support further integration of HIV prevention and care efforts; promote expansion of successful HIV testing and service delivery models; encourage innovative approaches to addressing barriers to accessing testing and treatment; and ensure that Federal resources are appropriately focused on implementing evidence-based interventions that improve outcomes along the HIV care continuum.

***

Section 3. Establishment of the HIV Care Continuum Working Group.

There is established the HIV Care Continuum Working Group (Working Group) to support the Initiative. The Working Group shall coordinate Federal efforts to improve outcomes nationally across the HIV care continuum. . . . The Working Group shall:

(i) request and review information from agencies describing efforts to improve testing, care, and treatment outcomes, and determine if there is appropriate emphasis on addressing the HIV care continuum in relation to other work concerning the domestic epidemic;

(ii) review research on improving outcomes along the HIV care continuum;

(iii) obtain input from Federal grantees, affected communities, and other stakeholders to inform strategies to improve outcomes along the HIV care continuum;

(iv) identify potential impediments to improving outcomes along the HIV care continuum, including for populations at greatest risk for HIV infection, based on the efforts undertaken pursuant to paragraphs (i), (ii), and (iii) of this subsection;

(v) identify opportunities to address issues identified pursuant to paragraph (iv) of this subsection, and thereby improve outcomes along the HIV care continuum;

(vi) recommend ways to integrate efforts to improve outcomes along the HIV care continuum with other evidence-based strategies to combat HIV; and

(vii) specify how to better align and coordinate Federal efforts, both within and across agencies, to improve outcomes along the HIV care continuum.

BARACK OBAMA

Judicial Branch

As discussed in Chapter 4, the courts play vital roles in health policymaking. They play specific roles in modifying health policy. The federal courts have responsibilities regarding how laws are interpreted and enforced. State courts are involved in interpreting and enforcing state laws and other policies in their jurisdictions. Teitelbaum and Wilensky (2013, 5) see the courts' focus in the healthcare domain as being on individuals' access to care, the quality of that care, and the financing of the care. In their view, the courts' focus in the public health domain "is on why and how the government regulates private individuals and corporations in the name of protecting the health, safety, and welfare of the general public."

One of the more important ways courts have modified policy is through their involvement in the implementation of the nation's environmental protection and occupational health and safety laws. For example, the Occupational Safety and Health Act (P.L. 91-596) set into motion a massive federal program of standard setting and enforcement that sought to improve safety and health conditions in the nation's workplaces under the Occupational Safety and Health Administration (OSHA) of the US Department of Labor. States are permitted under the law to manage their own occupational safety and health programs if they meet certain requirements. In California, the occupational safety and health program is known as the Cal/OSHA program and is operated under the state's Department of Industrial Relations.

Cal/OSHA

California is typical of the so-called state plan states. As such, California seeks to protect workers from health and safety hazards in almost every workplace in the state. Cal/OSHA operates four interrelated units (California Department of Industrial Relations 2014):

1. The Occupational Safety and Health Standards Board adopts, amends, or repeals occupational safety and health standards.
2. The Division of Occupational Safety and Health (DOSH) enforces the occupational safety and health standards by issuing citations, orders, and notices; by proposing civil penalties; and by specifying the abatement changes that must be made to correct an unsafe condition.
3. The Occupational Safety and Health Appeals Board hears appeals from citations and orders issued by DOSH.
4. The DOSH Consultation Service provides free on-site consultations to employers as well as advice and information regarding occupational safety and health to employers and employee groups.

The Appeals Board has three members, all of whom are administrative law judges. The appeals process is elaborate and designed to be fair, including a provision for reconsideration by the board of an order or decision by an administrative law judge. Beyond this provision, any party to an appeal who disagrees with a decision after reconsideration or the denial of reconsideration can apply to the California Superior Court for a judicial review. As you can see from this information about the operation of Cal/OSHA, judicial decision making plays an important role in the modification of formulation and implementation of workplace health and safety in California. The same can be said of many other states and of the federal OSHA activities.

Although enough adverse judicial decisions growing out of a particular policy can lead to its amendment or even stimulate new legislation, the courts' most direct modifying effect is on policy implementation, especially in ensuring the appropriate application of laws and supporting rules and provisions. The courts' role in policy modification is complicated by the fact that the US court system is highly decentralized, as we discussed at length in Chapter 4. Although court autonomy is an important element in the American system of government, one consequence of this autonomy is the possibility of inconsistent treatment of policy-relevant issues. This limitation aside, however, the judicial branch is a vital and integral structural feature of the policymaking process and is especially significant in the modification phase.

Having seen that policy modification is a ubiquitous and largely incremental process, carried out in all three branches of government, we are now ready to examine a second important fact about the mechanics of policy modifications: how modification occurs at multiple points throughout the policy formulation and implementation phases of policymaking.

Modification Occurs Throughout the Policymaking Process

As illustrated by the feedback arrows in Exhibit 9.1, policies can be modified at multiple points in the policymaking process: in the agenda-setting and legislation development stages that occur in the formulation phase and in the designing, rulemaking, operating, and evaluating activities that occur in the implementation phase.

Although modification can occur at any point in the policymaking process, it is not an evenly distributed activity. Modifications are far more likely to take place in the legislation development activity, where amendments to existing laws are made, and in the rulemaking activity, where modifications needed to smooth out implementation by improving the rules that guide implementation are revised, than in other components of the process. However, modification occurs throughout the process. We begin our discussion of these modifications in the formulation phase.

Modification in the Policy Formulation Phase

Modification of policies in the formulation phase, which means amending existing policies, occurs in agenda setting and legislation development. Recall from Chapter 3 that policy formulation—making the decisions that result in initial or amended public laws—entails two distinct and sequential sets of activities: agenda setting and legislation development. The result of the formulation phase of policymaking is new public laws or the far more likely case of amendments to existing laws.

The ability of legislators to modify existing laws means that when a new law emerges, or when an amendment to an existing law is made, the legislators can view this as an opportunity to change the change that has just been made. When the ACA was enacted, for example, those who opposed it immediately began the battle to repeal, replace, or at least to amend those parts of the law they found especially offensive. Because decisions by legislative bodies are not typically unanimous, these decisions invariably trigger thoughts and actions to modify them by legislators and those who seek to influence them in new rounds of policy formulation.

As we have noted throughout this book, initial public laws that pertain to health and subsequent amendments to them stem from the interactions of (1) a diverse array of health-related problems, (2) possible solutions to those problems, and (3) dynamic political circumstances that relate to both. The creation of an entirely new legislative proposal or the amendment of previously enacted public laws occurs through legislation development. The only significant difference is that previously enacted legislation already has a developmental history and an implementation experience, both of which can influence its amendment.

Modification at Agenda Setting

Policy modification routinely begins at agenda setting, because problems already receiving attention through existing policies become more sharply defined and better understood in light of the ongoing implementation of the related policies. Possible solutions to problems can be assessed and clarified in the same context, especially when operational experience and the results of evaluations and demonstration projects provide concrete evidence of the performance of potential solutions. In addition, interactions among the branches of government and health-related organizations and interest groups involved with and affected by ongoing policies become important components of the political circumstances surrounding their reformulation and the initial formulation of future policies. People learn from their experiences with policies, and those in a position to do so may act on what they learn.

Leaders in health-related organizations and interest groups, by virtue of their keen interest in certain health policies—an interest driven by the fact that they, and their organizations and groups, are directly affected by these policies—may be among the first to observe the need to modify a policy. They can use their experience to help policymakers better define or document problems that led to the original policy. These leaders can gather, catalog, and correlate facts that more accurately depict the actual state of a problem and can then share this information with policymakers.

Similarly, these leaders are well positioned to observe the actual consequences of a policy. Leaders can devise and assess possible new solutions or alterations to existing ones through the operational experience of the organizations and groups they lead. Finally, their experiences with ongoing policies may become a basis for their attempts to change the political circumstances involved in a particular situation. When the confluence of problems, possible solutions, and political circumstances that led to an original policy is altered, a new window of opportunity may open, this time permitting the amendment of previously enacted legislation.

Modification at Legislation Development

Health policies in the form of public laws are routinely amended, some of them repeatedly and over many years. Such amendments reflect, among other occurrences, the emergence of new technologies, change in federal budgetary conditions, and evolution of beneficiary demands. These and other stimuli for change often gain the attention of policymakers through routine activities and reporting mechanisms in implementation. Pressure to modify policy through changes in existing public laws may also come from the leaders of health-related organizations and interest groups—including those that represent individual memberships—who feel the policy consequences. When modifications occur at the point of legislation development, they follow the same procedures as the original legislative proposals or bills as we discussed in depth in Chapter 6.

In some instances, the impetus to modify an existing law arises from changes in another law. For example, policies intended to reduce the federal budget deficit have typically impinged on other policies, which often results in their modification. Implementation of the Deficit Reduction Act of 1984 (P.L. 98-369) required a temporary freeze on physicians' fees paid under the Medicare program, and implementation of the Emergency Deficit Reduction and Balanced Budget Act of 1985 (P.L. 99-177), also known as the Gramm-Rudman-Hollings Act, required budget cuts in defense and certain domestic programs, including a number of health programs. As was noted earlier, enactment of the ACA meant amendments to such existing laws as the Public Health Services Act; Employment Retirement Income Security Act; Internal Revenue Code; Social Security Act; and the Medicare Prescription Drug, Improvement, and Modernization Act.

Modification Through the Cyclical Relationship Between Agenda Setting and Legislation Development

As can be seen in Exhibit 9.1, there is a feedback loop between agenda setting and the development of legislation in the policy formulation phase. This feedback loop is an important relationship in terms of policy modification. When policies are developed, especially those that are enacted and implemented, people who opposed the legislation or preferred a different version from that developed can immediately take the result back into the agenda-setting activity. As we noted earlier, efforts to repeal or modify the ACA started immediately after the policy's enactment and continue today. Recall that between 2011 and early 2015, there were 56 attempts in the Republican-controlled House of Representatives to completely repeal, with or without replacement, or modify specific provisions of the ACA, including health insurance marketplaces, the individual mandate, taxes on medical device companies, and many others.

Given the complexity of public laws and the fact that they never satisfy everyone, it can be expected that one of the places where modification efforts routinely begin is between legislation development and the opportunity to circle back to try to modify the agenda so that the subject can be revisited and perhaps modified through new or amended legislation.

Modification in the Policy Implementation Phase

Modification of policies in the implementation phase can occur in any of the implementing activities of designing, rulemaking, operating, and evaluating. However, most substantive modifications of policies that occur in the implementation phase occur in rulemaking and operating activities. Feedback from the consequences of formulated and implemented policies routinely trigger modification of rules and operations, often in both concurrently. Because modification can occur in any of the activities that comprise the implementation phase of policymaking, however, we will note some of the ways it happens in each activity.

Modification Through Designing

The designing activity involves efforts to establish the agenda of an implementing organization, plan how to address the agenda, and organize to carry out the plans. Modification in designing may be necessitated by an implementing organization being given major new responsibilities, such as the case of the Centers for Medicare & Medicaid Services (CMS) and its implementation responsibilities for the ACA. As we saw in Chapter 8, implementing the ACA requires that CMS coordinate with states to set up health insurance marketplaces, expand Medicaid, and regulate private health insurance plans. It also greatly expanded the organization's role in cost containment and quality improvements in the nation's healthcare system. These modifications in the responsibilities of CMS will stimulate modification in the structure and functioning of the organization.

Modification in designing may also occur when a change is made in a law or in how it is to be implemented, which may include the timing of implementation. For example, a major provision of the ACA is the mandate for employers with more than 50 employees to provide health insurance coverage to their workers. Originally scheduled to take effect in 2014, rules written by the Treasury Department delayed the requirement until 2015. The delay was made in response to concerns expressed by employers about the challenges of meeting the requirement. Similarly, there was another one-year delay in some of the functions of the health insurance marketplaces pertaining to small businesses. Such modifications are examples of how designing implementation can be used by executive branch organizations to modify laws.

Modification Through Rulemaking

As we discussed in Chapter 8, rulemaking is a necessary precursor to the operation and full implementation of new or amended public laws, because enacted legislation is rarely explicit enough to completely guide its implementation. Newly enacted or amended policies are often vague on implementation details, usually intentionally so, and implementing organizations are left to promulgate the rules needed to guide operation of the policies. Public policies are modified most frequently through changes in the rules or regulations used to guide their implementation.

The practice of modifying policies by updating or changing the rules for their implementation pervades policymaking. As we discussed in Chapter 8, rules that are promulgated by executive branch agencies and departments to guide policy implementation possess the force of law. The rules themselves are policies. As implementation occurs, rulemaking becomes a means to modify policies and their implementation over time. In the process, rulemaking creates new policies. Changed rules are modified policies.

In view of the fact that certain policy modifications through rulemaking are recurrent, often annually, it is not surprising that the policymaking process includes features that institutionalize some routine modification activities. A good example of routine modification activities can be found in the context of payments to providers of services or products to Medicare beneficiaries. As we have noted elsewhere, these expenditures are substantial and growing. Total Medicare spending is projected to almost double from $592 billion in 2013 to $1.1 trillion in 2023 (Congressional Budget Office 2013). From the outset of Medicare, payments for services have been an ongoing process of modification and one of the most dynamic areas of policy modification in the entire health policymaking process.

Institutionalizing and Routinizing Aspects of Policy Modification

Congress established the Medicare Payment Advisory Commission (www.medpac.gov) in 1997 to provide advice, especially to Congress, on issues affecting Medicare. Its mandate includes questions of payments to private health plans participating in Medicare and to participants in Medicare's traditional fee-for-service (FFS) program. Medicare payments to providers on behalf of the beneficiaries enrolled in the traditional FFS Medicare program who receive inpatient hospital care are made to more than 3,500 facilities that contract with Medicare to provide acute inpatient care and agree to accept the program's predetermined payment rates as payment in full. Payments for skilled nursing care, home health care, inpatient rehabilitation hospital care, long-term care hospitals, inpatient psychiatric hospitals, and hospice are made under separate prospective payment systems. Much of the rulemaking for payment decisions in all of these services is highly routinized.

Payments made under the acute inpatient prospective payment system (IPPS) account for about 25 percent of Medicare spending. IPPS is an example of a special mechanism to institutionalize the process and to make the ongoing modifications in payment rates to 3,500 facilities that take care of millions of Medicare beneficiaries more routine and predictable. IPPS payment rates are intended to cover the costs that reasonably efficient providers would incur in furnishing high-quality care. The payment rates are determined through a complex, but widely known, formula.

IPPS pays hospitals for discharged Medicare inpatients using two national base payment rates, one covering operating expenses and the other covering capital expenses. These rates are adjusted to take into account the patient's condition and related treatment strategy as well as market conditions in the facility's geographic location. These adjustments to the national base payment rates are made as follows (Medicare Payment Advisory Commission 2014, 1):

> To account for the patient's needs, Medicare assigns discharges to Medicare severity diagnosis related groups (MS–DRGs), which group patients with similar clinical problems that are expected to require similar amounts of hospital resources. Each MS–DRG has a relative weight that reflects the expected relative costliness of inpatient treatment for patients in that group. To account for local market conditions, the payment rates for MS–DRGs in each local market are determined by adjusting the national base payment rates to reflect the relative input-price level in the local market.
>
> In addition to these two factors, the operating and capital payment rates are increased for facilities that operate an approved resident training program or that treat a disproportionate share of low-income patients. Conversely, rates are reduced for certain transfer cases, and outlier payments are added for cases that are extraordinarily costly.

This formulistic approach to determining payment rates is far from perfect. However, it does take some of the mystery out of the rulemaking process as it pertains to determining payment rates and makes the process more predictable from year to year. Illustrative of how ubiquitous policy modification is, however, provisions of the ACA mandate reductions in the Medicare payment rates as a means of reducing Medicare expenditures. In effect, an approach to routinize the annual determination of payment rates through IPPS is modified by another policy, the ACA.

Modification Through Operating

Policy operation, as we also discussed in Chapter 8, involves the actual running of the programs embedded in public laws. The appointees and civil servants who staff the government, particularly those who manage the implementing departments and agencies, are primarily responsible for the operating activities of the policymaking process. The managers responsible for operating a public law have significant opportunities to modify the policy—especially in terms of its effect on and consequences for those affected by the law—through the management of its operation.

Policies implemented by managers who are committed to the objectives of those policies and who have the talent and resources to vigorously implement them are qualitatively different from policies operated by managers who are not as committed or who lack adequate talent and resources. Modification of policies through changes in their operation is a routine occurrence in the ongoing policymaking process.

Stimulus for modification in the operation of policies comes from two principal sources, one internal and the other external. Internally, the managers responsible for operating policies can seek to control the results of operations. To accomplish this, they establish standards or operating objectives. Examples are to serve so many clients, to process so many reports, to distribute benefits to certain categories of beneficiaries, and to assess compliance with certain regulations by so many firms. Operations ensue, results are monitored, and when results do not measure up to the predetermined standards or operating objectives, changes are made in operations, objectives, or both (Longest 2015). Such routine operational modifications are part of the daily work that occurs in organizations that implement health policies.

Pressures for Change in Operating Policies

In addition to the internal pressures to modify policy operation, there are external pressures. These pressures come from individuals and especially health-related organizations and interest groups that experience the consequences of implemented policies. As we have noted, those who feel the consequences of policies may seek to modify them. One avenue open to them is the opportunity to influence the modification of policies through influencing those who manage their operation.

These opportunities for policy modification arise from the (sometimes close) working relationships that can develop between those responsible for implementing public policies and those directly affected by their decisions and activities. Opportunities to build these relationships are enhanced by a prominent feature of the careers of bureaucrats: longevity (Gormley and Balla 2013). Elected policymakers come and go, but the bureaucracy endures. Leaders of health-related organizations and interest groups can and do build long-standing working relationships with some of the people responsible for implementing the public policies that are of strategic importance to them.

The most solid base for these relationships is the exchange of useful information and expertise. The leader of a health-related organization or interest group, speaking from an authoritative position and imparting relevant information based on actual operational experience with the implementation of a policy, can influence the policy's further implementation. If the information supports change, especially if it is buttressed by similar information from others who are experiencing the effect of a particular policy, it may influence reasonable implementers to make needed changes. This type of influence is especially likely if there is a well-established working relationship based on mutual respect for the roles of each party and the challenges they face in fulfilling their responsibilities.

Sometimes those who experience the consequences of policies, usually working through their interest groups, and those responsible for implementing the policies are joined by members of the legislative committees or subcommittees with jurisdiction over the policies to form especially powerful alliances. This triad of mutual interests is prevalent in the defense policy arena. The widely divergent interests of so many organizations and groups have made the formation of such alliances more difficult and rarer in the health policy domain.

An obvious and limiting problem for those who wish to modify health policies through influencing their operation and the rulemaking that precedes it is the sheer enormity of the bureaucracy with which they might need to interact. Consider the number of components of the federal government involved in health policy rulemaking and operation. The number increases when relevant units of state and local government are added. The challenge of keeping track of where working relationships might be useful—to say nothing of actually developing and maintaining the relationships—begins to come into focus. Obviously, selectivity is necessary in determining which of these relationships are most strategically important.

Modification Through the Cyclical Relationship Between Rulemaking and Operating Activities

An important aspect of the implementation phase is the relationship between the rulemaking and operating activities. There is a distinctly cyclical relationship between rulemaking and the operating activities involved in a public law's implementation. Although rulemaking initially precedes operation, the experiences gained in operation feeds back directly into rulemaking (see Exhibit 9.1).

This cyclical relationship means that experience gained with operating policies and changes in the environments in which policies are operated—such as biomedical, cultural, and technological changes—can influence the modification of rules or regulations subsequently used in their operation. Appendix 29 illustrates the situation by showing how the Food and Drug Administration recently proposed a rule to update the nutrition facts label for packaged foods to reflect scientific advances, including the link between diet and chronic diseases such as obesity and heart disease. The proposed label would replace out-of-date serving sizes to better align with how much people actually eat, and it features a design highlighting key parts of the label such as calories and serving sizes. Practically, the cyclical relationship between rulemaking and operating means that rules promulgated to implement policies undergo revision—which is sometimes extensive and continual—and that new rules can be adopted or existing ones changed or dropped as experience and circumstances dictate.

Modification Through Evaluating

The evaluating activity, which brings the other activities in the implementation phase full circle, leads to modifications primarily through its impact on the other activities in the implementation phase—that is, through its impact on designing, rulemaking, and operating activities. Evaluations and other assessments and policy analyses can also help guide modification in the formulation phase of policymaking, although other factors often play stronger roles in shaping these decisions.

Large-scale experimental designs that include random assignments of individuals and control groups are the best analytical means of assessing policy impact. Randomized clinical trials, for example, are the standard in medical and scientific studies. Because of expense and degree of difficulty they are rare in social policy research. This approach has been used to help guide public policy in such areas as criminal justice, education, and welfare to some extent, but it is used less in health policy, although there have been some notable successes. An early example is the health insurance experiment conducted by the RAND Corporation in the 1970s (Newhouse 1974). More recently, the Oregon Health Insurance Experiment is producing useful guidance for policymaking (Finkelstein et al. 2012; Taubman et al. 2014).

The Oregon Health Insurance Experiment is a randomized controlled design to evaluate the impact of Medicaid. It includes information about the effect of expanding public health insurance on healthcare utilization, health outcomes, and the well-being of low-income adults. Because a major feature of the ACA is Medicaid expansion, information from the Oregon study is relevant to potential modifications of the act. For example, the study has shown that having Medicaid coverage actually *increases* hospital emergency department usage (Taubman et al. 2014).

A far more common approach to evaluations in health policy has been the use of demonstration projects. As we discussed in Chapter 8, CMI relies heavily on demonstrations that might lead to better understanding of what works and doesn't work in improving quality and reducing costs. The results of demonstration projects can trigger and guide modification in policies (Moran, Rein, and Goodin 2008). The most efficacious modification of policies is generally based on solid information, including that obtained through formal analysis.

Analyzing policies, especially in terms of demonstrating their results and outcomes, can be approached in a variety of ways. These include before-and-after comparisons, with-and-without comparisons, actual-versus-planned performance comparisons, and cost-oriented analytical approaches (Patton, Sawicki, and Clark 2012).

Analyses based on before-and-after comparisons, as the name suggests, involve comparing conditions or situations before a policy is implemented with conditions or situations after it has had an opportunity to affect individuals, organizations, and groups. This approach is the most widely used approach to policy analysis. A variation on this approach, known as with-and-without comparisons, involves assessing the consequences of the policy for individuals, organizations, or groups and comparing them to situations in which the policy does not exist.

Analyses based on with-and-without comparisons prevail in the health policy domain, because variation in the nation's states provides a natural laboratory in which such comparisons are possible. For example, the states differ in terms of seizing the opportunity the ACA affords them for federal funding to expand their Medicaid programs. As of 2014, 26 states (including DC) were expanding, 6 were still debating the decision, and 19 states were not participating (Kaiser Family Foundation 2014).

States may try policies initially or uniquely, and the results can inform consideration of these policies by other states and at the national level. In 2006, Massachusetts undertook major health reform intended to make comprehensive health insurance coverage available and affordable for its residents (Long 2010). Many of its features found their way into the ACA.

Another useful approach to assessing policy performance, actual-versus-planned performance comparisons, involves comparing policy objectives (e.g., health status improvements, dollars saved, people inoculated, tons of solid waste removed) with actual post-implementation results. The principal limitation of demonstrations, no matter their type, is that they do not support the unassailable assignment of causation to the policies being assessed or evaluated. This limitation is a significant weakness of this approach to evaluation or assessment. Nevertheless, this approach is widely used because it tends to be easily implemented and costs relatively little. The results of demonstrations must be interpreted and used carefully.

A final approach to policy analysis is one based on cost-oriented assessments or evaluations. This approach can be especially important in the search for policies that provide value for public dollars. Cost–benefit analysis (CBA) and cost-effectiveness analysis (CEA) are the two most widely used forms of cost-oriented policy evaluation (Glennerster and Takavarasha 2013). In CBA, the evaluation is based on the relationship between the benefits and costs of a particular policy, where all costs and benefits are expressed in monetary terms. Such analyses can help answer the fundamental question of whether a policy's benefits are worth its costs. In CEA, performance assessment is based on the desire to achieve certain policy objectives in the least costly way. This form of analysis compares alternative policies that might be used to achieve the same or similar objectives.

As we noted at the beginning of this chapter, and as we have seen throughout this book, policymaking is not a perfect process. It is not typically a rational decision-making process. As a result, the decisions made during this process must be routinely reviewed and changed as necessary by policymakers.

Furthermore, health policies have huge consequences for individuals, populations, and health-related organizations and interest groups. This means that these stakeholders, to varying degrees depending on their abilities and resources, seek to analyze and understand this process and to influence it. When policies have positive consequences, such as more services, higher incomes, less pollution, or more support for biomedical research, those enjoying the benefits will likely seek to maintain or increase them through modification of the existing policies that affect these benefits. Similarly, those who are negatively affected by policies will likely seek to remedy the negative effects through modification.

Those with policymaking responsibilities and those affected by their decisions are encouraged by the modifiability of policies and of the process by which they are made. The constant modification of existing policies is an important hallmark of policymaking in the United States. This aspect of policymaking permits the results of the process to be corrected or improved over time—an important attribute, given the complexity of the world in which the policymaking process plays out and the human fallibility of the participants in the process.

Summary

The modification phase of public policymaking brings the process full circle. Policy modification occurs because the performance and impact—and perceptions about performance and impact—of existing policies feeds back into the formulation and implementation phases of the policymaking process and stimulates changes in legislation or its implementation. This process is shown as the feedback arrows from modification to formulation and implementation in Exhibit 9.1.

As depicted in Exhibit 9.1, policy modification occurs in the agenda-setting and legislation development stages of policy formulation and in the designing, rulemaking, operating, and evaluating activities of policy implementation. As we have discussed in this chapter, all three levels of government participate actively in policy modification, although in different ways.

The modification phase is extremely important to the health policymaking process, because it provides continuing opportunities for the performance of policies and experiences with them to stimulate modifications. As we pointed out in Chapter 3 and reemphasized in this chapter, the modification phase of policymaking exists because perfection cannot be achieved in the other phases and because policies are established and exist in a dynamic world.

Review Questions

1. Briefly describe the roles played by each branch of government in policy modification.
2. Discuss the distinction between policy initiation and policy modification.
3. Discuss the concept of incrementalism in public policymaking.
4. Describe modification in agenda setting.
5. Discuss how modification occurs in legislation development.
6. Discuss how modification occurs in the designing, rulemaking, operating, and evaluating activities of policy implementation.
7. Discuss the cyclical relationship between rulemaking and operating and how it affects modification.

References

Anderson, J. E. 2014. *Public Policymaking*, eighth edition. Mason, OH: Cengage Learning.

California Department of Industrial Relations. 2014. "Overview of Appeal Process." Accessed February 27. www.dir.ca.gov/oshab/oshabappealpro.html.

Congressional Budget Office. 2013. "CBO's February 2013 Medicare Baseline." Washington, DC: Congressional Budget Office.

Finkelstein, A., S. Taubman, B. Wright, M. Bernstein, J. Gruber, J. P. Newhouse, H. Allen, K. Baicker, and the Oregon Health Study Group. 2012. *Quarterly Journal of Economics* 127 (3): 1057–105.

Glennerster, R., and K. Takavarasha. 2013. *Running Randomized Evaluations: A Practical Guide*. Princeton, NJ: Princeton University Press.

Gormley, W. T., and S. J. Balla. 2013. *Bureaucracy and Democracy: Accountability and Performance*. Thousand Oaks, CA: Sage.

Gruber, J. 2008. "Incremental Universalism for the United States: The States Move First?" *Journal of Economic Perspectives* 22 (4): 51–68.

Kaiser Family Foundation. 2014. "Status of State Action on the Medicaid Expansion Decision, 2014." Published August 28. http://kff.org/health-reform/state

-indicator/state-activity-around-expanding-medicaid-under-the-affordable
-care-act/.

Lindblom, C. E. 1969. "The Science of 'Muddling Through'." In *Readings in Modern Organizations*, edited by A. Etzioni, 154–65. Englewood Cliffs, NJ: Prentice Hall.

Long, S. 2010. "What Is the Evidence on Health Reform in Massachusetts and How Might the Lessons from Massachusetts Apply to National Health Reform?" Published June. www.urban.org/uploadedpdf/412118-massachusetts-national health-reform.pdf.

Longest, B. B., Jr. 2015. *Health Program Management: From Development Through Evaluation*. San Francisco: Jossey-Bass.

Medicare Payment Advisory Commission. 2014. *Hospital Acute Inpatient Services Payment System*. Published October. www.medpac.gov/documents/payment -basics/hospital-acute-inpatient-services-payment-system-14.pdf.

Moran, M., M. Rein, and R. E. Goodin (eds.). 2008. *The Oxford Handbook of Public Policy*. New York: Oxford University Press.

Newhouse, J. P. 1974. "A Design for a Health Insurance Experiment." *Inquiry* 11 (1): 5–27.

Oberlander, J. 2003. *The Political Life of Medicare*. Chicago: University of Chicago Press.

Patton, C. V., D. S. Sawicki, and J. J. Clark. 2012. *Basic Methods of Policy Analysis and Planning*, third edition. Upper Saddle River, NJ: Pearson Education.

Pear, R. 2015. "House G.O.P. Again Votes to Repeal Health Care Law." *New York Times*, February 4, A16.

Social Security Administration. 2014. "Medicare." In *Annual Statistical Supplement to the Social Security Bulletin, 2013*. SSA Publication No. 13-11700. Published February. www.ssa.gov/policy/docs/statcomps/supplement/2013 /supplement13.pdf.

Starr, P. 2013. *Remedy and Reaction: The Peculiar American Struggle Over Health Care Reform*, revised edition. New Haven, CT: Yale University Press.

Starr, P., and W. A. Zelman. 1993. "Bridge to Compromise: Competition Under a Budget." *Health Affairs* 12 (Suppl.): 7–23.

Taubman, S., H. Allen, B. Wright, K. Baicker, A. Finkelstein, and the Oregon Health Study Group. 2014. "Medicaid Increases Emergency-Department Use: Evidence from Oregon's Health Insurance Experiment." *Science* 343 (17): 263–68.

Teitelbaum, J. B., and S. E. Wilensky. 2013. *Essentials of Health Policy and Law*, second edition. Burlington, MA: Jones and Bartlett Learning.

BUILDING POLICY COMPETENCE FOR HEALTH PROFESSIONALS

Learning Objectives

After reading this chapter, you should be able to

- define *policy competence* and describe how it is useful to health professionals;
- describe four philosophical principles that can guide ethical policymaking;
- discuss the five steps health professionals can use to be influential in policymaking;
- discuss each step separately:
  - observing, including deciding what to observe;
  - assessing, including how to decide what policy information is important;
  - monitoring, including the benefits of careful monitoring;
  - forecasting, including common forecasting techniques;
  - influencing, including the role of social power and focus in general terms;
- describe the relationship between social power (including sources) and influence in policymaking;
- describe the relationship between focus and influence in policymaking;
- discuss the use of a map to guide focus of efforts to be influential;
- identify the health policy interests of health services provider organizations, resource providing organizations, and health-related interest groups; and
- discuss organization design to support policy competence.

Professionals in all domains are concerned about public policies as they affect them and their work. The same is true for health professionals, whether their work is predominantly clinical or managerial. The reason for their concern about policies is the relationship between policies and the central professional goals of health professionals: improved health for the individuals and populations they serve. This relationship is straightforward. As we have discussed, health in humans is determined by a number of variables—the physical environments in which people live and work; their behaviors and genetics; social factors, including economic circumstances, socioeconomic position, income distribution, discrimination based on factors such as race/ethnicity, gender, or sexual orientation, and the availability of social networks or social support; and the type, quality, and timing of health services that people receive—all of which can be affected by public policy. Thus, health professionals need a degree of working knowledge of policy and policymaking to do their core work—improving the health of those they serve—most effectively. The contemporary word for a working knowledge of something is competence, the subject of this chapter.

Policy Competence Defined

In any work setting, *competence* means "a cluster of related abilities, commitments, knowledge, and skills that enable a person or an organization to act effectively in a job or situation" (BusinessDictionary.com 2014). *Policy competence* simply means competence in relation to policy and the policymaking process. *Health policy competence*, by extension, means competence in relation to health policy and the process through which health policy is formulated, implemented, and modified over time. Thus, a degree of health policy competence is beneficial for health professionals because they can use this competence to further their work in improving human health.

There are of course other reasons for health professionals to possess policy competence. It can lead to higher incomes, more or less professional autonomy, higher or lower student loan burdens, and so on. For this chapter, however, we will focus on the fact that policy competence can help health professionals have greater impact on human health. Specifically, policy competence can help health professionals influence policymaking and the decisions reached through this process so that the decisions contribute to improved health.

So, how much policy competence do health professionals need? Obviously, they need enough to do their jobs effectively. As with other areas of professional competence, policy competence comes in degrees. Some people have more; some have less. Health professionals need enough policy competence to perform their jobs well. They do not have to be the most brilliant policy analysts nor the most skilled lobbyists. However, they will be more effective health professionals if they understand the policymaking process to the point that they can exert some influence in the process toward achieving higher levels of human health. This idea acknowledges that a manager, physician, nurse, or other health professional can positively affect health by improving access to and the quality of appropriate health services, preventing further degradation of the physical and social environments in which people live, educating people about healthier lifestyles and choices, conducting or supporting the conduct of research, and participating in a host of other health-enhancing activities.

As we have discussed throughout this book, health policies—the authoritative decisions made in government—affect people, including health professionals and those they serve as individuals and populations. This chapter focuses on how health professionals can exert influence in the policymaking process. Possessing policy competence for a health professional means having enough knowledge of the policy market and the policymaking process to be able to exert some influence toward shaping public policies that improve health in some way.

The single most important contributor to policy competence is to understand the public policymaking process as a decision-making process that occurs in the context of policy markets. As has been said repeatedly in this book, public policies, including health policies, are decisions. Policy competence requires an understanding of the context, participants, and processes of this particular type of decision making. Remembering the discussion of policy markets in Chapter 2 and the fact that these markets are controlled by humans, an appropriate place to begin thinking about how health professionals can effectively participate and be influential in the policy market is to consider the ethical questions involved.

The Ethics of Influencing Policymaking

Because humans control policy markets, and the decisions made in those markets, various mixes of altruism and egoism influence policymaking. The operation and outcomes, and largely the consequences, of the public policymaking process are directly affected by the ethics of those who participate in it.

Ethical considerations shape and guide the development of new policies and the modification of existing policies by contributing to the definition of problems, the development of possible solutions, and the political circumstances that may lead to new or amended policies. The ethical behavior of all participants in the market where policymaking occurs should be guided by four philosophical principles: respect for the autonomy of other people, justice, beneficence, and nonmaleficence. The implications of each principle for ethical policymaking and efforts to influence the process are discussed in the following sections.

Respect for Persons

The ethical principle of respect for persons is based on the concept that individuals have the right to their own beliefs and values and to the decisions and choices that further these beliefs and values. This ethical principle undergirds much of the formal system of government that the nation's founders envisioned. Beauchamp and Childress (2012) point out that no fundamental inconsistency or incompatibility exists between the autonomy of individuals and the authority of government so long as government's authority does not exceed the limits set by those who are governed.

In the context of seeking to influence policymaking, respect for persons pertains to the rights inherent in citizenship. Specifically, it relates to the rights of individuals to independent self-determination regarding how they live their lives and to their rights regarding the integrity of their bodies and minds. Respect for persons in seeking to influence health policymaking reflects issues that pertain to privacy and individual choice, including behavioral or lifestyle choices.

Respect for persons as autonomous beings can sometimes be better understood in contrast to its opposite: paternalism. Paternalism implies that someone else determines what is best for people. Policies guided by a preference for the autonomy of people limit paternalism. A vivid example of such a policy is the 1990 Patient Self-Determination Act (P.L. 101-508). This policy gives individuals the right to make decisions concerning their medical care, including the right to accept or refuse treatment and the right to formulate advance directives regarding their care.

Advance directives allow competent individuals to give instructions about their healthcare, to be implemented at some later date should they then lack the capacity to make medical decisions. In concept, this policy gives people the right to exercise their autonomy in advance of a time when they might no longer be able to exercise that right actively. In the absence of such directives, decisions may fall to the courts. On occasion they have done so, generating national attention. Well-known cases include Karen Ann Quinlan (in 1976, a New Jersey court ruled in favor of the removal of a respirator from the brain-damaged woman); Nancy Cruzan (in 1990, the US Supreme Court ruled that a feeding tube could be withdrawn); and Terri Schiavo (in 2005, a Florida court judge ruled that the feeding tube keeping her alive in a persistent vegetative state could be removed).

The principle of respect for persons includes several other elements that are important in guiding ethical policymaking behavior. One is telling the truth. Respect for people as autonomous beings implies honesty in relationships. Closely related to honesty is confidentiality. Confidences broken in policymaking can impair the process. A third element of respect for persons that is important to the policymaking process is fidelity, which means doing one's duty and keeping one's word. Fidelity is often equated with keeping promises. When policymakers and those trying to influence their decisions tell the truth, honor confidences, and keep promises, they are behaving in a more ethically sound manner.

Justice

Another ethical principle of importance to public policymaking is justice. The degree of adherence to this principle directly affects the policymaking process and policies themselves. Much of this principle's effect on policies and policymaking hinges on defining justice as fairness (Rawls and Kelly 2001). Justice also includes the concept of just deserts, which holds that justice is done when a person receives that which he deserves (Beauchamp and Childress 2012).

The principle of justice provides much of the underpinning for all health policies, whether allocative or regulatory. Gostin (2014, xiii), for example, referring to the global health context, says, "By global health with justice, I mean achieving the highest attainable standard of physical and mental health, fairly distributed." Just allocative policies distribute benefits and burdens according to the provisions of a morally defensible system rather than through arbitrary or capricious decisions. Just regulatory policies affect those to whom the regulations are targeted fairly and equitably. The nation's legal system exists in part to ensure that the principle of justice is respected in the formulation and implementation of public policies and to serve as an appeals mechanism for those who believe that the process has not adequately honored this principle.

The practical implications for health policymaking are felt largely in terms of distributive justice—that is, in terms of fairness in the distribution of health-related benefits and burdens in society. Gostin (2008, 69) argues that

> public health policy conforms to the principle of social justice (it is fair) when, to the extent possible, it provides services to those in need and imposes burdens and costs on those who endanger the public health. Services provided to those without need are wasteful and, given scarce resources, may deny benefits to those with genuine need. Regulation aimed at persons or businesses where there is no danger imposes costs and burdens without a corresponding public benefit. Ideally, services should be allocated on the basis of need and burdens imposed only where necessary to prevent a serious health risk.

The most difficult policy question deriving from application of the ethical principle of justice is, of course, what is fair? The opinions of participants in policy markets and in the health policymaking process vary on the issue of fair distribution of the benefits and burdens involved in the pursuit of health in American society. The three most prominent perspectives on justice provide useful insight into the range of possible views on this matter.

Egalitarian Perspective

The egalitarian perspective of justice holds that everyone should have equal access to the benefits and burdens arising from the pursuit of health and that fairness requires recognition of different levels of need. The influence of the egalitarian view is evident in, for example, policies intended to remove discrimination in the provision of health services and those intended to provide more resources to people who need them most (e.g., Medicare for elderly individuals, Medicaid for low-income people, charging more for Medicare prescription coverage of higher-income people, providing different levels of subsidy for insurance purchased in the Affordable Care Act's [ACA's] health insurance marketplaces).

Libertarian Perspective

The libertarian perspective of fairness requires a maximum of social and economic liberty for individuals. Policies that favor unfettered markets as the means of distributing the benefits and burdens associated with the pursuit of health reflect the libertarian theory of justice. This perspective is not a widely popular one in the United States.

Utilitarian Perspective

The utilitarian view of fairness is best served when public utility is maximized. This view is sometimes expressed as the greatest good for the greatest number. Many health policies, including those pertaining to restricting pollution, ensuring safe workplaces, and controlling the spread of communicable diseases, have been heavily influenced by a utilitarian view.

Beneficence

Beneficence in policymaking means that participants in the process act with charity and kindness; that is, they overtly seek to do good. This principle is widely reflected in policies that provide tangible benefits. Thus, beneficence characterizes such allocative policies as Medicare and Medicaid. It plays an especially prominent role in the ACA, where so much of the policy is intended to mitigate the problem of lack of health insurance coverage in the population. The expansion of Medicaid and the subsidization of health insurance premiums are clear examples of beneficent health policy. But beneficence also includes the complex concept of balancing benefits and burdens.

Participants in the policy market who seek to influence policymaking to produce policies that benefit them or their interests exclusively, while burdening others, violate the principle of beneficence. Those who seek to influence policymakers—as well as policymakers themselves—who are guided by the principle of beneficence make decisions that maximize the net benefits to society as a whole and balance fairly the benefits and burdens of their decisions.

Nonmaleficence

A fourth principle with deep roots in medical ethics but applicability to health policy is nonmaleficence. This principle is exemplified in the dictum *primum non nocere*—first, do no harm. Policymakers who are guided by the principle of nonmaleficence make decisions that minimize harm. The principles of beneficence (do good) and nonmaleficence (do no harm) are clearly reflected in health policies that seek to ensure the quality of health services and products. Similarly, policies such as those the Food and Drug Administration (FDA) uses to ensure the safety of pharmaceuticals and the policies that established and maintain the Agency for Healthcare Research and Quality are also examples of policies that reflect the principles of beneficence and nonmaleficence.

With the understanding that policy competence for health professionals means the ability to influence policymaking toward the goal of improving health for individuals and populations and to exert this influence ethically, we are now ready to consider the specifics of how professionals can be influential in the policy market and policymaking process. These specifics are the focus of the next section.

Policy Competence for Health Professionals: Influencing Policymaking

Possessing policy competence for a health professional requires having enough knowledge of the policy market and the policymaking process to be able to exert some influence toward shaping public policies that improve health in some way. Such competence is acquirable through education and other learning and experiences. For example, the information in this book about policy markets and the policymaking process contributes to policy competence.

Whatever the source of policy competence, however, a systematic approach to being influential in the public policy domain for health professionals is useful. A series of steps that health professionals can take to increase their likelihood of being influential—or having policy competence—is described in the following sections.

These steps are built on several key aspects of policy competence. First, policy competence requires sufficient knowledge of the context and process of policymaking to be able to observe in a systematic, at least somewhat ana-lytical way, much about what goes on in the context and process. Context and process were the focus of Chapters 2 and 3. Armed with information gained by systematic observation, health professionals then need to use the information to guide their efforts to exert influence for the purpose of help-ing shape decisions that contribute to health.

We can think of gaining and using information to guide influenc-ing activities as the practice of influence. The premise here is that being effective at this practice can support health professionals in their work of improving health. The five steps in the actual practice of influencing poli-cymaking are

1. observe the policy market and policymaking process to identify public policy information that is possibly relevant and important to the professional's goals;
2. assess the level of importance of identified public policy information;
3. monitor public policy information identified as important;
4. forecast the future direction of important public policy information; and
5. influence policymaking.

Each of these steps is examined in the following sections.

Observing to Identify Public Policy Information That Is Possibly Important to the Professional

Health professionals are accustomed to observing relevant developments in their professional domains. This practice is simply "keeping up" with their professional domains. It is accomplished through reading the relevant litera-ture, interacting with knowledgeable colleagues, and participating in con-tinuing professional education programs. This first step in developing policy competence is closely akin to typical efforts to stay abreast with developments in a professional's domain of expertise. As with all efforts to keep up in one's professional domain, effectively observing the health policy market and policymaking process provides a number of benefits to attentive professionals who want to develop policy competence. It helps them

- classify and organize complex information about the policy market and the public policymaking process and the forces and pressures that affect the process;

- identify current public policies that do or will affect their goal accomplishment;
- identify the formulation of emerging public policies—including new laws, amendments, and changes in rules—that might eventually affect their goal accomplishment;
- speculate in a systematic way about potential future relevant public policies; and
- link information about public policies to their professional goals and strategies, and thus to their performance.

These potential benefits can be offset by several limitations inherent in any attempt to observe and analyze complex public policy markets and the policymaking process. These limitations in the ability of individuals, no matter how talented they are or how well supported their endeavors may be, include some of the following facts:

- Health professionals cannot foretell the future through observation and analyses of public policy markets and the policymaking process; at best, they can develop informed opinions and guesses about the future.
- Professionals cannot possibly see every aspect of the policy market or the policymaking process, nor can they be aware of every detail of public policies that will affect them.
- Professionals may discern relevant public policy information but be unable to correctly interpret its effect on them or their professional goals and strategies.
- Professionals may discern and interpret the effect of public policy information but find that they are unable to respond appropriately.

Efforts to effectively observe a public policy market and the policymaking process face limitations, but the benefits that may be derived from doing so may justify the efforts. The fact that organizations and interest groups have more resources for this purpose is a good reason for health professionals, when possible, to rely on these entities for help in this observational task. Whether undertaken by individual professionals or by well-resourced organizations and interest groups, the effective observation of policy markets and the policymaking is a good place to begin development of policy competence.

Observation properly begins with careful consideration by health professionals of what they believe to be important public policy information. In guiding the focus of observation, it is useful to remember that public policies are a large set of decisions, shaped by many variables. Some of these decisions are codified in the statutory language of specific public laws. Others are the rules or regulations established to implement public laws or to operate government and its various programs. Still others are decisions made in the judicial branch.

Relevant public policies, however, represent only part of what should be observed. Problems, potential solutions, and political circumstances that might lead to new or modified policies must also be considered important. Thus, effective observation involves identifying relevant policies and emerging problems, possible solutions, and the political circumstances that surround them, which could eventually lead to relevant policies.

Consideration about what policy information is relevant for the health professional is largely judgmental and idiosyncratic. Obviously, the quality of the judgments about what to observe is important. Typically, more than one person should decide what should be observed. The opinions of colleagues can be helpful, as can judgments made by others as to what is relevant in the policy markets and policymaking process. Formal and informal interactions with colleagues with similar policy interests are excellent sources of information about what might be productively observed. The use of social media for this purpose can be helpful.

Newsletter content from professional societies and associations can reflect the collective judgment of other people and may be useful for this reason. General health policy–content newsletters may also be useful. For example, the *Morning Briefing* produced by Kaiser Health News and available at http://kaiserhealthnews.org/latest-morning-briefing/, free to its users, is an excellent source of health policy–related information.

As noted earlier, the starting point in observing is the question of who or what to observe. The appropriate foci include the policymakers in federal, state, and local governments and those who can influence their decisions. Those who can influence policymakers' decisions may do so through helping shape conceptualizations of problems and their potential solutions or through the political circumstances that help drive the policymaking process.

In effect, the focus of observation is on the suppliers of public policies and those who can influence them. As we discussed in Chapter 1, members of each branch of government supply policies in the policy market, although the role of each branch is different. Each should receive attention in this step. Because policies are made in all three branches of government, the list of potential policymakers is lengthy, and adding those who can influence them makes it even longer.

Effectively observing the policy markets and policymaking process identifies specific policies that are of relevance and importance. Effective observation also identifies the emerging problems, possible solutions to them, and the political circumstances that surround them that could eventually lead to important policies. But observing is only the first step in analyzing policy markets and the policymaking process.

Assessing the Level of Importance of Identified Public Policy Information for the Professional

Observation may identify possibly important information in the policy market and policymaking process. Assessment determines which of the many possibilities is worthy of continuing interest. The health professional may observe a large amount of activity and information, but only some of it is important and relevant to that person. Determining the importance of public policy information is subjective to a large extent, and never easy.

One useful device in assessing importance is to characterize information as opportunity or threat. If something is clearly a threat or opportunity, it probably bears continuing interest. Such assessments, however, are far from exact. Sound human judgment may well be the best technique for making these determinations, although the importance of public policy information can be considered on several bases.

Experience with similar issues is frequently a useful basis for assessing the importance of public policy information. Like all competence, policy competence grows with experience. The experience may have been acquired firsthand, or it may come from contact with colleagues who have encountered similar public policy issues and situations and who are willing to share their experiences.

Public policies that affect the pursuit of health vary among the states; this variety can be instructive. For example, much was learned from the Massachusetts experience that was useful in developing the ACA (Long 2010). Valuable lessons are being learned in the Oregon Health Insurance Experiment (Finkelstein et al. 2012; Taubman et al. 2014). Similarly, professionals can draw insight from experiences in other countries. Other bases for assessments include intuition or best guesses about what particular public policy information might mean and advice from well-informed and experienced others. When possible, quantification, modeling, and simulation of the potential effects of the issues being assessed can be useful, but this is often beyond the realistic capability of the individual professional.

Making the appropriate determination is rarely simple, even when all the bases we have suggested are considered. Aside from the difficulties in collecting and properly analyzing enough information to inform the assessment fully, problems sometimes derive from the personal biases of those making the assessment. Such problems can force assessments that fit some preconceived notions about what is important rather than accurately reflecting a particular situation (Lindgren and Bandhold 2009).

Using Underlying Theory and Logic Models to Assess Importance

As we have noted, many policies contain, at least implicitly, an underlying theory, rationale, or logic. They are not written as logic models, but a logic model is inherent in many policies, whether they take the form of public laws, rules or regulations, other implementation decisions, or judicial decisions. Essentially, a policy's underlying theory or logic model is an expression of how resources are meant to be used or processed to achieve the policy's objectives. As such, the theory or logic model can be useful in assessing whether or not a policy being observed is relevant and important to the health professional.

Logic Models in Assessing Policies

Any mechanism that can help better assess policies has utility. Logic models were developed in the context of program evaluation (Knowlton and Phillips 2013) and were subsequently found to be useful in managing programs more effectively. Regarding programs, logic models depict what resources will be used in various processes to yield results. They can be used in the same manner to depict the relationships among the results sought from a policy and the resources and processes necessary to attain those results. In fact, such models could help policymakers more carefully conceptualize policies as they are being formulated. Unfortunately, these models are rarely used in this way.

Although logic models are not widely used in drafting policies and they are not made explicit in the language of policies, they could be useful. Consider the possible benefit when someone is drafting a policy of simply saying in clear language, "These are the results I hope the policy will achieve, and these are the necessary resources that will be processed in the following ways to achieve the results." This logical thinking could certainly improve many policies if used by those drafting the policies. However, the purpose here is not to consider how useful logic models might be in drafting policies, but rather to consider their potential usefulness to health professionals in assessing policies. If the implicit logic model of a policy can be developed, the result likely will help the professional determine the policy's relevance and importance. Usefulness could emerge simply because the results and the resources and processes involved in pursuing them will have been more clearly specified. It is a modest next step to determine if the results or the resources used by a policy are relevant to an interest of the health professional. If either or both are relevant, then the policy is a good candidate for the professional's continuing interest and attention.

One way to visualize the purpose of a public policy is to think of it as a theory. A policy's theory is a plausible model of how the policy is supposed to work. A good policy theory is based on an underlying rationale or logic. For example, one can theorize about a proposed policy as follows: If resources a, b, and c are assembled and then processed by doing m, n, and o with the resources, the results will be x, y, and z. For example, one element of theory inherent in the ACA was that increasing federal resources for states to use in expanding their Medicaid program enrollments by loosening eligibility requirements, modernizing and simplifying enrollment processes, and increasing outreach efforts would result in greater enrollment in the program. This theory has been realized, as the ACA has resulted in "very strong enrollment growth relative to historic trends" (Wachino, Artiga, and Rudowitz 2014, 1).

The relationships among resources, processes, and results form a policy's underlying theory, which can be used to draw a logic model of how the policy is intended to operate. Exhibit 10.1 depicts a basic logic model template for a policy.

The Logic Model Concept

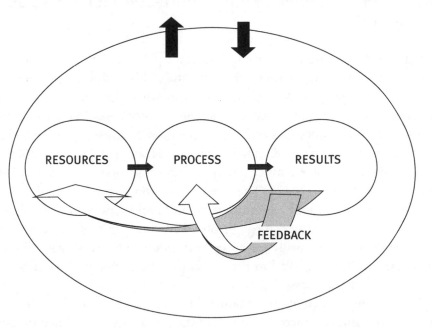

External Environment of the Policy (including the situations and preferences of individuals, organizations, and groups, as well as biological, biomedical, cultural, demographic, ecological, economic, ethical, legal, psychological, science, social, and technological variables)

RESOURCES → PROCESS → RESULTS

FEEDBACK

EXHIBIT 10.1
Logic Model Template for a Policy

This model shows that resources are used in processes to accomplish the policy's results. The model includes feedback in the form of loops from results to resources and processes to indicate that policies can be adjusted as they are implemented. The logic model also shows that a policy exists in an external environment.

The external environment of a policy typically includes many factors that can influence operation and performance. These are illustrated in Exhibit 10.1 by the top arrows that flow between external environment and the logic model. Biological, biomedical, cultural, demographic, ecological, economic, ethical, legal, psychological, science, social, and technological variables that can influence formulation and implementation are shown.

Public policies do not exist in isolation. All policies affect and are affected by their external environments. Resources needed for implementation flow from the external environment. A policy's results flow out into the external environment, where they affect individuals, organizations, and groups as well as other variables such as the economy and science.

When done well, observing and assessing the importance of policy information will yield a set of information drawn from the policy market and the policymaking process that the health professional should then routinely monitor over time.

Monitoring the Public Policy Information Identified as Important

Monitoring is tracking or following important public policy information over time. Health professionals should monitor the public policy information they believe to be important. Monitoring, especially when the information is complex, poorly structured, or ambiguous, permits the professional to assemble more information so that questions and uncertainties can be answered or clarified and their importance can be more fully determined (Heath and Palenchar 2009).

Monitoring takes a much narrower focus than does observing (Ginter, Duncan, and Swayne 2013). The purpose of monitoring is to build a base of knowledge and insight around relevant and important public policy information that was identified through observation or verified through earlier monitoring. Fewer—usually far fewer—pieces of information will be monitored than will be observed in the analysis of the public policy market and the policymaking process.

The importance of public policy information can be difficult to determine. Uncertainty characterizes much of the public policy information being observed, assessed, and monitored. Monitoring information over time will not eliminate uncertainty, but it will likely reduce it significantly as more detailed and sustained information is acquired.

As with the observing and assessing steps, multiple perspectives and expert opinions can help professionals determine what should be monitored and what the information being monitored means. Furthermore, monitoring public policy information will affirm for the professional that the vast majority of contemporary health policies spring from a relatively few earlier policies. Monitoring affirms that public policies have histories. Many of them continually, although incrementally, evolve through modification. As professionals monitor these changes, they tend to become intimately familiar with the policies' evolutionary paths. Such familiarity can serve as a background for the next step: forecasting changes.

Forecasting the Future Direction of Important Public Policy Information

Effective observing, assessing, and monitoring cannot provide all the public policy information that is relevant to health professionals. Being able to use public policy information to prepare for or respond to future changes in policy or to influence the policymaking process typically requires lead time. Observing, assessing importance, and monitoring relevant public policy information involves searching for signals, sometimes distant and faint, that may be the forerunners of important future circumstances. Forecasting or projecting involves extending the information and its impact beyond its current state.

For some public policy information (e.g., the impact on health insurance coverage for individuals and populations of a change in Medicaid eligibility requirements such as those included in the ACA), adequate forecasts can be made by extending past trends or applying a formula. In other situations, forecasting must rely on conjecture and speculation or, at the other extreme, on more formal forecasting methods. However, some degree of uncertainty characterizes the results of all forecasting techniques.

Other challenges with forecasts include the fact that important public policy information never exists in a vacuum and typically involves many issues and circumstances simultaneously. Existing forecasting techniques and models do not fully account for either condition. That aside, there are some useful forecasting techniques that individual professionals might constructively use in projecting where the public policy information they are focused on might be going.

Trend Extrapolation

The most widely used technique for forecasting changes in public policy information is trend extrapolation (Hanke and Wichern 2008). When properly used, this technique is relatively simple and can be remarkably effective. Trend extrapolation is simply tracking particular information and its path or trajectory to predict future changes. Public policies do not emerge *de novo*. Instead, they result from chains of activities that can and typically do span many years. Understanding the history of policies and related policy information makes the results of the policymaking process easier to predict.

Even so, trend extrapolation must be handled carefully. It works best under highly stable conditions; under other conditions it has significant limitations. When used to forecast changes in public policy information, it usually predicts some general trend—such as a directional trend in the number of people served by a program or in a funding stream—rather than quantifies the trend with great specificity.

Significant policy changes and changes in technology, demographics, or other variables can render the extrapolation of a trend meaningless or misleading. However, predictions based on extrapolation can be useful to health professionals as they seek to predict the paths of important policy information. For those who exercise caution in its use and who factor in the effect of major changes such as the introduction of a new or modified policy or a shift in political control of a legislative body, trend extrapolation can be useful in forecasting certain aspects of public policy information.

Scenario Development

Another technique for forecasting public policy information is the development, usually in writing, of future scenarios (Chermack 2011; Selsky, Ramirez, and van der Heijden 2012). In this context, a scenario is simply a plausible story about the future. This technique is especially appropriate for analyzing policy markets and the policymaking process because they contain many uncertainties and imponderables.

The essence of scenario development is to define several alternative scenarios, or states of affairs. These can be used as the basis for developing contingent responses to the public policy information being analyzed; alternatively, the professional can select the most likely from among the scenarios and prepare accordingly.

Scenarios of the future can pertain to a single piece of policy information (e.g., the federal government's policy regarding approval procedures for new medical technology) or to broader-based sets of policy information (e.g., the federal government's policies on regulation of health plans, funding for medical education or research, or a preventive approach to improved health). Scenarios can, and in practice do, vary considerably in scope and depth (Lindgren and Bandhold 2009).

As a general rule, forecasters will find it useful to develop several scenarios. Multiple scenarios permit the breadth of future possibilities to be explored. After the full range of possibilities has been reflected in a set of scenarios, one can be chosen as the most likely. However, the most common mistake in scenario development is envisioning one particular scenario too early in the process and basing a response on it. Health professionals who think they know which scenario will prevail and who prepare only for the one they select may find that the price of guessing incorrectly can be high indeed.

Influencing Policymaking

The previous four steps are analytical, serving the purpose of providing information about the public policy market and policymaking process to guide efforts to influence policymaking. In this fifth step, the health professional actually seeks to exert influence in the policy market and policymaking process for the purpose of helping shape decisions that contribute to health.

Mostly because of the abusive and inappropriate use of social power to exert influence in the policy market, influencing has acquired a negative connotation among some people. However, there is nothing innately wrong with a health professional seeking to influence health policymaking. After all, policy can affect the determinants of health and, ultimately, the health of individuals and populations in many ways. The health professional seeking to influence health policy to improve the health of individuals or populations is behaving appropriately. Because influencing activities can easily be tainted by self-serving purposes, however, adherence to the ethical principles described earlier is especially important.

Effectively exerting influence in the public policy market and policymaking process is not a simple matter. However, a great deal is known about influence and its exertion in policymaking. Being able to exert influence depends on two variables: (1) possession and use of social power and (2) knowing where and when to focus efforts to exert influence. We consider both social power and focus in the following sections.

Social Power and Influence in Policymaking

As we discussed in detail in Chapter 2, social power is the basis of influence in public policy markets and policymaking processes. *Social power* means the degree of influence that an individual, organization, or group possesses. *Influence* means the capacity to have an effect on decisions and actions of others. A health professional, or anyone else wanting to exert influence in policymaking, has three sources of social power: position in society; the ability to provide or withhold rewards; and the possession of information, knowledge, or expertise. Each source can be useful to the health professional.

Positional Social Power

Health professionals may possess social power by virtue of their place or role in the larger society. Health professionals have some degree of positional social power simply because they exist as health professionals and are recognized as legitimate participants in the policy market and policymaking process.

Policymakers entertain the opinions and consider the preferences of health professionals, in part because they recognize them as legitimate participants in the health policy domain. Positional social power is not limited to individuals. Organizations and interest groups, often in the person of their leaders, also possess positional social power. This power is a good reason for individuals to associate themselves with organizations or groups that share their policy preferences as a means of increasing their ability to be influential in policymaking. Examples of organizations and groups with positional social power in health policymaking are Baxter International, Inc., a global healthcare company involved in medical devices, pharmaceuticals, and biotechnology, and America's Health Insurance Plans, a national trade association whose members provide health insurance and supplemental benefits to more than 200 million people.

An important aspect of using positional social power to influence policymaking is the ability of individuals, but especially of organizations and interest groups, to bring legal actions as part of their efforts to exert influence. Positional social power alone may gain a hearing for particular views or preferences. The exertion of influence, however, usually requires social power of other kinds.

Reward-Based Social Power

Some social power is based on the capacity to reward policymakers' compliance or punish their noncompliance with preferred decisions. Such rewards include campaign contributions, votes, and the organization and mobilization of grassroots activities designed to persuade other people on particular issues. Rewards can also be withheld if policymakers' decisions are not popular with those who hold reward-based social power.

Expert Social Power

Another source of influence in policymaking is based on possession of expertise, knowledge, or information that is valued by policymakers. In public policy markets and policymaking processes, useful information and expertise may pertain to the definition or clarification of problems or to the development of solutions. Expertise in the intricacies of the political circumstances that also help shape the public policymaking process is also valuable.

Health professionals, who can marshal the bases of social power, and especially those who can integrate the three, can be influential. The degree of influence, of course, varies. Relative influence is determined by the amount of social power one possesses, reputation for exerting influence ethically and effectively, and the strength of ideological convictions held by those who seek to exert influence. Whatever the bases, however, social power is only one part of the complex equation that determines influence. Social power must be effectively used if it is to translate into influence.

Focus and Influence in Policymaking

In addition to marshaling enough social power to influence policymaking, health professionals must also consider the focus of their efforts to influence policymaking. Typically, focus is guided by the identification of policies that are important or may become so and of problems, potential solutions, and political circumstances that might eventually lead to such policies. Possible foci include relevant policymakers in all three branches and all levels of government and others who have influence with these policymakers.

In addition to influencing policymakers' decisions directly, those who want to influence policymaking can help shape the conceptualizations of problems, the development of potential solutions to the problems, and the political circumstances that help drive the policymaking process. The suppliers of relevant public policies and those who can influence them form the appropriate focus for health professionals seeking to influence public policymaking.

A "Map" Can Sharpen Focus

The graphic of the three phases of the policymaking process shown in Exhibit 3.1 can serve as something of a map to direct influencing efforts to where they can be most useful. Depending on the circumstances, the proper focus may be one or more of the phases of the policymaking process, or the components of the process during the phases. Influence can be exerted in the initiation of policy, or the more likely circumstance of policy modification. Thinking of Exhibit 3.1 as a map of sorts yields many examples of opportunities for focusing efforts to influence policymaking, such as the following:

- Influencing policy formulation
  - At agenda setting
    ○ Defining and documenting problems
    ○ Developing and evaluating possible solutions
    ○ Shaping political circumstances through lobbying and the courts

- At legislation development
  - ○ Participating in drafting legislation
  - ○ Testifying at legislative hearings
- Influencing policy implementation
  - At designing
    - ○ Collaborating with policy implementers to make programs succeed
    - ○ Serving as demonstration sites for testing new approaches
  - At rulemaking
    - ○ Providing formal comments on proposed rules
    - ○ Serving on and providing input to rulemaking advisory bodies
  - At operating
    - ○ Interacting with and giving feedback to policy implementers
    - ○ Documenting the case for modification through operational experience
  - At evaluating
    - ○ Conducting formal evaluations and sharing results
    - ○ Participating in evaluations conducted by others

Opportunities for Health Professionals to Exert Influence in Policymaking

Combining the sources of social power, which permits health professionals to be influential, with the places where influence might be constructively exerted yields a large array of opportunities for health professionals to be influential in policymaking and to further their health-enhancing roles. Exhibit 10.2 shows this pattern of opportunities based on intersections of sources of social power and places to use the power to exert influence. This exhibit shows that opportunities to be influential occur in policy initiation and modification.

As we have stated several times in this book, the vast majority of health policies result from the modification of existing policies in modest, incremental steps. Policy modification occurs when the experiences with existing policies feed back into the agenda-setting and legislation development stages of the formulation phase and into the activities of the implementation phase and stimulate changes in legislation, and in the designing, rulemaking, operating, and evaluating activities of its implementation. Opportunities for health professionals, and others, to influence policies continually arise as experiences with them and preferences for alternatives trigger modification. Those who would influence policies have an opportunity to do so in the initial iteration of any particular policy, but many more additional opportunities arise during the subsequent modification of existing policies.

EXHIBIT 10.2
Matrix of Opportunities to Influence Policymaking (by initiation or modification)

Social Power Bases	Policy Formulation				Policy Implementation			
	Problem Definition	Solution Development	Shaping of Political Circumstances	Legislation Development	Designing	Rulemaking	Operating	Evaluating
Positional	cell (1)	(2)	(3)	(4)	(5)	(6)	(7)	(8)
Capacity to reward	(9)	(10)	(11)	(12)	(13)	(14)	(15)	(16)
Expertise	(17)	(18)	(19)	(20)	(21)	(22)	(23)	(24)

Examples of Health Professionals Influencing Policymaking

As Exhibit 10.2 illustrates, health professionals, whether clinical or managerial, have many opportunities to exert influence in policymaking. Some concrete examples will further illustrate these opportunities and are categorized as those focused on policy formulation and those focused on implementation, including examples of policy initiation and modification.

Influencing Policy Formulation

In the policy formulation phase, where the health policy agenda is shaped by the interaction of problems, possible solutions to the problems, and political circumstances, health professionals with relevant expertise (cells 17 and 18 in Exhibit 10.2) could influence policymaking by helping define the problems that eventually become the focus of public policymaking or by participating in the design of possible solutions to these problems. Clinicians, IT specialists, or managers responsible for reimbursements in hospitals can help define problems and identify possible solutions in their domains of expertise. A senior manager with a national reputation might influence the political circumstances around an issue (cell 3). Professionals with sufficient positional or reward-based power can help shape the political circumstances necessary to convert potential solutions into actual policies (cells 3 and 11), although, as is discussed in a later section, they are more likely to do so when individuals work through interest groups.

In short, influencing the factors that establish the policy agenda itself can have a powerful influence on policies, and there are opportunities for health professionals to do so. Because agenda setting involves the confluence of problems, possible solutions, and political circumstances, health professionals and others can exert influence by making certain that problems become more sharply defined and better understood through the experiences of those affected by the policies. In fact, health professionals and others directly involved in healthcare are often excellent sources of feedback on a policy's performance, including its effects on the people, communities, and populations they serve. Similarly, potential new solutions to problems can be conceived and assessed through experiences with particular policies, especially when demonstrations and evaluations provide concrete evidence of their performance and impact. Health professionals—guided by their experiences and interactions with ongoing policies—become important components of the political circumstances surrounding the modification of these policies.

Once issues achieve a prominent place on the policy agenda, they can but do not always proceed to the next stage of the policy formulation phase, development of legislation. At this stage, specific legislative proposals go through a carefully prescribed set of steps that can, but do not often, lead to policies in the form of new legislation or amendments to previously enacted legislation (see Chapter 6). Although this path is long and arduous, it is replete with opportunities to influence legislation development. Both as individuals and through the organizations and interest groups to which they may belong, health professionals can participate directly in the drafting of legislative proposals and the hearings associated with the development of legislation. For example, at the April 3, 2014, Subcommittee on Health of the Committee on Energy and Commerce of the US House of Representatives hearing on H.R. 3717, the Helping Families in Mental Health Crisis Act of 2013, testimony was provided by an executive of Mental Health America, an executive of the National Alliance on Mental Illness, a psychiatrist, and a patient advocate, among others. Their testimony can be read at http://docs .house.gov/Committee/Calendar/ByEvent.aspx?EventID=102059. Experience with existing policies positions health professionals to identify needed modifications in policies that affect them and their patients and communities (cells 4 and 20). The long evolution of Medicare legislation is a good example of this phenomenon. Over this policy's life, services have been added and deleted; premiums and copayment provisions have been changed; reimbursement mechanisms have been changed; features to ensure quality and medical necessity of services have been added, changed, and deleted; and so on. Feedback from directly affected health professionals (cells 4, 12, and 20) and others played a role in amending the original legislation, although other influences certainly contributed.

Influencing Policy Implementation

Health professionals and others can actively participate in policymaking in the implementation phase of the process. As we discussed in Chapters 7 and 8, enacted legislation is rarely explicit enough to fully guide its implementation. Rather, laws and amendments are often vague on implementation details, leaving to the implementing agencies and organizations the responsibility for designing, rulemaking, operating, and evaluating activities of policy implementation. Implementation is the domain of the appointees and civil servants who staff the government and whose implementation decisions are also policies. There are numerous and significant opportunities for health professionals to influence these decisions, especially using expertise as the basis for exerting influence (cells 21, 22, 23, and 24). In fact, the implementation phase of policymaking literally invites the participation of those with a stake in policy in a number of ways. Some concrete examples of this participation follow.

Many implementing organizations support demonstration projects as a means of discovering ways to improve implementation (cells 22 and 24). For example, the Centers for Medicare & Medicaid Services (CMS) operates an extensive program of demonstrations in which health professionals with

Participating in Demonstration Projects

appropriate expertise can participate. As we discussed more fully in Chapter 8, CMS's Innovation Center has three current priorities:

1. Testing new payment and service delivery models
2. Evaluating results and advancing best practices
3. Engaging a broad range of stakeholders to develop additional models for testing

The Innovation Center is running numerous demonstrations involving many health professionals in seven categories as follows (CMS 2014a):

1. Accountable Care
2. Bundled Payments for Care Improvement
3. Primary Care Transformation
4. Initiatives Focused on the Medicaid and Children's Health Insurance Program Population
5. Initiatives Focused on the Medicare–Medicaid Enrollees
6. Initiatives to Speed the Adoption of Best Practices
7. Initiatives to Accelerate the Development and Testing of New Payment and Service Delivery Models

Health professionals participating in these demonstrations have a direct impact on the shape of future health policy. The CEO of the Greater Baltimore Medical Center HealthCare System, a participant in one of the demonstrations, the Shared Savings Program, said, "We are delighted to be participating in the Shared Savings Program because of its goal to reduce costs while simultaneously increasing the quality of care and services we provide to our patients and community. The Shared Savings Program is a tangible reminder of the historic transformation taking place in our health care system and we are pleased to be a part of it" (CMS 2014c, 1).

Participating in Rulemaking

Another way that health professionals actively participate in policy implementation is through involvement in rulemaking (cell 22). Rulemaking as an important policy implementation activity was discussed extensively in Chapter 8. Rulemaking is an especially promising place for health professionals to seek to exert influence because they are literally invited to participate. With appropriate expertise, health professionals can be effective in helping shape the rules that guide policy implementation. For example, CMS solicited comments on its development of payment methodologies for certain durable medical equipment and enteral nutrition in an advance notice of federal rulemaking published in the *Federal Register* as follows:

This advance notice of proposed rulemaking (ANPRM) solicits public comments on different methodologies we may consider using with regard to applying information from the durable medical equipment, prosthetics, orthotics, and supplies (DMEPOS) competitive bidding programs to adjust Medicare fee schedule payment amounts or other Medicare payment amounts for DMEPOS items and services furnished in areas that are not included in these competitive bidding programs. In addition, we are also requesting comments on a different matter regarding ideas for potentially changing the payment methodologies used under the competitive bidding programs for certain durable medical equipment and enteral nutrition. (CMS 2014b)

A website, www.regulations.gov, has been established to facilitate participation in the rulemaking process. Health professionals and others can use this site to submit comments on proposed rules electronically. The site offers the following advice for submitting effective comments (Regulations.gov 2014):

1. Comment periods close at 11:59 ET on the date comments are due—begin work well before the deadline.
2. Attempt to fully understand each issue; if you have questions or do not understand a part of the regulatory document, you may ask for help from the agency contact listed in the document.
3. Clearly identify the issues within the regulatory action on which you are commenting. If you are commenting on a particular word, phrase or sentence, provide the page number, column, and paragraph citation from the federal register document.
   a. If you chose to comment on the comments of others, identify such comments using their comment ID's before you respond to them.
4. If a rule raises many issues, do not feel obligated to comment on every one—select those issues that concern you the most, affect you the most, and/or you understand the best.
5. Agencies often ask specific questions or raise issues in rulemaking proposals on subjects where they are actively looking for more information. While they will still accept comments on any part of the proposed regulation, please keep these questions and issues in mind while formulating your comment.
6. Although agencies receive and appreciate all comments, constructive comments (either positive or negative) are the most likely to have an influence.
7. If you disagree with a proposed action, suggest an alternative (including not regulating at all) and include an explanation and/or analysis of how the alternative might meet the same objective or be more effective.

8. The comment process is not a vote. The government is attempting to formulate the best policy, so when crafting a comment it is important that you adequately explain the reasoning behind your position.

9. Identify credentials and experience that may distinguish your comments from others. If you are commenting in an area in which you have relevant personal or professional experience say so.

10. Agency reviewers look for sound science and reasoning in the comments they receive. When possible, support your comment with substantive data, facts, and/or expert opinions. You may also provide personal experience in your comment, as may be appropriate. By supporting your arguments well you are more likely to influence the agency decision making.

11. Consider including examples of how the proposed rule would impact you negatively or positively.

12. Comments on the economic effects of rules that include quantitative and qualitative data are especially helpful.

13. Include the pros and cons and trade-offs of your position and explain them. Consider other points of view, and respond to them with facts and sound reasoning.

14. Keep a copy of your comment in a separate file—this practice helps ensure that you will not lose your comment if you have a problem submitting it using the Regulations.gov web form.

Participating with Policy Advisory Bodies and Commissions

Health professionals can also exert influence by serving on or by interacting with health policy advisory bodies and commissions. The Medicare Payment Advisory Commission (MedPAC) is one such body. Operationally, MedPAC meets publicly to discuss policy issues and formulate its recommendations to Congress. In the course of these meetings, commissioners consider the results of staff research, presentations by policy experts, and comments from interested parties, such as staff from congressional committees and CMS, health services researchers, health professionals and other health services providers, and beneficiary advocates. In addition to input obtained at public meetings, MedPAC invites stakeholders to comment on its deliberations on its website (www.medpac.gov/-public-meetings-).

The MedPAC commissioners include healthcare executives, clinicians, and academicians. Their biographies can be read at www.medpac.gov/-about-medpac-/commission-members. Although opportunities for direct service on such commissions are limited to few people, others can influence their thinking. Health professionals can, and sometimes do, influence commission members and thus the advice that commission members ultimately provide about formulating and implementing policy.

Another implementing organization that provides extensive opportunities for health professionals to directly influence policymaking is the FDA (www.fda.gov). The FDA uses 50 advisory committees and panels, which are listed in Exhibit 10.3. Exhibit 10.4 lists the health professionals involved on one of these panels, the Ophthalmic Devices Panel of the Medical Devices Committee. Appendix 30 shows the Summary of the Ophthalmic Devices Panel Meeting held on March 14, 2014, and is representative of the actual work of the FDA's advisory committees and panels. (For a much more in-depth picture of the work of this committee, the 334-page transcript of the March 14, 2014, meeting is available at www.fda.gov/downloads/Advisory Committees/CommitteesMeetingMaterials/MedicalDevices/Medical DevicesAdvisoryCommittee/OphthalmicDevicesPanel/UCM392476.pdf.) Many other federal and state implementing organizations routinely use such advisory groups, representing an important avenue for participation by health professionals in policymaking.

More generally, policies can be influenced through personal interactions with those who have implementation responsibilities. Significant opportunities to exert influence can arise from the sometimes close working relationships that may develop between those responsible for policy implementation and those whom their decisions and activities affect directly, including health professionals.

Participating Through Personal Interactions

Opportunities to build these relationships are supported by the longevity of bureaucrats' careers (Gormley and Balla 2013). Elected policymakers come and go, but the bureaucracy endures. Health professionals can—and many do—build long-standing working relationships with people responsible for implementing the public policies that are important to them and to the health of their patients and communities.

The most solid base for these working relationships is the exchange of useful information and expertise. A health professional, speaking from an authoritative position based on operational experience with the implementation of a policy, for example, can influence the policy's further implementation. If the information provided supports change, especially if it is buttressed by similar information from others who are experiencing the policy's effect, reasonable implementers may be influenced to make needed changes. This is especially likely in the context of a well-established working relationship based on mutual respect for the roles of each party and the challenges each faces.

An obvious—and limiting—problem for those wanting to influence the policymaking process though the designing, rulemaking, operating, and evaluating activities of policy implementation is the enormity of the bureaucracy with which they might need to interact. Consider how many components of the federal government are involved in implementing health-related policies. Add to these components the relevant units of state and local government and the challenge of keeping track of where working relationships

EXHIBIT 10.3
Current FDA
Advisory
Committees
and Panels

Office of the Commissioner
Pediatric Advisory Committee
Risk Communication Advisory Committee
Science Board to FDA

Center for Biologics Evaluation and Research
Allergenic Products Advisory Committee
Blood Products Advisory Committee
Cellular, Tissue and Gene Therapies Advisory Committee
Transmissible Spongiform Encephalopathies Advisory Committee
Vaccines and Related Biological Products Advisory Committee

Center for Drug Evaluation and Research
Anesthetic and Analgesic Drug Products Advisory Committee
Anti-Infective Drugs Advisory Committee
Antiviral Drugs Advisory Committee
Arthritis Advisory Committee
Cardiovascular and Renal Drugs Advisory Committee
Dermatologic and Ophthalmic Drugs Advisory Committee
Drug Safety and Risk Management Advisory Committee
Endocrinologic and Metabolic Drugs Advisory Committee
Gastrointestinal Drugs Advisory Committee
Medical Imaging Drugs Advisory Committee
Nonprescription Drugs Advisory Committee
Oncologic Drugs Advisory Committee
Peripheral and Central Nervous System Drugs Advisory Committee
Advisory Committee for Pharmaceutical Science and Clinical Pharmacology
Pharmacy Compounding Advisory Committee
Psychopharmacologic Drugs Advisory Committee
Pulmonary-Allergy Drugs Advisory Committee
Advisory Committee for Reproductive Health Drugs

(continued)

Center for Devices and Radiological Health
Medical Devices Advisory Committee (Comprised of 18 Panels)
Anesthesiology and Respiratory Therapy Devices Panel
Circulatory System Devices Panel
Clinical Chemistry and Clinical Toxicology Devices Panel
Dental Products Panel
Ear, Nose, and Throat Devices Panel
Gastroenterology-Urology Devices Panel
General and Plastic Surgery Devices Panel
General Hospital and Personal Use Devices Panel
Hematology and Pathology Devices Panel
Immunology Devices Panel
Medical Devices Dispute Resolution Panel
Microbiology Devices Panel
Molecular and Clinical Genetics Panel
Neurological Devices Panel
Obstetrics and Gynecology Devices Panel
Ophthalmic Devices Panel
Orthopaedic and Rehabilitation Devices Panel
Radiological Devices Panel
Device Good Manufacturing Practice Advisory Committee
National Mammography Quality Assurance Advisory Committee
Technical Electronic Product Radiation Safety Standards Committee
Center for Food Safety and Applied Nutrition
Food Advisory Committee
Center for Tobacco Products
Tobacco Products Scientific Advisory Committee
National Center for Toxicological Research (NCTR)
Science Advisory Board to NCTR

EXHIBIT 10.3
Current FDA
Advisory
Committees
and Panels
(continued)

Source: FDA (2014a).

EXHIBIT 10.4
Panel Roster
of the FDA's
Ophthalmic
Devices Panel
of the Medical
Devices
Advisory
Committee
Meeting of
March 14, 2014

Eve J. Higginbotham, S.M., M.D. (Panel Chair)
University of Pennsylvania, Perelman School of Medicine

Winston D. Chamberlain, M.D., Ph.D.
Oregon Health & Science University, Casey Eye Institute

Richard J. Chappell, Ph.D.
University of Wisconsin–Madison, Department of Biostatistics

Anne L. Coleman, M.D., Ph.D.
UCLA, Jules Stein Eye Institute

David B. Glasser, M.D.
Patapsco Eye MDs, LLC

Andrew J.W. Huang, M.D., M.P.H.
Washington University, School of Medicine

Bennie H. Jeng, M.D., M.S.
University of Maryland, School of Medicine

Marian S. Macsai-Kaplan, M.D.
Evanston Northwestern Health Care

Hady Saheb, M.D., M.P.H.
McGill University

Jayne S. Weiss, M.D.
LSU Health Science Center

Ronald J. Zabransky, Ph.D.
Case Western Reserve University, School of Medicine

Jody A. Latimer, RN, BSN, M.P.H. (Consumer Representative)
Woodward Incorporated

Michael E. Pfleger, J.D. (Industry Representative)
Alcon, Inc.

Jennifer Schwartzott (Patient Representative)
Center for Biologics Evaluation and Research Patient Representative

Malvina B. Eydelman, M.D.
Food and Drug Administration, Division of Ophthalmic and Ear, Nose and Throat
Devices

Natasha G. Facey (Designated Federal Officer)
Food and Drug Administration, Center for Devices and Radiological Health

Source: FDA (2014b).

might be useful in influencing policymaking in the implementation phase is great. There is also the challenge of actually developing and maintaining the relationships. Obviously, selectivity is required in determining which of these relationships should be cultivated.

Using Organizational Relationships to Increase Influence in Policymaking

As noted earlier, individual health professionals are rarely as influential in policymaking as organizations and interest groups. This relative lack of influence is primarily a matter of resource availability, including the time required to engage effectively in the policy market and policymaking process. The organizational aspect of policy competence is important. It takes policy competence beyond what individuals may possess and into the realm of organizational policy competence. Many organizations actively participate in the nation's pursuit of health. People who are employed in these organizations, who govern them, or who independently practice their professions within them have an interest in health policies that affect the mission and purpose of these organizations, their day-to-day operations, and, ultimately, their successes and failures. In addition, individuals associated with organizations and groups can gain synergy from these relationships in their own efforts to exert influence in policymaking. We explore how in this section.

The individual professionals and the organizations in which many of them work that have the greatest or most concentrated interest in the policymaking process are most likely to become involved with formal interest groups to more effectively address their policy concerns and interests. Remember from extensive discussion of the topic in Chapters 5 and 6 that interest groups are groups of people or organizations with similar policy goals who band together to pursue those goals. Thus, it is useful to consider the policy competence of health professionals, of organizations that participate in the pursuit of health, and of health-related interest groups to which individual professionals and organizations can belong.

From the perspectives of health professionals, organizations, and interest groups, policy competence means the same thing. Policy competence means being influential in the policymaking process. One of the ways that individual health professionals can increase their competence in influencing policymaking is by joining effective organizations and groups, which typically have greater resources, in the shared pursuit of influence. Greater resources mean that organizations and groups are more likely to be influential in the policymaking process in cells 1–8 of Exhibit 10.2 using the positional power of their leaders and by using reward-based power in cells 9–16 as a source of influence. Many health-related organizations and groups have strong incentives driving their involvement in influencing policymaking.

Health Policy and Health-Related Organizations and Interest Groups

The performance of many organizations and interest groups are affected by health policies. Although the missions, objectives, and internal structures and resources of these organizations and groups help shape and determine how they perform, their performance levels—whether measured in terms of contribution to health outcomes for people, financial strength, reputation, growth, competitive position, scope of services provided, or some other parameter—are also heavily influenced by the opportunities and threats posed by their external environments.

The external environments that health-related organizations and interest groups face have all of the variables surrounding the policymaking process, although the variables are different in some respects. That is, their external environments include the situations and preferences of individuals, organizations, and groups, as well as biological, biomedical, cultural, demographic, ecological, economic, ethical, legal, psychological, science, social, and technological variables.

Differences between the external environments of the policymaking process and health-related organizations and groups arise, for example, because the individuals, organizations, and groups are constituents for policymakers but also customers and perhaps even competitors for other organizations and groups. Also, for the health-related organizations and groups, policies become important variables in their external environments. Policies may determine existence and routinely determine degrees of success and failure achieved. As Exhibit 10.5 illustrates, policies, along with the other variables in the external environment, present a health-related organization or interest group with a set of opportunities and threats to which it can choose to respond.

The organization or interest group can respond to these threats and opportunities with strategies and structures created to carry them out. The ability of the strategies and structures to respond appropriately results in organizational performance. But these opportunities and threats are the direct result of conditions in the external environment, including the public policies that affect the organization or group.

The organizations that populate the health sector defy easy categorization, but they are all affected by and have interests in health policies. For this discussion, we divide the organizations and groups into three categories and describe their policy interests: health services provider organizations, resource producers, and interest groups.

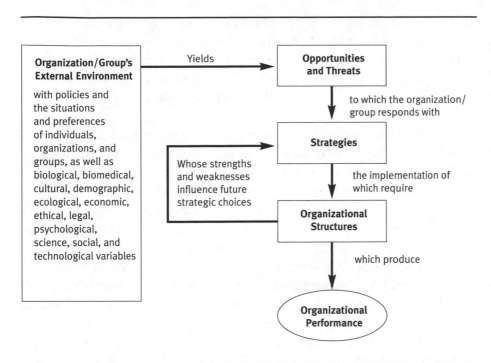

EXHIBIT 10.5
The Relation-
ship Between a
Health-Related
Organization
or Interest
Group's External
Environment
and Its
Performance

Policy Interests of Health Services Provider Organizations

Hospitals, state or county health departments, health maintenance organizations, hospices, and nursing homes are examples of health services providers whose policy interests are identifiable. The policy interests of health services provider organizations vary, but their leaders share certain generic interests. Those in charge of provider organizations tend to focus, for example, on policies that might affect access to their services, the costs of those services, or their revenues from them. These executives and governing board members also are typically concerned about policies that relate to the availability of insurance coverage and the structure of the healthcare system, including antitrust issues involved in mergers and consolidations; policies that relate to meeting the needs of special populations that they may serve; policies pertaining to quality assurance; and a number of ethical and legal issues related to providing access to affordable health services of an appropriate quality to all who need them.

Policy Interests of Resource-Producing Organizations

Related to the organizations that provide health services directly are those that produce resources for providers to use in conducting their work or that facilitate this work in some way. Such organizations include educational institutions that produce the healthcare system's workforce; insurance companies and health plans that organize and facilitate payment for health services (at least those insurers and plans that are not integrated into provider systems); and organizations, such as pharmaceutical, medical device, and biomedical technology companies, whose products are used in providing health services.

The policy interests of resource-producing organizations are also identifiable. Educational organizations and programs involved in producing the health workforce are interested in policies that affect the resources used in their educational missions, such as faculty, buildings, and equipment. Interest is also keen in policies that relate to licensure and practice guidelines and those that may influence the demand for their programs' graduates, including policies that affect coverage under public insurance programs. They are also interested in policies that affect people's ability to pay for education.

Health plans and insurance organizations are vitally interested in policies that affect their operations and decisions. Because these organizations are licensed by the states, they are affected by federal and state policies. Similarly, pharmaceutical and biotechnology firms and medical supply companies have wide-ranging health policy interests, including specific interests in policies that affect their markets, products, and profits.

Policy Interests of Health-Related Interest Groups

Health services provider organizations and resource-producing organizations, as we discussed in the previous sections, are not the only entities with health policy concerns and interests. A wide variety of health-related interest groups exist because of the collective interests of their members in health policymaking and the resulting policies.

As we discussed in Chapter 2, a significant feature of the health policy market and policymaking process is the presence of interest groups that exist to serve the collective interests of their members. These groups analyze the policymaking process to discern policy changes that might affect their members and inform them about such changes. They also seek to influence the process to provide the group's members with some advantage. The interests of their constituent members define the health policy interests of these groups. We examine the policy interests of some of these groups next.

Interest Groups of Health Services Providers   Some interest groups have health services provider organizations or individual professionals as their members. As we discussed in Chapter 5, hospitals can join the American Hospital Association (www.aha.org), long-term care organizations can join the American Health Care Association (www.ahca.org) or the American Association of Homes and Services for the Aging, now known as LeadingAge (www.leadingage.org), and health insurers and health plans can join America's Health Insurance Plans (www.ahip.org).

Other interest groups represent individual health professionals and are of specific relevance to them. Physicians can join the American Medical Association (www.ama-assn.org). In addition, physicians have the opportunity to affiliate with groups based on medical specialty such as the American College of Surgeons (www.facs.org) and the American Academy of Pediatrics (AAP; www.aap.org). Other personal membership groups include the American College of Healthcare Executives (www.ache.org), the American Nurses Association (www.ana.org), and the American Dental Association (www.ada.org).

The organizations that produce resources for the health services providers have their own interest groups. Examples include the following:

Interest Groups of Resource-Producing Organizations

- Association of American Medical Colleges (www.aamc.org)
- Association of University Programs in Health Administration (www.aupha.org)
- Biotechnology Industry Organization (www.bio.org)
- Pharmaceutical Research and Manufacturers of America (www.phrma.org)

Like groups whose members are health services providers, these groups focus particularly on policies that affect their members directly.

Indeed, all health services providers and resource-producing organizations and health-related interest groups are interested in health policy, if only because policy affects their performance levels. Decades ago, Mesch (1984) constructed a list of questions that senior-level managers can use to determine their relative interest in public policies. The questions, in an adapted form, are as follows:

- Do public policies influence your organization or group's capital allocation decisions or its strategic plans for services and markets?
- Have previous strategic plans been scrapped or substantially altered because of changes in public policy?
- Does the interplay of public policies and the other variables in your organization or group's external environment seem to be influencing strategic decisions?
- Are you and other senior-level managers in your organization or group displeased because of surprises resulting from changes in public policies that affected your organization or group's performance?

If the manager of a health-related organization or group, whether a health services provider, a producer of resources, or an interest group, can answer yes to even one of these questions, the manager is likely to be interested in the public policymaking process and in relevant policies. If the answer to most or all of the questions is yes, as is typical for contemporary health-related organizations and groups, they will consider interest in their public policy environment to be imperative and will make strong operational commitments to understanding and effectively responding to the threats and opportunities public policy presents to their organization or group's constituents (Longest and Darr 2014). They will establish units and employ expertise devoted to influencing policymaking as described briefly in the next section.

Organization Design to Support Policy Competence

The resources of organizations and interest groups can enhance the policy competence of their individual members beyond that of individuals acting alone. As part of their organizing or structuring responsibilities, managers in these organizations and groups must establish the patterns of relationships among human and other resources within their domains of responsibility. These patterns are called organization designs (Longest 2015). Intentional patterns of relationships established by managers are formal organization designs. This distinction is important because existing within the bounds of formal organization designs are informal structures—relationships and interactions that lie outside the boundaries of the formal structure—that people working together invariably establish. All organization designs have formal aspects, which are developed by managers, and informal aspects, which reflect the wishes and preferences of other participants.

Management literature is replete with recommendations for creating specialized administrative units to analyze and influence the public policy market and policymaking process (Ginter, Duncan, and Swayne 2013). When a health-related organization or interest group wants to rigorously analyze and be influential in the policy market and policymaking process, its leaders typically establish a specialized department or unit—usually called the public affairs department, government affairs department, or government relations department—to perform the actual work.

Some large organizations and many interest groups divide government relations into separate departments or units in a department, one for the federal government and another for state government. The directors of such departments often report to the CEO, because CEOs have vital interests in public policy and its impact on their organizations or groups. Departments or units devoted to government affairs mainly serve to enhance the policy competence of an entity's senior-level managers, especially its CEO. If these units are well designed and staffed with policy-competent people, they can give an entity and its leaders the enormous advantage of lead time in dealing with policy market and policymaking process. When the leaders of organizations or groups are able to anticipate policy changes months—or better still, years—in advance, their responses can be more effective and more appropriate.

Beyond giving themselves more lead time, those who understand emerging policies or modifications in existing policies can better influence emerging policies to the advantage of their entities. They foresee the emergence of relevant public policies and the consequences on their domains of responsibility. This foresight—derived from policy competence—serves as a basis for efforts to participate in shaping policies that will affect their organizations or groups.

But how is such prescience achieved? The answer lies in the approach to policy analysis. People who look beyond specific policies to the larger public policy market and policymaking process have a great advantage over those who merely wait until a policy is determined and then react to it. Former hockey player Wayne Gretzky is commonly known to have said, "Most players skate to the puck. I skate to where the puck will be. This has made all the difference in my success." People benefit when they focus on the policies that affect their domains, but they gain much greater advantage when they consider why and how these policies emerge. Those who focus broadly on the public policy environment of their domain increase their chances of anticipating policy changes.

This anticipatory focus—thinking about where the puck is going, not simply where it is now—provides an opportunity to influence policies in their emergent states. Leaders of entities who understand public policy environments, with all their complex interplay of actors, actions, inactions, and other variables, are better equipped to anticipate and influence policies than their less policy-competent counterparts. They are prepared to ask more anticipatory, "what if" questions.

Leading an entity based on solid predictions of future policies differs significantly from reacting to announced changes, or even to soon-to-be-announced changes. Proactive preparation and the opportunity to influence the ultimate shape of policies are possible with enough foreknowledge. After policy changes occur, only reaction is possible, typically with inadequate time for thoughtful responses.

An Example of Effective Organization Design for Policy Competence

Entities with policy interests and sufficient resources can build formal structures for effectively influencing policymaking. An example of an effective organization design of this type is the New York University Langone Medical Center. This design, as described on the organization's website (www.nyulangone.org) and adapted with permission, is as follows:

The NYU Langone Medical Center, a world-class, patient-centered, integrated, academic medical center, is one of the nation's premier centers for excellence in clinical care, biomedical research and medical education. Located in the heart of Manhattan, NYU Langone is composed of four hospitals—Tisch Hospital, its flagship acute care facility; Rusk Rehabilitation; the Hospital for Joint Diseases, one of only five hospitals in the nation dedicated to orthopaedics and rheumatology; and Hassenfeld Children's Hospital, a comprehensive pediatric hospital supporting a full array of children's health services across the medical center.

The Center also includes the NYU School of Medicine, which since 1841 has trained thousands of physicians and scientists who have helped to shape the course of medical history. The medical center's tri-fold mission to serve, teach and discover is achieved 365 days a year through the seamless integration of a culture devoted to excellence in patient care, education and research.

Among its administrative offices is the Office of Government Affairs, headed by the Vice President for Government Affairs. This Office is largely responsible for promoting NYU Langone Medical Center's advocacy agenda and in that sense can be seen as the "lobbying arm" of the institution. The Office closely monitors and analyzes important proposed federal, state, and city legislation, rules/regulations and budget proposals as they affect NYU Langone Medical Center. As part of its advocacy efforts, the Office of Government Affairs drafts correspondence to government officials from the Dean/CEO, Vice Deans, faculty members and other NYU staff on issues of importance to the Medical Center.

The Office routinely meets with elected officials and their staff in New York City, Albany and Washington, DC. The Office of Government Affairs also arranges for Medical Center personnel to meet with elected officials and their staff, as well as government agency representatives to promote the Medical Center's advocacy agenda or to pursue specific projects. This often involves coordinating visits to the Medical Center for federal, state, and city officials to meet with Leadership and tour areas of interest.

The Office of Government Affairs secures government funding for various Medical Center programs and projects when city, state or federal funds are available. The Office is also responsible for ensuring compliance with lobbying laws at the city, state and federal levels. There are strict requirements for reporting lobbying efforts made by any employee, and this Office must be made aware of any lobbying interactions so that they may be captured in lobbying reports for NYU Hospitals Center and NYU School of Medicine. There are also strict laws concerning meetings with government officials regarding policy issues or projects. The staff of the Office of Government Affairs is available to assist Center employees or representatives with any interactions with government officials to ensure that we comply with all applicable regulations.

The Office performs a wide array of additional functions to meet the advocacy needs of the NYU Langone Medical Center. Members of the Office attend City, State, and Federal hearings, councils, and agency meetings. In addition, the Office of Government Affairs serves as a liaison to health-trade associations such as the Associated Medical Schools of New York (AMS), the American Hospital Association (AHA), the Hospital Association of New York State (HANYS), Greater New York Hospital Association (GNYHA), and Association of American Medical Colleges (AAMC). The Office maintains working relationships with local Community Boards and takes on specific projects as issues arise. (New York University Langone Medical Center 2014a, 2014b)

Any organization or interest group's approach to organization design is likely to be unique to its situation, as the following additional examples suggest. In each example, responsibility for seeking to influence policymaking rests predominantly with senior-level managers and governing board members. These leaders, especially in large entities, may be assisted by specialized staff organized to fulfill these responsibilities.

Additional Examples of Organization Designs

1. *American Academy of Pediatrics* (www.aap.org). The academy's Department of Federal Affairs is its link to federal policymaking. Pediatricians who wish to make a difference in child and adolescent health through Congress or federal agencies receive the information and tools they need to become effective child advocates. This office prepares them to offer testimony in legislation development or meet with representatives or senators. AAP's policy agenda includes access to healthcare for all children, immunizations, disaster preparedness, and childhood obesity and injury prevention. Its other interests include legislation and regulations involving Medicaid, the education of new physicians, the ethics of medical practice, biomedical research, and clinical laboratory testing.

2. *Wisconsin Medical Society* (www.wismed.org). The society's mission is to "improve the health of the people of Wisconsin by supporting and strengthening physicians' ability to practice high-quality patient care in a changing environment." The society's Government Relations Department is responsible for legislative affairs (lobbying), policy research and development, and WISMedPAC, the society's political action committee. Members of the lobbying team represent the society before the state and federal governments. At the state level, government includes the legislature and a variety of government agencies. The policy staff assists the lobbyists in seeking to affect legislation and rule changes. The society regularly submits testimony to

the state legislature. The department staff collaborates with a variety of patient advocacy organizations to strengthen mutual political agendas. In addition, staff communicates with other medical societies, including the American Medical Association and state and national specialty societies, to learn from related legislative activities in other states.

3. *Council on Governmental Relations* (COGR; www.cogr.edu). The council is an association of 150 leading research-intensive universities that receive a significant share of the federal funds available to higher education through contracts and grants for research and scholarship. COGR concerns itself with the influence of government regulations, policies, and practices on research conducted at colleges and universities. COGR's primary function is to help develop policies and practices that fairly reflect the mutual interest and separate obligations of federal agencies and universities in federal research and training. COGR deals mainly with policies and technical issues involved in the administration of federally sponsored programs at universities. COGR provides advice and information to its membership and makes certain that federal agencies understand academic operations and the burden their proposed regulations might impose on colleges and universities.

4. *Hospital & Healthsystem Association of Pennsylvania* (HAP; www.haponline.org). The association's mission is to "be the leading advocate for improving the health and well-being of Pennsylvanians." The Policy and Regulatory Advocacy staff, which includes a senior vice president and a senior director, is responsible for the association's policy development activities and for state and federal regulatory advocacy. The association's presence in the national and state capitals is intended to "keep hospital priorities at the forefront as policymakers decide key health care issues." The association's current advocacy initiatives are federal funding, healthcare facility licensure, health insurance coverage expansion, hospital oversight and regulation of operations, insurer market conduct, medical liability reform, hospital tax-exempt status, state funding, and policies that support a stable and effective workplace. The association maintains HAPAC and HAPAC-Federal as political action committees.

The Human Element in Influencing Public Policy Environments

The fact that public policymaking is largely controlled by humans complicates efforts at influencing the process, even for those with high levels of policy competence. The diverse preferences, objectives, priorities, levels of understanding of issues, and other variables among the people in the policy market makes accurate analysis or successful influence difficult. The widely divergent positions held by policymakers regarding the ACA, for example, illustrate the nature of this challenge.

The ACA, and before it other policies such as Medicare, have from their inception been the focus of contention among policymakers, including legislators responsible for formulating these policies and for the staff at CMS, who are responsible for implementation. Constant and sometimes intense pressure from organizations and groups with vested interests in policies such as the ACA and Medicare, and many others, fuel the policy battles over their funding and operation.

Taking Medicare as a simpler example than the ACA, we can note that policymakers' perspectives on Medicare are affected by the program's massive size. Medicare expenditures could reach about $1 trillion by 2020 (CMS 2012). As they look to the continued growth in the elderly population, policymakers see a widening gap between program revenues and program expenditures. They know this gap creates a looming government financial crisis. Policymakers, especially those who stand for periodic reelection, detest difficult fiscal choices because of the political consequences such choices impose. They find themselves attempting to balance the preferences of hospitals and other providers for generous reimbursements against the understandable desires of beneficiaries for expanding benefits, all the while keeping a lid on escalating program costs and seeking new revenues. They have options in this balancing act, but none of them are politically palatable. The variety of strongly held opinions among policy suppliers and demanders makes it more difficult to effectively analyze and anticipate the results of the policymaking process regarding this policy, or to influence the outcome.

Summary

In any work setting, competence means "a cluster of related abilities, commitments, knowledge, and skills that enable a person or an organization to act effectively in a job or situation" (BusinessDictionary.com 2014). Policy competence simply means competence in relation to policy and the policymaking process. Health policy competence, by extension, means competence in relation to health policy and the process through which health policy is formulated, implemented, and modified over time. An important reason for health professionals to possess a degree of policy competence is that it can be used by them to further human health.

Because humans control policy markets and the policymaking process, ethical considerations are important. Four philosophical principles that can help guide ethical behavior are presented: respect for the autonomy of other people, justice, beneficence, and nonmaleficence. The implications of each principle for ethical policymaking and efforts to influence the process are discussed in the chapter.

The heart of this chapter is a presentation of a series of steps that health professionals can take to increase their likelihood of being influential—or having policy competence. These steps are built on several key aspects of policy competence. First, policy competence requires sufficient knowledge of the context and process of policymaking to be able to observe in a systematic, at least somewhat analytical way, much about what goes on in the context and process. This context and process was the focus of Chapters 2 and 3. Armed with information gained by systematic observation, health professionals then need to use the information to guide their efforts to exert influence to help shape decisions that contribute to health. We can think of gaining and using information to guide influencing activities as the practice of influence. The premise here is that being effective at this practice can support health professionals in their work of improving health. The five steps in the actual practice of influencing policymaking are to

1. observe the policy market and policymaking process to identify public policy information that is possibly relevant and important to the professional's goals;
2. assess the level of importance of identified public policy information;
3. monitor public policy information identified as important;
4. forecast the future direction of important public policy information; and
5. influence policymaking.

Effective influence in the public policy market and policymaking process depends on two variables: possession and use of social power, and knowing where and when to focus efforts to exert influence. Both social power, including its sources, and focus are considered in this chapter.

A health professional, or anyone else wanting to exert influence in policymaking, has three sources of social power: position in society; the ability to provide or withhold rewards; and the possession of information, knowledge, or expertise. Each source of social power is discussed.

In addition to marshaling enough social power to influence policymaking, health professionals must also consider the focus of their efforts to influence policymaking. The graphic of the three phases of the policymaking process shown in Exhibit 3.1 can serve as a map to direct influencing efforts to where they can be most useful. Exhibit 10.3 offers another way to consider where in the policymaking process to exert influence and suggests some specific ways to do so.

The chapter notes that individual health professionals are rarely as influential in policymaking as organizations and interest groups. This relative lack of influence is primarily a matter of resource availability, including the time required to engage effectively in the policy market and policymaking process. Individuals associated with organizations and groups can gain synergy from these relationships in their own efforts to exert influence in policymaking. The chapter concludes with a discussion of how organizations and groups design themselves to effectively influence policymaking, and specific examples of these designs are provided.

Review Questions

1. Define *policy competence*.
2. Discuss the way policy competence can help health professionals improve health in individuals and populations.
3. Discuss four philosophical principles that can guide ethical policymaking.
4. Discuss the five steps health professionals can use to be influential in policymaking.
5. Effectively observing the health policy market and policymaking process provides a number of benefits to attentive professionals. Describe these benefits.
6. How can health professionals assess the importance of policy information they are observing? Include the role of policy theory and logic models in your response.
7. How can health professionals approach the task of forecasting policy information? Include specific forecasting techniques in your response.
8. Describe the relationship between social power (including sources) and influence in policymaking.
9. Describe the relationship between focus and influence in policymaking. Include the use of a map to guide the focus of efforts to be influential.
10. Discuss the health policy interests of health services provider organizations, resource-producing organizations, and health-related interest groups.

References

Beauchamp, T. L., and J. F. Childress. 2012. *Principles of Biomedical Ethics*, seventh edition. New York: Oxford University Press.

BusinessDictionary.com. 2014. "Competence." Accessed March 4. www.business dictionary.com/definition/competence.html.

Centers for Medicare & Medicaid Services (CMS). 2014a. "Innovation Models." Accessed April 11. www.innovation.cms.gov/initiatives/index.html #views=models.

———. 2014b. "Medicare Program; Methodology for Adjusting Payment Amounts for Certain Medical Equipment, Prosthetics, Orthotics, and Supplies (DME-POS) Using Information From Competitive Bidding Programs." *Federal Register* 79 (38): 10754–60.

———. 2014c. "Medicare's Delivery System Reform Initiatives Achieve Significant Savings and Quality Improvements—Off to a Strong Start." Press release. Published January 30. www.cms.gov/Newsroom/MediaReleaseDatabase /Press-releases/2014-Press-releases-items/2014-01-30.html.

———. 2012. "National Health Expenditure Projections 2012–2022." Accessed April 13, 2014. www.cms.gov/Research-Statistics-Data-and-Systems /Statistics-Trends-and-Reports/NationalHealthExpendData/downloads /proj2012.pdf.

Chermack, T. J. 2011. *Scenario Planning in Organizations*. San Francisco: Berrett-Koehler.

Finkelstein, A., S. Taubman, B. Wright, M. Bernstein, J. Gruber, J. P. Newhouse, H. Allen, K. Baicker, and the Oregon Health Study Group. 2012. *Quarterly Journal of Economics* 127 (3): 1057–105.

Food and Drug Administration (FDA). 2014a. "Advisory Committees." Accessed April 11. www.fda.gov/AdvisoryCommittees/default.htm.

———. 2014b. "Panel Roster: Ophthalmic Devices Panel of the Medical Devices Advisory Committee, March 14, 2014." www.fda.gov/downloads/Advisory Committees/CommitteesMeetingMaterials/MedicalDevices/Medical DevicesAdvisoryCommittee/OphthalmicDevicesPanel/UCM388674.pdf.

Ginter, P. M., W. J. Duncan, and L. E. Swayne. 2013. *Strategic Management of Health Care Organizations*, seventh edition. San Francisco: Jossey-Bass.

Gormley, W. T., and S. J. Balla. 2013. *Bureaucracy and Democracy: Accountability and Performance*, third edition. Thousand Oaks, CA: CQ Press.

Gostin, L. O. 2014. *Global Health Law*. Cambridge, MA: Harvard University Press.

———. 2008. *Public Health Law: Power, Duty, Restraint*, second edition. Berkeley, CA: University of California Press/Milbank Memorial Fund.

Hanke, J. E., and D. Wichern. 2008. *Business Forecasting*, ninth edition. Essex, UK: Pearson Education Limited.

Heath, R. L., and M. J. Palenchar. 2009. *Strategic Issues Management: Organizations and Public Policy Challenges*. Thousand Oaks, CA: Sage.

Knowlton, L. W., and C. C. Phillips. 2013. *The Logic Model Guidebook*, second edition. Thousand Oaks, CA: Sage.

Lindgren, M., and H. Bandhold. 2009. *Scenario Planning: The Link Between Future and Strategy*. Basinstroke, Hampshire, UK: Palgrave Macmillan.

Long, S. 2010. "What Is the Evidence on Health Reform in Massachusetts and How Might the Lessons from Massachusetts Apply to National Health Reform?" Urban Institute. Published June. www.urban.org/uploadedpdf/412118-massachusetts-national-health-reform.pdf.

Longest, B. B., Jr. 2015. *Health Program Management: From Development Through Evaluation*. San Francisco: Jossey-Bass.

Longest, B. B., Jr., and K. Darr. 2014. *Managing Health Services Organizations and Systems*, sixth edition. Baltimore, MD: Health Professions Press.

Mesch, A. H. 1984. "Developing an Effective Environmental Assessment Function." *Managerial Planning* 32 (1): 17–22.

New York University Langone Medical Center. 2014a. "About Us." Accessed March 11. www.med.nyu.edu/about-us.

———. 2014b. "Office of Government Affairs." Accessed December 12. http://govtaffairs.med.nyu.edu.

Rawls, J., and E. Kelly. 2001. *Justice as Fairness: A Restatement*. Cambridge, MA: Harvard University Press.

Regulations.gov. 2014. "Tips for Submitting Effective Comments." Accessed April 11. www.regulations.gov/docs/Tips_For_Submitting_Effective_Comments.pdf.

Selsky, J. W., R. Ramirez, and K. van der Heijden (eds). 2012. *Business Planning for Turbulent Times: New Methods for Applying Scenarios*. New York: Routledge.

Taubman, S., H. Allen, B. Wright, K. Baicker, A. Finkelstein, and the Oregon Health Study Group. 2014. "Medicaid Increases Emergency-Department Use: Evidence from Oregon's Health Insurance Experiment." *Science* 343 (17): 263–68.

Wachino, V., S. Artiga, and R. Rudowitz. 2014. "How Is the ACA Impacting Medicaid Enrollment?" Henry J. Kaiser Family Foundation. Published May. www.kaiserfamilyfoundation.files.wordpress.com/2014/05/8584-how-is-the-aca-impacting-medicaid-enrollment2.pdf.

OVERVIEW OF THE PATIENT PROTECTION AND AFFORDABLE CARE ACT

The 111th Congress passed major health reform legislation, the Patient Protection and Affordable Care Act (ACA; P.L. 111-148), which was substantially amended by the health provisions in the Health Care and Education Reconciliation Act of 2010 (HCERA; P.L. 111-152).

Overview of Health Reform Law

The primary goal of ACA is to increase access to affordable health insurance for the millions of Americans without coverage and make health insurance more affordable for those already covered. In addition, ACA makes numerous changes in the way health care is financed, organized, and delivered. Among its many provisions, ACA restructures the private health insurance market, sets minimum standards for health coverage, creates a mandate for most U.S. residents to obtain health insurance coverage, and provides for the establishment by 2014 of state-based insurance marketplaces (previously called exchanges) for the purchase of private health insurance. Certain individuals and families will be able to receive federal subsidies to reduce the cost of purchasing coverage through the insurance marketplaces. The new law also expands eligibility for Medicaid; amends the Medicare program in ways that are intended to reduce the growth in Medicare spending; imposes an excise tax on insurance plans found to have high premiums; and makes numerous other changes to the tax code, Medicare, Medicaid, the State Children's Health Insurance Program (CHIP), and many other federal programs.

ACA is projected to have a significant impact on federal spending and revenues. The law includes spending to subsidize the purchase of health insurance coverage through the state health insurance marketplaces, as well as increased outlays for the expansion of the Medicaid program. ACA also includes numerous mandatory appropriations to fund temporary programs to increase access and funding for targeted groups, provide funding to states to plan and establish health insurance marketplaces, and support many other research and demonstration programs and activities. The costs of expanding public and private health insurance coverage and other spending are offset by revenues from new taxes and fees, and by savings from payment and health care delivery system reforms designed to reduce spending on Medicare and other federal health care programs.

Coverage Expansions and Market Reforms: Pre-2014

The law creates several temporary programs to increase access and funding for targeted groups. They include (1) temporary high-risk pools for uninsured individuals with preexisting conditions; (2) a reinsurance program to reimburse employers for a portion of the health insurance claims' costs for their 55- to 64-year-old retirees; and (3) small business tax credits for firms with fewer than 25 full-time equivalents (FTEs) and average wages below $50,000 that choose to offer health insurance. Additionally, prior to 2014, states may choose voluntarily to expand their Medicaid programs.

Some private health insurance market reforms have already taken effect, such as extending dependent coverage to children under age 26, and not allowing children under age 19 to be denied insurance and benefits based on preexisting health conditions. Major medical plans can no longer impose any lifetime dollar limits on essential health benefits, and plans may only restrict annual dollar limits on essential benefits to defined amounts (such annual limits will be prohibited altogether beginning in 2014). Plans must cover preventive care with no cost-sharing, and they cannot rescind coverage, except in cases of fraud. They must also establish an appeals process for coverage and claims. Insurers must also limit the ratio of premiums spent on administrative costs compared to medical costs, referred to as medical loss ratios, or MLRs.

Coverage Expansions and Market Reforms: Beginning in 2014

The major expansion and reform provisions in ACA take effect beginning in 2014. States are expected to establish health insurance marketplaces that provide access to private health insurance plans with standardized benefit and cost-sharing packages for eligible individuals and small employers. In 2017, states may allow larger employers to purchase health insurance through the marketplaces, but are not required to do so. The Secretary of Health and Human Services (HHS) will establish marketplaces in states that do not create their own approved marketplace. Premium credits and cost-sharing subsidies will be available to individuals who enroll in marketplace plans, provided their income is generally at or above 100 percent and does not exceed 400 percent of the federal poverty level (FPL) and they meet certain other requirements.

Also beginning in 2014, most individuals will be required to have insurance or pay a penalty (an individual mandate). Certain employers with more than 50 employees who do not offer health insurance may be subject to penalties.

While most of these employers who offer health insurance will meet the law's requirements, some also may be required to pay a penalty if any of their full-time workers enroll in marketplace plans and receive premium tax credits.

ACA's market reforms are further expanded in 2014, with no annual dollar limits allowed on essential health benefits, and no coverage exclusions for preexisting conditions allowed regardless of age. Plans offered within the marketplaces and certain other plans must meet essential benefit standards and cover emergency services, hospital care, physician services, preventive services, prescription drugs, and mental health and substance use treatment, among other services. Premiums for individual and small group coverage may vary by limited amounts, but only based on age, family size, geographic area, and tobacco use. Additionally, plans must sell and renew policies to all individuals and may not discriminate based on health status.

In addition to the expanding private health insurance coverage, ACA, as enacted, requires state Medicaid programs to expand coverage to all eligible non-pregnant, non-elderly legal residents with incomes up to 133 percent of the FPL, or risk losing their federal Medicaid matching funds. The federal government will initially cover all the costs for this group, with the federal matching percentage phased down to 90 percent of the costs by 2020. The law also requires states to maintain the current CHIP structure through FY2019, and provides federal CHIP appropriations through FY2015 (thus providing a two-year extension on CHIP funding).

In *National Federation of Independent Business v. Sebelius*, the Supreme Court found that the Medicaid expansion violated the Constitution by threatening states with the loss of their existing federal Medicaid matching funds if they fail to comply with the expansion (see discussion below under "U.S. Supreme Court Decision").

Health Care Quality and Payment Incentives

ACA incorporates numerous Medicare payment provisions intended to reduce the rate of growth in spending. They include reductions in Medicare Advantage (MA) plan payments and a lowering of the annual payment update for hospitals and certain other providers. ACA established an Independent Payment Advisory Board (IPAB) to make recommendations for achieving specific Medicare spending reductions if costs exceed a target growth rate. IPAB's recommendations will take effect unless Congress overrides them, in which case Congress would be responsible for achieving the same level of savings. Also, ACA provides tools to help reduce fraud, waste, and abuse in both Medicare and Medicaid.

Other provisions establish pilot, demonstration, and grant programs to test integrated models of care, including accountable care organizations (ACOs), medical homes that provide coordinated care for high-need individuals, and bundling payments for acute-care episodes (including hospitalization and follow-up care). ACA creates the Center for Medicare and Medicaid Innovation (CMMI) to pilot payment and service delivery models, primarily for Medicare and Medicaid beneficiaries. The law also establishes new pay-for-reporting and pay-for-performance programs within Medicare that will pay providers based on the reporting of, or performance on, selected quality measures.

Additionally, ACA creates incentives for promoting primary care and prevention; for example, by increasing primary care payment rates under Medicare and Medicaid, covering some preventive services without cost-sharing, and funding community-based prevention and employer wellness programs, among other things. The law increases funding for community health centers and the National Health Service Corps to expand access to primary care services in rural and medically underserved areas and reduce health disparities. Finally, ACA requires the HHS Secretary to develop a national strategy for health care quality to improve care delivery, patient outcomes, and population health.

***

Implementation and Oversight

Implementation of ACA, which began upon the law's enactment in 2010 and will continue to unfold over the next few years, involves all the major health care stakeholders, including the federal and state governments, as well as employers, insurers, and health care providers. The HHS Secretary is tasked with implementation and oversight of many of ACA's key provisions. Other federal agencies, notably the Internal Revenue Service (IRS), also have substantial regulatory and administrative responsibilities under the new law. For many of ACA's most significant reform provisions, the HHS Secretary and other federal officials are required to take certain actions, such as issuing regulations or interim final rules, by a specific date. As already noted, many of the key components of market reform and coverage expansion do not take effect until 2014. Implementing some parts of the law will entail extensive rulemaking and other actions by federal agencies; other changes will be largely self-executing, pursuant to the new statutory requirements. ACA also creates a variety of new commissions and advisory bodies, some with substantial decision-making authority (e.g., IPAB).

Under ACA, states are required to expand Medicaid coverage—though some may now elect not to do so without risk of losing federal matching funds for their existing Medicaid program—and are expected to take the lead in establishing the health insurance marketplaces, even as many of them struggle with budget shortfalls and weak economies. Employers, too, have a key role to play in ACA implementation. The law made changes to the employer-based system under which more than half of all Americans get health insurance coverage. Many small employers will face decisions on whether to use the new incentives to provide coverage to their employees, while larger employers must weigh the benefits and costs of continuing to offer coverage or paying the penalties for not doing so.

The federal subsidies and outlays for expanding insurance coverage represent mandatory spending under the new law. In addition, ACA included numerous mandatory appropriations (and transfers from the Medicare trust funds) that provide billions of dollars over the coming years to support new and existing grant programs and other activities authorized under the law. For example, funding is provided for states to plan and establish health insurance marketplaces (once established, marketplaces must become self-sustaining), and for CMMI to test innovative payment and service delivery models. ACA funded three multi-billion dollar trust funds to support health centers and health workforce programs, comparative effectiveness research, and public health programs. It also established the Health Insurance Reform Implementation Fund (HIRIF) and appropriated $1 billion to the Fund to cover federal regulatory and other administrative costs associated with ACA's implementation. The HIRIF funds, which have largely been used by HHS and the IRS, will all have been obligated by the end of FY2012. Consequently, the President's FY2013 budget requested more than $1 billion in new discretionary funding for HHS and the IRS to pay ACA-related administrative costs. It remains unclear, however, whether congressional appropriators will provide some or all of those funds.

Finally, the law established many new grant programs and provided for each an authorization of appropriations, and reauthorized funding for numerous existing programs whose authorization of appropriations had expired. Obtaining funding for all these discretionary programs requires action by the congressional appropriators.

Rules and Guidance Documents

ACA is being implemented in a variety of ways, including new agency programs, grants, demonstration projects, guidance documents, and regulations. Whereas regulations or rules have the force and effect of law, agency guidance documents do not. The federal rulemaking process is governed by the Administrative Procedure Act (APA), other statutes, and executive orders. Under the APA's informal rulemaking procedures, agencies generally are required to publish notice of a proposed rulemaking, provide opportunity for the submission of comments by the public, and publish a final rule and a general statement of basis and purpose in the *Federal Register* at least 30 days before the effective date of the rule. Agencies' compliance with the APA is subject to judicial review. The APA's rulemaking requirements do not apply to guidance documents. More than 40 provisions in ACA require or permit agencies to issue rules, with some allowing the agencies to "prescribe such regulations as may be necessary."

Congressional Oversight

Congress has a range of options as it oversees the implementation of ACA, including oversight hearings, confirmation hearings for agency officials, letters to and meetings with agency officials and the Office of Information and Regulatory Affairs regarding particular rules, comments on proposed rules, and new legislation regarding specific rules. Congress, committees, and individual Members can also request that the Government Accountability Office or federal offices of inspectors general (OIGs) evaluate agencies' actions to implement, or agency decisions not to implement, certain provisions of ACA. Congress can also include provisions in the text of agencies' appropriations bills directing or preventing the development or enforcement of particular regulations, or use the Congressional Review Act to disapprove an agency rule implementing ACA.

Legal Challenges

Following enactment of ACA, state attorneys general and others brought a number of lawsuits challenging provisions of the act on constitutional grounds. While some of these cases were dismissed for procedural reasons, others moved forward, eventually reaching the U.S. Supreme Court. During the last week of March 2012, the Court heard arguments in *HHS v. Florida*, a case in which attorneys general and governors in 26 states as well as others brought an action against the Administration, seeking to invalidate the individual mandate and other provisions of ACA.

U.S. Supreme Court Decision

On June 28, 2012, the United States Supreme Court issued its decision in *National Federation of Independent Business v. Sebelius*, finding that the individual mandate in ACA is a constitutional exercise of Congress's authority to levy taxes. However, the Court held that it was not a valid exercise of Congress's power under the Commerce Clause or the Necessary and Proper Clause.

With regard to the Medicaid expansion provision, the Court, in an opinion written by Chief Justice Roberts, accepted an argument that the scope of the changes imposed by the Medicaid expansion transformed the ACA requirements into a "new" Medicaid benefit program. As this "new" program was to be enforced by the threat of withholding of existing federal Medicaid matching funds, the Court found that the states were being "coerced" in violation of the Tenth Amendment into administering this new program. Chief Justice Roberts' opinion, however, went on to note that the Medicaid requirement in question was subject to other statutory language providing for severance of unconstitutional provisions. Since it was only the withholding of existing federal Medicaid matching funds that was unconstitutional, the Chief Justice held that severance under the statute could be limited to termination of those funds. Thus the federal government would still be allowed, under the statute and the Tenth Amendment, to provide federal matching funds associated with the expansion. In other words, states can now decline to participate in the Medicaid expansion without financial penalty, but, if they wish to participate, must comply with the new requirements in order to receive the expansion-related funds.

It is unclear how many states may now decide not to participate in the Medicaid expansion. In so doing, they would forgo a substantial amount of federal funding. As already noted, the federal government will provide 100 percent of the costs of the expansion for the first three years, phasing down to 90 percent in the years thereafter. Moreover, if a state were to decide not to implement the Medicaid expansion, low-income adults below the poverty line (i.e., 100 percent FPL) who were not covered by, or eligible for, the state's existing Medicaid program would in general be ineligible for the marketplace subsidies.

Source: Reprinted, with slight adaptation, from Redhead, C. S., H. Chaikind, B. Fernandez, and J. Staman. 2012. *ACA: A Brief Overview of the Law, Implementation, and Legal Challenges.* Washington, DC: Congressional Research Service, R41664.

The ACA can be read in Public Law form at www.congress.gov/111/plaws/publ148/PLAW-111publ148.pdf.

For additional information on the ACA, see:

Emanuel, E. J. 2014. *Reinventing American Health Care.* New York: PublicAffairs.

Kaiser Family Foundation. 2014. "Health Reform." Accessed March 13, 2014. www.kff.org/health-reform.

OVERVIEW OF MEDICARE

Title XVIII of the Social Security Act, designated "Health Insurance for the Aged and Disabled," is commonly known as Medicare. As part of the Social Security Amendments of 1965, the Medicare legislation established a health insurance program for aged persons to complement the retirement, survivors, and disability insurance benefits under Title II of the Social Security Act.

When first implemented in 1966, Medicare covered most persons aged 65 or older. In 1973, the following groups also became eligible for Medicare benefits: persons entitled to Social Security or Railroad Retirement disability cash benefits for at least 24 months, most persons with end-stage renal disease (ESRD), and certain otherwise noncovered aged persons who elect to pay a premium for Medicare coverage. Beginning in July 2001, persons with Amyotrophic Lateral Sclerosis (Lou Gehrig's Disease) are allowed to waive the 24-month waiting period. Beginning March 30, 2010, individuals in the vicinity of Libby, Montana who are diagnosed with an asbestos-related condition are Medicare-eligible. Medicare eligibility could also apply to individuals in other areas who are diagnosed with a medical condition caused by exposure to a public health hazard for which a future public health emergency declaration is made under the Comprehensive Environmental Response, Compensation, and Liability Act of 1980 (Public Law 96-510). This very broad description of Medicare eligibility is expanded in the next section.

Medicare originally consisted of two parts: Hospital Insurance (HI), also known as Part A, and Supplementary Medical Insurance (SMI), which in the past was also known simply as Part B. Part A helps pay for inpatient hospital, home health agency, skilled nursing facility, and hospice care. Part A is provided free of premiums to most eligible people; certain otherwise ineligible people may voluntarily pay a monthly premium for coverage. Part B helps pay for physician, outpatient hospital, home health agency, and other services. To be covered by Part B, all eligible people must pay a monthly premium (or have the premium paid on their behalf).

A third part of Medicare, sometimes known as Part C, is the Medicare Advantage program, which was established as the Medicare+Choice program by the Balanced Budget Act of 1997 (Public Law 105-33) and subsequently renamed and modified by the Medicare Prescription Drug, Improvement, and Modernization Act (MMA) of 2003 (Public Law 108-173). The Medicare Advantage program expands beneficiaries' options for participation in private-sector health care plans.

The MMA also established a fourth part of Medicare, known as Part D, to help pay for prescription drugs not otherwise covered by Part A or Part B. Part D initially provided access to prescription drug discount cards, on a voluntary basis and at limited cost to all enrollees (except those entitled to Medicaid drug coverage) and, for low-income beneficiaries, transitional limited financial assistance for purchasing prescription drugs and a subsidized enrollment fee for the discount cards. This temporary plan began in mid-2004 and phased out during 2006. In 2006 and later, Part D provides subsidized access to prescription drug insurance coverage on a voluntary basis for all beneficiaries upon payment of a premium, with premium and cost-sharing subsidies for low-income enrollees.

Part D activities are handled within the SMI trust fund but in an account separate from Part B. It should thus be noted that the traditional treatment of "SMI" and "Part B" as synonymous is no longer accurate, since SMI now consists of Parts B and D. The purpose of the two separate accounts within the SMI trust fund is to ensure that funds from one part are not used to finance the other.

When Medicare began on July 1, 1966, approximately 19 million people enrolled. In 2013, over 52 million are enrolled in one or both of Parts A and B of the Medicare program, and almost 15 million of them have chosen to participate in a Medicare Advantage plan.

Entitlement and Coverage

Part A is generally provided automatically and free of premiums to persons aged 65 or older who are eligible for Social Security or Railroad Retirement benefits, whether they have claimed these monthly cash benefits or not. Also, workers and their spouses with a sufficient period of Medicare-only coverage in federal, state, or local government employment are eligible beginning at age 65. Similarly, individuals who have been entitled to Social Security or Railroad Retirement disability benefits for at least 24 months, and government employees with Medicare-only coverage who have been disabled for more than 29 months, are entitled to Part A benefits. (As noted previously, the waiting period is waived for persons with Lou Gehrig's Disease, and certain persons in the Libby, Montana vicinity who are diagnosed with asbestos-related conditions are Medicare-eligible. It should also be noted that, over the years, there have been certain liberalizations made to both the waiting period requirement and the limit on earnings allowed for entitlement to Medicare coverage based on disability.) Part A coverage is also provided to insured workers with ESRD (and to insured workers' spouses and children with ESRD), as well as to some otherwise ineligible aged and disabled beneficiaries who voluntarily pay a monthly premium for their coverage. In 2012, Part A provided protection against the costs of hospital and specific other medical care to more than 50 million people (almost 42 million aged and almost 9 million disabled enrollees). Part A benefit payments totaled $262.9 billion in 2012.

The following health care services are covered under Part A:

- Inpatient hospital care. Coverage includes costs of a semiprivate room, meals, regular nursing services, operating and recovery rooms, intensive care, inpatient prescription drugs, laboratory tests, X-rays, psychiatric hospitals, inpatient rehabilitation, and long-term care hospitalization when medically necessary, as well as all other medically necessary services and supplies provided in the hospital. An initial deductible payment is required of beneficiaries who are admitted to a hospital, plus copayments for all hospital days following day 60 within a benefit period (described later).

- Skilled nursing facility (SNF) care. Coverage is provided by Part A only if the care follows within 30 days (generally) a hospitalization of 3 days or more and is certified as medically necessary. Covered services are similar to those for inpatient hospital care, and include rehabilitation services and appliances. The number of SNF days provided under Medicare is limited to 100 days per benefit period (described later), with a copayment required for days 21 through 100. Part A does not cover nursing facility care if the patient does not require skilled nursing or skilled rehabilitation services.

- Home health agency (HHA) care (covered by Parts A and B). The Balanced Budget Act transferred from Part A to Part B those home health services furnished on or after January 1, 1998, that are unassociated with a hospital or SNF stay. Part A will continue to cover the first 100 visits following a 3-day hospital stay or a SNF stay; Part B covers any visits thereafter. Home health care under Parts A and B has no copayment and no deductible.

- HHA care, including care provided by a home health aide, may be furnished part time by an HHA in the residence of a homebound beneficiary, if intermittent or part-time skilled nursing and/or certain other therapy or rehabilitation care is necessary. Certain medical supplies and durable medical equipment may also be provided, although beneficiaries must pay a 20 percent coinsurance for durable medical equipment, as required under Part B of Medicare. There must be a plan of treatment and periodic review by a physician. Full-time nursing care, food, blood, and drugs are not provided as HHA services.

- Hospice care. Coverage is provided for services to terminally ill persons with life expectancies of 6 months or less who elect to forgo the standard Medicare benefits for treatment of their illness and to receive only hospice care for it. Such care includes pain relief, supportive medical and social services, physical therapy, nursing services, and symptom management. However, if a hospice patient requires treatment for a condition that is not related to the terminal illness, Medicare will pay for all covered services necessary for that condition. The Medicare beneficiary pays no deductible for the hospice program but does pay small coinsurance amounts for drugs and inpatient respite care.

An important Part A component is the benefit period, which starts when the beneficiary first enters a hospital and ends when there has been a break of at least 60 consecutive days since inpatient hospital or skilled nursing care was provided. There is no limit to the number of benefit periods covered by Part A during a beneficiary's lifetime; however, inpatient hospital care is normally limited to 90 days during a benefit period, and copayment requirements (detailed later) apply for days 61 through 90. If a beneficiary exhausts the 90 days of inpatient hospital care available in a benefit period, the beneficiary can elect to use days of Medicare coverage from a nonrenewable "lifetime reserve" of up to 60 (total) additional days of inpatient hospital care. Copayments are also required for such additional days.

All citizens (and certain legal aliens) aged 65 or older, and all disabled persons entitled to coverage under Part A, are eligible to enroll in Part B on a voluntary basis by payment of a monthly premium. Almost all persons entitled to Part A choose to enroll in Part B. In 2012, Part B provided protection against the costs of physician and other medical services to more than 46 million people (almost 39 million aged and almost 8 million disabled enrollees). Part B benefits totaled $236.5 billion in 2012.

Part B covers certain medical services and supplies, including the following:

- Physicians' and surgeons' services, including some covered services furnished by chiropractors, podiatrists, dentists, and optometrists;
- Services provided by Medicare-approved practitioners who are not physicians, including certified registered nurse anesthetists, clinical psychologists, clinical social workers (other than in a hospital or SNF), physician assistants, and nurse practitioners and clinical nurse specialists in collaboration with a physician;
- Services in an emergency room, outpatient clinic, or ambulatory surgical center, including same-day surgery;

- Home health care not covered under Part A;
- Laboratory tests, X-rays, and other diagnostic radiology services;
- Certain preventive care services and screening tests;
- Most physical and occupational therapy and speech pathology services;
- Comprehensive outpatient rehabilitation facility services, and mental health care in a partial hospitalization psychiatric program, if a physician certifies that inpatient treatment would be required without it;
- Radiation therapy; renal (kidney) dialysis and transplants; heart, lung, heart-lung, liver, pancreas, and bone marrow transplants; and, as of April 2001, intestinal transplants;
- Approved durable medical equipment for home use, such as oxygen equipment and wheelchairs, prosthetic devices, and surgical dressings, splints, casts, and braces;
- Drugs and biologicals that are not usually self-administered, such as hepatitis B vaccines and immunosuppressive drugs (certain self-administered anticancer drugs are covered);
- Certain services specific to people with diabetes; and
- Ambulance services, when other methods of transportation are contraindicated.

To be covered, all services must be either medically necessary or one of several prescribed preventive benefits. Part B services are generally subject to a deductible and coinsurance (see next section). Certain medical services and related care are subject to special payment rules, including deductibles (for blood), maximum approved amounts (for Medicare-approved physical, speech, or occupational therapy services performed in settings other than hospitals), and higher cost-sharing requirements (such as those for certain outpatient hospital services). The preceding description of Part B-covered services should be used only as a general guide, due to the wide range of services covered under Part B and the quite specific rules and regulations that apply.

Medicare Parts A and B, as described above, constitute the original fee-for-service Medicare program. Medicare Part C, also known as Medicare Advantage, is an alternative to traditional Medicare. Although all Medicare beneficiaries can receive their benefits through the traditional fee-for-service program, most beneficiaries enrolled in both Part A and Part B can choose to participate in a Medicare Advantage plan instead. Medicare Advantage plans are offered by private companies and organizations and are required to provide at least those services covered by Parts A and B, except hospice services. These plans may (and in certain situations must) provide extra benefits (such as vision or hearing) or reduce cost sharing or premiums. The primary Medicare Advantage plans are:

- Local coordinated care plans (LCCPs), including health maintenance organizations (HMOs), provider-sponsored organizations, local preferred provider organizations (PPOs), and other certified coordinated care plans and entities that meet the standards set forth in the law. Generally, each plan has a network of participating providers. Enrollees may be required to use these providers or, alternatively, may be allowed to go outside the network but pay higher cost-sharing fees for doing so.
- Regional PPO plans, which began in 2006 and offer coverage to one of 26 defined regions. Like local PPOs, regional PPOs have networks of participating providers, and enrollees must use these providers or pay higher cost-sharing fees. However, regional PPOs are required to provide beneficiary financial protection in the form of limits on out-of-pocket cost sharing, and there are specific provisions to encourage regional PPO plans to participate in Medicare.
- Private fee-for-service (PFFS) plans, which were not required to have networks of participating providers through 2010. Beginning in 2011, this is still the case for PFFS plans in areas (usually counties) with fewer than two network-based LCCPs and/or regional PPOs, and members may go to any Medicare provider willing to accept the plan's payment. However, for PFFS plans in network areas with two or more network-based LCCPs and/or regional PPOs, provider networks are mandatory, and members may be required to use these participating providers.
- Special Needs Plans, which are restricted to beneficiaries who are dually eligible for Medicare and Medicaid, live in long-term care institutions, or have certain severe and disabling conditions.

For individuals entitled to Part A or enrolled in Part B (except those entitled to Medicaid drug coverage), the new Part D initially provided access to prescription drug discount cards, at a cost of no more than $30 annually, on a voluntary basis. For low-income beneficiaries, Part D initially provided transitional financial assistance of up to $600 per year for purchasing prescription drugs, plus a subsidized enrollment fee for the discount cards. This temporary plan began in mid-2004 and phased out in 2006.

Beginning in 2006, Part D provides subsidized access to prescription drug insurance coverage on a voluntary basis, upon payment of a premium, to individuals entitled to Part A or enrolled in Part B, with premium and cost-sharing subsidies for low-income enrollees. Beneficiaries may enroll in either a stand-alone prescription drug plan (PDP) or an integrated Medicare Advantage plan that offers Part D coverage. Enrollment began in late 2005. In 2012, Part D provided protection against the costs of prescription drugs to over 37 million people. Estimated Part D benefits totaled $66.5 billion in

2012. (This amount includes an estimated $5.2 billion in benefits financed by enrollee premiums paid directly to the Part D plans. These direct premium amounts are available only on an estimated basis.)

Part D coverage includes most FDA-approved prescription drugs and biologicals. (The specific drugs currently covered in Parts A and B remain covered there.) However, plans may set up formularies for their prescription drug coverage, subject to certain statutory standards. Part D coverage can consist of either standard coverage (defined later) or an alternative design that provides the same actuarial value. For an additional premium, plans may also offer supplemental coverage exceeding the value of basic coverage.

It should be noted that some health care services are not covered by any portion of Medicare. Noncovered services include long-term nursing care, custodial care, and certain other health care needs, such as dentures and dental care, eyeglasses, and hearing aids. These services are not a part of the Medicare program, unless they are a part of a private health plan under the Medicare Advantage program.

Program Financing, Beneficiary Liabilities, and Payments to Providers

All financial operations for Medicare are handled through two trust funds, one for Hospital Insurance (HI, Part A) and one for Supplementary Medical Insurance (SMI, Parts B and D). These trust funds, which are special accounts in the U.S. Treasury, are credited with all receipts and charged with all expenditures for benefits and administrative costs. The trust funds cannot be used for any other purpose. Assets not needed for the payment of costs are invested in special Treasury securities. The following sections describe Medicare's financing provisions, beneficiary cost-sharing requirements, and the basis for determining Medicare reimbursements to health care providers.

Program Financing

The HI trust fund is financed primarily through a mandatory payroll tax. Almost all employees and self-employed workers in the United States work in employment covered by Part A and pay taxes to support the cost of benefits for aged and disabled beneficiaries. The Part A tax rate is 1.45 percent of earnings, to be paid by each employee and a matching amount by the employer for each employee, and 2.90 percent for self-employed persons. Beginning in 1994, this tax is paid on all covered wages and self-employment income without limit. (Prior to 1994, the tax applied only up to a specified maximum amount of earnings.) Beginning in 2013, an additional Part A payroll tax of 0.9 percent will be collected on earned income in excess of

$200,000 (for those filing income tax singly) and $250,000 (for those filing jointly; the earnings thresholds are not indexed). The Part A tax rate is specified in the Social Security Act and cannot be changed without legislation.

Part A also receives income from the following sources:

- a portion of the income taxes levied on Social Security benefits paid to high-income beneficiaries;
- premiums from certain persons who are not otherwise eligible and choose to enroll voluntarily;
- reimbursements from the general fund of the U.S. Treasury for the cost of providing Part A coverage to (1) certain aged persons who retired when Part A began and thus were unable to earn sufficient quarters of coverage (the last surviving members of this group have died, and these reimbursements are complete) and (2) those federal retirees similarly unable to earn sufficient quarters of Medicare-qualified federal employment;
- interest earnings on its invested assets; and
- other small miscellaneous income sources.

Payroll taxes are used mainly to pay benefits for current beneficiaries.

The SMI trust fund differs fundamentally from the HI trust fund with regard to the nature of its financing. As previously noted, SMI is now composed of two parts, Part B and Part D, each with its own separate account within the SMI trust fund. The nature of the financing for both parts of SMI is similar, in that both parts are primarily financed by contributions from the general fund of the U.S. Treasury and (to a much lesser degree) by beneficiary premiums.

For Part B, the contributions from the general fund of the U.S. Treasury are the largest source of income, since beneficiary premiums are generally set at a level that covers 25 percent of the average expenditures for aged beneficiaries. The standard Part B premium rate will be $104.90 per beneficiary per month in 2014. There are, however, three provisions that can alter the premium rate for certain enrollees. First, penalties for late enrollment (that is, enrollment after an individual's initial enrollment period) may apply, subject to certain statutory criteria. Second, beginning in 2007, beneficiaries whose income is above certain thresholds are required to pay an income-related monthly adjustment amount, in addition to their standard monthly premium. Finally, a "hold-harmless" provision, which prohibits increases in the standard Part B premium from exceeding the dollar amount of an individual's Social Security cost-of-living adjustment, lowers the premium rate for certain individuals who have their premiums deducted from their Social Security checks.

The 2014 Part B income-related monthly adjustment amounts and total monthly premium amounts to be paid by beneficiaries, according to income level and filing status, are shown in the following table.

2014 Part B income-related monthly adjustment amounts and total monthly premium amounts to be paid by beneficiaries, by filing status and income level

Income	Income-related monthly adjustment (dollars)	Total monthly premium (dollars)
Beneficiaries who file individual tax returns and are single individuals, heads of households, qualifying widow(er)s with dependent children, or married individuals who lived apart from their spouse for the entire taxable year and file separately		
Less than or equal to $85,000	0	104.90
Greater than $85,000 and less than or equal to $107,000	42.00	146.90
Greater than $107,000 and less than or equal to $160,000	104.90	209.80
Greater than $160,000 and less than or equal to $214,000	167.80	272.70
Greater than $214,000	230.80	335.70
Beneficiaries who file joint tax returns		
Less than or equal to $170,000	0	104.90
Greater than $170,000 and less than or equal to $214,000	42.00	146.90
Greater than $214,000 and less than or equal to $320,000	104.90	209.80
Greater than $320,000 and less than or equal to $428,000	167.80	272.70
Greater than $428,000	230.80	335.70
Beneficiaries who are married and lived with their spouse at any time during the year but file separate tax returns		
Less than or equal to $85,000	0	104.90
Greater than $85,000 and less than or equal to $128,000	167.80	272.70
Greater than $128,000	230.80	335.70

For Part D, as with Part B, general fund contributions account for the largest source of income, since Part D beneficiary premiums are to represent, on average, 25.5 percent of the cost of standard coverage. The Part D base beneficiary premium for 2014 will be $32.42. The actual Part D premium paid by an individual beneficiary equals the base beneficiary premium adjusted by a number of factors. In practice, premiums vary significantly from one Part D plan to another and seldom equal the base beneficiary premium.

As of this writing, it is estimated that the average monthly premium for basic Part D coverage, which reflects the specific plan-by-plan premiums and the estimated number of beneficiaries in each plan, will be about $31 in 2014. Penalties for late enrollment may apply. (Late enrollment penalties do not apply to enrollees who have maintained creditable prescription drug coverage.) Beneficiaries meeting certain low-income and limited-resources requirements pay substantially reduced premiums or no premiums at all (and are not subject to late enrollment penalties).

Beginning in 2011, beneficiaries with income above certain thresholds are required to pay an income-related monthly adjustment amount, in addition to their monthly premium. The 2014 Part D income-related monthly adjustment amounts to be paid by beneficiaries, according to income level and filing status, are shown in the following table.

2014 Part D income-related monthly adjustment amounts to be paid by beneficiaries, by filing status and income level

Income	Income-related monthly adjustment (dollars)
Beneficiaries who file individual tax returns and are single individuals, heads of households, qualifying widow(er)s with dependent children, or married individuals who lived apart from their spouse for the entire taxable year and file separately	
Less than or equal to $85,000	0
Greater than $85,000 and less than or equal to $107,000	12.10
Greater than $107,000 and less than or equal to $160,000	31.10
Greater than $160,000 and less than or equal to $214,000	50.20
Greater than $214,000	69.30
Beneficiaries who file joint tax returns	
Less than or equal to $170,000	0
Greater than $170,000 and less than or equal to $214,000	12.10
Greater than $214,000 and less than or equal to $320,000	31.10
Greater than $320,000 and less than or equal to $428,000	50.20
Greater than $428,000	69.30
Beneficiaries who are married and lived with their spouse at any time during the year but file separate tax returns	
Less than or equal to $85,000	0
Greater than $85,000 and less than or equal to $129,000	50.20
Greater than $129,000	69.30

In addition to contributions from the general fund of the U.S. Treasury and beneficiary premiums, Part D also receives payments from the states. With the availability of prescription drug coverage and low-income subsidies under Part D, Medicaid is no longer the primary payer for prescription drugs for Medicaid beneficiaries who also have Medicare, and states are required to defray a portion of Part D expenditures for those beneficiaries.

During the Part D transitional period that began in mid-2004 and phased out during 2006, the general fund of the U.S. Treasury financed the transitional assistance benefit for low-income beneficiaries. Funds were transferred to, and paid from, a Transitional Assistance account within the SMI trust fund.

The SMI trust fund also receives income from interest earnings on its invested assets, as well as a small amount of miscellaneous income. It is important to note that beneficiary premiums and general fund payments for Parts B and D are redetermined annually and separately.

Payments to Medicare Advantage plans are financed from both the HI trust fund and the Part B account within the SMI trust fund in proportion to the relative weights of Part A and Part B benefits to the total benefits paid by the Medicare program.

Beneficiary Payment Liabilities

Fee-for-service beneficiaries are responsible for charges not covered by the Medicare program and for various cost-sharing aspects of Parts A and B. These liabilities may be paid (1) by the Medicare beneficiary; (2) by a third party, such as an employer-sponsored retiree health plan or private Medigap insurance; or (3) by Medicaid, if the person is eligible. The term "Medigap" is used to mean private health insurance that pays, within limits, most of the health care service charges not covered by Parts A or B of Medicare. These policies, which must meet federally imposed standards, are offered by Blue Cross and Blue Shield and various commercial health insurance companies.

In Medicare Advantage plans, the beneficiary's payment share is based on the cost-sharing structure of the specific plan selected by the beneficiary, since each plan has its own requirements. Most plans have lower deductibles and coinsurance than are required of fee-for-service beneficiaries. Such beneficiaries, in general, pay the monthly Part B premium. However, some Medicare Advantage plans may pay part or all of the Part B premium for their enrollees as an added benefit. Depending on the plan, enrollees may also pay an additional premium for certain extra benefits provided (or, in a small number of cases, for certain Medicare-covered services).

For hospital care covered under Part A, a beneficiary's fee-for-service payment share includes a one-time deductible amount at the beginning of each benefit period ($1,216 in 2014). This deductible covers the beneficiary's part of the first 60 days of each spell of inpatient hospital care. If continued inpatient care is needed beyond the 60 days, additional coinsurance payments ($304 per day in 2014) are required through the 90th day of a benefit period. Each Part A beneficiary also has a "lifetime reserve" of 60 additional hospital days that may be used when the covered days within a benefit period have been exhausted. Lifetime reserve days may be used only once, and coinsurance payments ($608 per day in 2014) are required.

For skilled nursing care covered under Part A, Medicare fully covers the first 20 days of SNF care in a benefit period. But for days 21 through 100, a copayment ($152.00 per day in 2014) is required from the beneficiary. After 100 days per benefit period, Medicare pays nothing for SNF care. Home health care requires no deductible or coinsurance payment by the beneficiary. In any Part A service, the beneficiary is responsible for fees to cover the first 3 pints or units of nonreplaced blood per calendar year. The beneficiary has the option of paying the fee or of having the blood replaced.

There are no premiums for most people covered by Part A. Eligibility is generally earned through the work experience of the beneficiary or of the beneficiary's spouse. However, most aged people who are otherwise ineligible for premium-free Part A coverage can enroll voluntarily by paying a monthly premium, if they also enroll in Part B. For people with fewer than 30 quarters of coverage as defined by the Social Security Administration (SSA), the Part A monthly premium rate will be $426 in 2014; for those with 30 to 39 quarters of coverage, the rate will be reduced to $234. Penalties for late enrollment may apply. Voluntary coverage upon payment of the Part A premium, with or without enrolling in Part B, is also available to disabled individuals for whom coverage has ceased because earnings are in excess of those allowed.

The Part B beneficiary's payment share includes the following: one annual deductible ($147 in 2014), the monthly premiums, the coinsurance payments for Part B services (usually 20 percent of the remaining allowed charges with certain exceptions noted below), a deductible for blood, certain charges above the Medicare-allowed charge (for claims not on assignment), and payment for any services not covered by Medicare. For outpatient mental health services, the beneficiary is liable for 20 percent of the approved charges beginning in 2014. This percentage was 50 percent through 2009, then phased down in the intervening years. For services reimbursed under the outpatient hospital prospective payment system, coinsurance percentages vary by service and currently fall in the range of 20 percent to 50 percent. There are no deductibles or coinsurance for certain services, such as clinical lab tests, HHA services, and some preventive care services (including an initial,

"Welcome to Medicare" preventive physical examination and, beginning in 2011, an annual wellness visit to develop or update a prevention plan).

For the standard Part D benefit design, there is an initial deductible ($310 in 2014). After meeting the deductible, the beneficiary pays 25 percent of the remaining costs, up to an initial coverage limit ($2,850 in 2014). A coverage gap starts after an individual's drug costs reach the initial coverage limit and stops when the beneficiary incurs a certain threshold of out-of-pocket costs ($4,550 in 2014). Previously, the beneficiary had to pay the full cost of prescription drugs while in this coverage gap. However, under the Patient Protection and Affordable Care Act (Public Law 111-148) as amended by the Health Care and Education Reconciliation Act of 2010 (Public Law 111-152)—collectively referred to as the Affordable Care Act—a beneficiary (excluding low-income enrollees eligible for cost-sharing subsidies) who entered the coverage gap in 2010 received a $250 rebate; a beneficiary entering in 2011 received a 50-percent manufacturer discount for applicable prescription drugs and a 7-percent benefit from his or her plan for nonapplicable drugs; a beneficiary entering in 2012 received a 50-percent manufacturer discount for applicable prescription drugs and a 14-percent benefit from his or her plan for nonapplicable drugs; and a beneficiary entering in 2013 received a 50-percent manufacturer discount and a 2.5-percent benefit from his or her Part D plan for applicable prescription drugs and a 21-percent benefit from his or her plan for nonapplicable drugs. A beneficiary entering the coverage gap in 2014 will receive a 50-percent manufacturer discount and a 2.5-percent benefit from his or her Part D plan for applicable prescription drugs and a 28-percent benefit from his or her plan for nonapplicable drugs. "Applicable" drugs are generally covered brand-name Part D drugs (including insulin and Part D vaccines); "nonapplicable" drugs are generally nonbrand-name (that is, generic) Part D drugs (including supplies associated with the delivery of insulin). Additional reductions in beneficiary cost sharing in the coverage gap continue in future years such that, by 2020, the coverage gap will be fully phased out, with the beneficiary responsible for 25 percent of prescription drug costs. The 2014 out-of-pocket threshold of $4,550 is equivalent to estimated average total covered drug spending of $6,690.77 under the defined standard benefit design, during the initial coverage period and the coverage gap, for enrollees not eligible for low-income cost-sharing subsidies. This estimated amount is based on an average blend of usage of applicable and nonapplicable drugs by enrollees while in the coverage gap. In determining out-of-pocket costs, the dollar value of the 50-percent manufacturer discount for applicable drugs is included, even though the beneficiary does not pay it. The dollar values of the 28-percent drug plan benefit on nonapplicable drugs and the 2.5-percent drug plan benefit on applicable drugs do not count toward out-of-pocket spending. Under the defined standard benefit design, the out-of-pocket threshold of $4,550 for 2014 is equivalent to $6,455.00 in total covered drug costs for enrollees eligible for low-income cost-sharing subsidies.

For costs incurred after reaching the out-of-pocket threshold, catastrophic coverage is provided, which requires the enrollee to pay the greater of 5 percent coinsurance or a small defined copayment amount ($2.55 in 2014 for generic or preferred multisource drugs and $6.35 in 2014 for other drugs). The benefit parameters are indexed annually to the growth in average per capita Part D costs. Beneficiaries meeting certain low-income and limited-resources requirements pay substantially reduced cost-sharing amounts. In determining out-of-pocket costs, only those amounts actually paid by the enrollee or another individual (and not reimbursed through insurance) are counted; the exceptions to this "true out-of-pocket" provision are cost-sharing assistance from the low-income subsidies provided under Part D and from State Pharmacy Assistance programs and, starting in 2011, the 50-percent manufacturer discount on applicable brand-name drugs purchased by enrollees in the Part D coverage gap.

Many Part D plans offer alternative coverage that differs from the standard coverage described above. In fact, the majority of beneficiaries are not enrolled in the standard benefit design but rather in plans with low or no deductibles, flat payments for covered drugs, and, in some cases, additional partial coverage in the coverage gap. The monthly premiums required for Part D coverage are described in the previous section.

Payments to Providers

Before 1983, Part A payments to providers were made on a reasonable cost basis. Medicare payments for most inpatient hospital services are now made under a reimbursement mechanism known as the prospective payment system (PPS). Under the PPS for acute inpatient hospitals, each stay is categorized into a diagnosis-related group (DRG). Each DRG has a specific predetermined amount associated with it, which serves as the basis for payment. A number of adjustments are applied to the DRG's specific predetermined amount to calculate the payment for each stay. In some cases the payment the hospital receives is less than the hospital's actual cost for providing Part A–covered inpatient hospital services for the stay; in other cases it is more. The hospital absorbs the loss or makes a profit. Certain payment adjustments exist for extraordinarily costly inpatient hospital stays and other situations. Payments for skilled nursing care, home health care, inpatient rehabilitation hospital care, long-term care hospitals, inpatient psychiatric hospitals, and hospice are made under separate prospective payment systems.

For nonphysician Part B services, home health care is reimbursed under the same prospective payment system as Part A, most hospital outpatient services are reimbursed on a separate prospective payment system, and most payments for clinical laboratory and ambulance services are based on fee schedules. A fee schedule is a comprehensive listing of maximum fees used to pay providers. Most durable medical equipment has also been paid on a fee schedule in recent years but is paid based on a competitive bidding process in some areas beginning January 1, 2011. This competitive bidding process will be expanded to all areas within the next several years.

In general, the prospective payment systems and fee schedules used for Part A and non-physician Part B services are increased each year either by indices related to the "market basket" of goods and services that the provider must purchase or by indices related to the Consumer Price Index (CPI). These indices vary by type of provider. The Affordable Care Act mandates reductions in most of these payment updates. In most cases, the payment updates are reduced by stipulated amounts for 2010–2019 and are further and permanently reduced by growth in economy-wide productivity. Starting dates and amounts of reductions vary by provider. It is likely that the lower payment increases will not be viable in the long range. The best available evidence indicates that most health care providers cannot improve their productivity to this degree because of the labor-intensive nature of most of these services.

For Part B, before 1992, physicians were paid on the basis of reasonable charge. This amount was initially defined as the lowest of (1) the physician's actual charge, (2) the physician's customary charge, or (3) the prevailing charge for similar services in that locality. Since January 1992, allowed charges have been defined as the lesser of (1) the submitted charges or (2) the amount determined by a fee schedule based on a relative value scale. In practice, most allowed charges are based on the fee schedule, which is supposed to be updated each year by a Sustainable Growth Rate (SGR) system prescribed in the law. However, over the past 10 years, the SGR system would have required significant fee reductions for physicians, and Congress has passed a series of bills to override the reductions.

If a doctor or supplier agrees to accept the Medicare-approved rate as payment in full ("takes assignment"), then payments provided must be considered as payments in full for that service. The provider may not request any added payments (beyond the initial annual deductible and coinsurance) from the beneficiary or insurer. If the provider does not take assignment, the beneficiary will be charged for the excess (which may be paid by Medigap insurance). Limits now exist on the excess that doctors or suppliers can charge. Physicians are "participating physicians" if they agree before the beginning of the year to accept assignment for all Medicare services they furnish during the year. Since beneficiaries in the original Medicare fee-for-service program may select their doctors, they can choose participating physicians.

Medicare Advantage plans and their precursors have generally been paid on a capitation basis, meaning that a fixed, predetermined amount per month per member is paid to the plan, without regard to the actual number and nature of services used by the members. The specific mechanisms to determine the payment amounts have changed over the years. In 2006, Medicare began paying capitated payment rates to plans based on a competitive bidding process.

For Part D, each month for each plan member, Medicare pays stand-alone PDPs and the prescription drug portions of Medicare Advantage plans their risk-adjusted bid, minus the enrollee premium. Plans also receive payments representing premiums and cost-sharing amounts for certain low-income beneficiaries for whom these items are reduced or waived. Under the reinsurance provision, plans receive payments for 80 percent of costs in the catastrophic coverage category.

To help them gain experience with the Medicare population, Part D plans are protected by a system of "risk corridors" that allow Medicare to assist with unexpected costs and share in unexpected savings. The risk corridors became less protective after 2007.

Under Part D, Medicare provides certain subsidies to employer and union PDPs that continue to offer coverage to Medicare retirees and meet specific criteria in doing so. These retiree drug subsidy (RDS) payments are tax-exempt, but will be taxable under the Affordable Care Act beginning in 2013.

Claims Processing

Since the inception of Medicare, fee-for-service claims have been processed by nongovernment organizations or agencies under contract to serve as the fiscal agent between providers and the federal government. These entities apply the Medicare coverage rules to determine appropriate reimbursement amounts and make payments to the providers and suppliers. Their responsibilities also include maintaining records, establishing controls, safeguarding against fraud and abuse, and assisting both providers and beneficiaries as needed.

Before the enactment of the MMA in 2003, contractors known as fiscal intermediaries processed Part A claims for institutional services, including claims for inpatient hospital, SNF, HHA, and hospice services. They also processed outpatient hospital claims for Part B. Similarly, contractors known as carriers handled Part B claims for services by physicians and medical suppliers. By law, the Centers for Medicare & Medicaid Services (CMS) was required to select fiscal intermediaries from among companies that were nominated by health care provider associations and to select carriers from among health insurers or similar companies.

The MMA mandated the replacement of that system with a new system of entities known as Medicare Administrative Contractors (MACs). Each MAC processes and pays fee-for-service claims for both Part A and Part B services to all providers and suppliers within its geographic jurisdiction. MACs are selected through a competitive procedure. This new system is intended to improve Medicare services to beneficiaries, providers, and suppliers, who now have a single point of contact for all claims-related business. CMS will evaluate MACs based in part on customer satisfaction with their services. The new system enables the Medicare fee-for-service program to benefit from economies of scale and competitive performance contracting.

The transition from fiscal intermediaries and carriers to MACs began in 2005, and the last intermediary and carrier contracts ended in September 2013. Under the initial implementation of the MAC system, Part A and Part B claims were processed by fifteen "A/B MACs," with the exception of (1) durable medical equipment claims, which were processed by four specialty MACs, and (2) home health and hospice claims, which were processed by four other specialty MACs. CMS is in the process of consolidating the A/B MAC jurisdictions from fifteen to ten. As of November 2013, there are twelve A/B MACs, and the four home health and hospice MACs have been integrated into A/B MAC jurisdictions.

Claims for services provided by Medicare Advantage plans (that is, claims under Part C) are processed by the plans themselves.

Part D plans are responsible for processing their claims, akin to Part C. However, because of the "true out-of-pocket" provision discussed previously, CMS has contracted the services of a facilitator, who works with CMS, Part D drug plans (stand-alone PDPs and the prescription drug portions of Medicare Advantage plans), and carriers of supplemental drug coverage to coordinate benefit payments and track the sources of cost-sharing payments. Claims under Part D also have to be submitted by the plans to CMS, so that certain payments based on actual experience (such as payments for low-income cost-sharing and premium subsidies, reinsurance, and risk corridors) can be determined.

Because of its size and complexity, Medicare is vulnerable to improper payments, ranging from inadvertent errors to outright fraud and abuse. Although providers are responsible for submitting accurate claims, and MACs are responsible for ensuring that only such claims are paid, there are additional groups whose duties include the prevention, reduction, and recovery of improper payments.

Quality improvement organizations (QIOs, formerly called peer review organizations or PROs) are groups of practicing health care professionals who are paid by the federal government to improve the effectiveness, efficiency, economy, and quality of services delivered to Medicare beneficiaries. One function of QIOs is to ensure that Medicare pays only for services and goods that are reasonable and necessary and that are provided in the most appropriate setting.

The ongoing effort to address improper payments intensified after enactment of the Health Insurance Portability and Accountability Act (HIPAA) of 1996 (Public Law 104-191), which created the Medicare Integrity Program (MIP). The MIP provides CMS with dedicated funds to identify and combat improper payments, including those caused by fraud and abuse, and, for the first time, allows CMS to award contracts competitively with entities other than carriers and intermediaries to conduct these activities. MIP funds are used for (1) audits of cost reports, which are financial documents that hospitals and other institutions are required to submit annually to CMS; (2) medical reviews of claims to determine whether services provided are medically reasonable and necessary; (3) determinations of whether Medicare or other insurance sources have primary responsibility for payment; (4) identification and investigation of potential fraud cases; and (5) education to inform providers about appropriate billing procedures. In addition to creating the MIP, HIPAA established a fund to provide resources for the Department of Justice—including the Federal Bureau of Investigation—and the Office of Inspector General (OIG) within the Department of Health and Human Services (HHS) to investigate and prosecute health care fraud and abuse.

The Deficit Reduction Act (DRA) of 2005 (Public Law 109-171) established and funded the Medicare-Medicaid Data Match Program, which is designed to identify improper billing and utilization patterns by matching Medicare and Medicaid claims information. As is the case under the MIP, CMS can contract with third parties. The funds also can be used (1) to coordinate actions by CMS, the states, the Attorney General, and the HHS OIG to prevent improper Medicaid and Medicare expenditures and (2) to increase the effectiveness and efficiency of both Medicare and Medicaid through cost avoidance, savings, and the recoupment of fraudulent, wasteful, or abusive expenditures.

The Affordable Care Act includes many provisions intended to improve the accuracy of payments and to link those payments to quality and efficiency in the Medicare program. One of the most important provisions establishes the Center for Medicare and Medicaid Innovation (CMMI) in CMS to test innovative payment and service delivery models, with the goal of reducing Medicare, Medicaid, and the Children's Health Insurance Program (CHIP) expenditures while preserving or enhancing quality of care.

Administration

HHS has the overall responsibility for administration of the Medicare program. Within HHS, responsibility for administering Medicare rests with

CMS. The Social Security Administration (SSA) assists, however, by initially determining an individual's Medicare entitlement, by withholding Part B premiums from the Social Security benefit checks of most beneficiaries, and by maintaining Medicare data on the Master Beneficiary Record, which is SSA's primary record of beneficiaries.

The MMA requires SSA to undertake a number of additional Medicare-related responsibilities, including making low-income subsidy determinations under Part D, notifying individuals of the availability of Part D subsidies, withholding Part D premiums from monthly Social Security cash benefits for beneficiaries who request such an arrangement, and, for 2007 and later, determining the individual's Part B premium if the Part B income-related monthly adjustment applies. For 2011 and later, the Affordable Care Act requires SSA to determine the individual's Part D premium if the Part D income-related monthly adjustment applies. The Internal Revenue Service (IRS) in the Department of the Treasury collects the Part A payroll taxes from workers and their employers. IRS data, in the form of income tax returns, play a role in determining which Part D enrollees are eligible for low-income subsidies (and to what degree) and which Part B and Part D enrollees are subject to the income-related monthly adjustment amounts in their premiums (and to what degree).

A Medicare Board of Trustees, composed of two appointed members of the public and four members who serve by virtue of their positions in the federal government, oversees the financial operations of the HI and SMI trust funds. The Secretary of the Treasury is the managing trustee. Each year, around the first day of April, the Board of Trustees reports to Congress on the financial and actuarial status of the Medicare trust funds.

State agencies (usually state health departments under agreements with CMS) identify, survey, and inspect provider and supplier facilities and institutions wishing to participate in the Medicare program. In consultation with CMS, these agencies then certify the facilities that are qualified.

Medicare Financial Status

Medicare is the largest health care insurance program—and the second-largest social insurance program—in the United States. Medicare is also complex, and it faces a number of financial challenges in both the short term and the long term. These challenges include:

- The solvency of the HI trust fund, which fails the Medicare Board of Trustees' test of short-range financial adequacy, as annual expenditures are projected to exceed annual assets within 10 years.

- The long-range health of the HI trust fund, as the trust fund fails the Trustees' long-range test of close actuarial balance.
- The rapid growth projected for SMI costs as a percent of Gross Domestic Product. (The Part B and Part D accounts in the SMI trust fund are automatically in financial balance—in both the short range and the long range—since premiums and general revenue financing rates are reset each year to match estimated costs.)
- The substantial reductions in Part B physician payment rates required under the Sustainable Growth Rate system in current law. In recent years, Congress has consistently passed legislation that overrides the reductions (also discussed above).
- The likelihood that the lower payment rate updates to most categories of Medicare providers for 2011 and later, as mandated by the Affordable Care Act, will not be viable in the long range (also discussed above).

A detailed description of these issues is beyond the scope of this summary. For more information, see the Medicare Trustees Report (www.cms .gov/Research-Statistics-Data-and-Systems/Statistics-Trends-and-Reports /ReportsTrustFunds/index.html).

Data Summary

The Medicare program covers 95 percent of our nation's aged population, as well as many people who receive Social Security disability benefits. In 2012, Part A covered over 50 million enrollees with benefit payments of $262.9 billion, Part B covered over 46 million enrollees with benefit payments of $236.5 billion, and Part D covered over 37 million enrollees with benefit payments of $66.5 billion. Administrative costs in 2012 were about 1.5 percent, 1.6 percent, and 0.6 percent of expenditures for Part A, Part B, and Part D, respectively. Total expenditures for Medicare in 2012 were $574.2 billion.

Source: Reprinted from Klees, B. S., and C. J. Wolfe. 2014. *Medicare Program Description and Legislative History.* Office of the Actuary, Centers for Medicare and Medicaid Services (CMS), US Department of Health and Human Services. Accessed March 13, 2014. www.ssa .gov/policy/docs/statcomps/supplement/2013/medicare.html#mn1.

For additional information on Medicare, see:

Kaiser Family Foundation. 2013. *Policy Options to Sustain Medicare for the Future.* Accessed March 13, 2014. http://kaiserfamilyfoundation.files.wordpress.com/2013/02/8402.pdf.

OVERVIEW OF MEDICAID

Title XIX of the Social Security Act is a federal and state entitlement program that pays for medical assistance for certain individuals and families with low incomes and resources. This program, known as Medicaid, became law in 1965 as a cooperative venture jointly funded by the federal and state governments (including the District of Columbia and the territories) to assist states in furnishing medical assistance to eligible needy persons. Medicaid is the largest source of funding for medical and health-related services for America's poorest people.

Within broad national guidelines established by federal statutes, regulations, and policies, each state establishes its own eligibility standards; determines the type, amount, duration, and scope of services; sets the rate of payment for services; and administers its own program. Medicaid policies for eligibility, services, and payment are complex and vary considerably, even among states of similar size or geographic proximity. Thus, a person who is eligible for Medicaid in one state may not be eligible in another state, and the services provided by one state may differ considerably in amount, duration, or scope from services provided in a similar or neighboring state. In addition, state legislatures may change Medicaid eligibility, services, and/or reimbursement at any time.

Title XXI of the Social Security Act, the Children's Health Insurance Program (CHIP, known from its inception until March 2009 as the State Children's Health Insurance Program, or SCHIP), is a program initiated by the Balanced Budget Act (BBA) of 1997 (Public Law 105-33). The BBA provided $40 billion in federal funding through fiscal year 2007 to furnish health care coverage for low-income children—generally those in families with income below 200 percent of the federal poverty level (FPL)—who did not qualify for Medicaid and would otherwise be uninsured. Subsequent legislation, including the Children's Health Insurance Program Reauthorization Act (CHIPRA) of 2009 (Public Law 111-3) and the Patient Protection and Affordable Care Act (Public Law 111-148) as amended by the Health Care and Education Reconciliation Act of 2010 (Public Law 111-152)—collectively referred to as the Affordable Care Act—extended CHIP funding through fiscal year 2015. Under CHIP, states may elect to provide coverage to qualifying children by expanding their Medicaid programs or through a state program separate from Medicaid. A number of states have also been granted waivers to cover parents of children enrolled in CHIP.

Medicaid Eligibility

Until 2014, when the Affordable Care Act will expand Medicaid eligibility, Medicaid does not provide medical assistance for all poor persons. Under the broadest provisions of the federal statute, Medicaid does not currently provide health care services even for very poor persons unless they are in one of the groups designated below. Low income is only one test for Medicaid eligibility for most of those within these groups; their financial resources also are tested against threshold levels (as determined by each state within federal guidelines).

States generally have broad discretion in determining which groups their Medicaid programs will cover and the financial criteria for Medicaid eligibility. To be eligible for federal funds, however, states are required to provide Medicaid coverage for certain individuals who receive federally assisted income-maintenance payments, as well as for related groups not receiving cash payments. In addition to their Medicaid programs, most states have additional "state-only" programs to provide medical assistance for specified poor persons who do not qualify for Medicaid. Federal funds are not provided for state-only programs. The following enumerates the mandatory Medicaid "categorically needy" eligibility groups for which federal matching funds are provided:

- Limited-income families with children, as described in section 1931 of the Social Security Act, are generally eligible for Medicaid if they meet the requirements for the Aid to Families with Dependent Children (AFDC) program that were in effect in their state on July 16, 1996.
- Children under age 6 whose family income is at or below 133 percent of the FPL. (As of January 2013, the FPL has been set at $23,550 for a family of four in the continental U.S.; Alaska and Hawaii's FPLs are $29,440 and $27,090, respectively.)
- Pregnant women whose family income is below 133 percent of the FPL. (Services to these women are limited to those related to pregnancy, complications of pregnancy, delivery, and postpartum care.)
- Infants born to Medicaid-eligible women, for the first year of life with certain restrictions.
- Supplemental Security Income (SSI) recipients in most states (or aged, blind, and disabled individuals in states using more restrictive Medicaid eligibility requirements that pre-date SSI).

- Recipients of adoption or foster care assistance under Title IV-E of the Social Security Act.
- Special protected groups (typically individuals who lose their cash assistance under Title IV-A or SSI because of earnings from work or from increased Social Security benefits, but who may keep Medicaid for a period of time).
- All children under age 19, in families with incomes at or below the FPL.
- Certain Medicare beneficiaries (described later).

States also have the option of providing Medicaid coverage for other "categorically related" groups. These optional groups share characteristics of the mandatory groups (that is, they fall within defined categories), but the eligibility criteria are somewhat more liberally defined. The broadest optional groups for which states can receive federal matching funds for coverage under the Medicaid program include the following:

- Infants up to age 1 and pregnant women not covered under the mandatory rules whose family income is no more than 185 percent of the FPL. (The percentage amount is set by each state.)
- Children under age 21 who meet criteria more liberal than the AFDC income and resources requirements that were in effect in their state on July 16, 1996.
- Institutionalized individuals, and individuals in home and community-based waiver programs, who are eligible under a "special income level." (The amount is set by each state—up to 300 percent of the SSI federal benefit rate.)
- Individuals who would be eligible if institutionalized, but who are receiving care under home and community-based services waivers.
- Certain aged, blind, or disabled adults who have incomes above those requiring mandatory coverage, but below the FPL.
- Aged, blind, or disabled recipients of state supplementary income payments.
- Certain working-and-disabled persons with family income less than 250 percent of the FPL who would qualify for SSI if they did not work.
- Tuberculosis-infected persons who would be financially eligible for Medicaid at the SSI income level if they were in a Medicaid-covered category. (Coverage is limited to tuberculosis-related ambulatory services and tuberculosis drugs.)

- Certain uninsured or low-income women who are screened for breast or cervical cancer through a program administered by the Centers for Disease Control and Prevention. The Breast and Cervical Cancer Prevention and Treatment Act of 2000 (Public Law 106-354) provides these women with medical assistance and follow-up diagnostic services through Medicaid.
- "Optional targeted low-income children" included in the CHIP (formerly SCHIP) program established by the BBA.
- "Medically needy" persons (described below).

The medically needy (MN) option allows states to extend Medicaid eligibility to additional persons. These persons would be eligible for Medicaid under one of the mandatory or optional groups, except that their income and/or resources are above the eligibility level set by their state for those groups. Persons may qualify immediately or may "spend down" by incurring medical expenses greater than the amount by which their income exceeds their state's MN income level.

Medicaid eligibility and benefit provisions for the medically needy do not have to be as extensive as for the categorically needy, and may be quite restrictive. Federal matching funds are available for MN programs. However, if a state elects to have an MN program, it must meet federal requirements that certain groups (including children under age 19 and pregnant women) be covered and that certain services (including prenatal and delivery care for pregnant women and ambulatory care for children) be provided. A state may elect to provide MN eligibility to certain additional groups and may elect to provide certain additional services as part of its MN program. As of 2010, 34 states plus the District of Columbia have elected to have an MN program and are providing services to at least some MN beneficiaries. All remaining states utilize the "special income level" option to extend Medicaid to the "near poor" in medical institutional settings.

The Personal Responsibility and Work Opportunity Reconciliation Act of 1996 (Public Law 104-193)—known as the "welfare reform" bill—made restrictive changes regarding eligibility for SSI coverage that affected the Medicaid program. For example, legal resident aliens and other qualified aliens who entered the United States on or after August 22, 1996 are ineligible for Medicaid for 5 years. States have the option of providing Medicaid coverage for most aliens entering before that date and coverage for those eligible after the 5-year ban; emergency services, however, are mandatory for both of these alien coverage groups. For aliens who lose SSI benefits because of these restrictions regarding SSI coverage, Medicaid benefits can continue only if these persons can be covered under some other eligibility status (again with the exception of emergency services, which are mandatory). Public

Law 104-193 also affected a number of disabled children, who lost SSI as a result of the restrictive changes; however, their eligibility for Medicaid was reinstituted by Public Law 105-33, the BBA.

In addition, welfare reform repealed the open-ended federal entitlement program known as Aid to Families with Dependent Children (AFDC) and replaced it with Temporary Assistance for Needy Families (TANF), which provides states with grants to be spent on time-limited cash assistance. TANF generally limits a family's lifetime cash welfare benefits to a maximum of 5 years and permits states to impose a wide range of other requirements as well—in particular, those related to employment. However, the impact on Medicaid eligibility has not been significant. Under welfare reform, persons who would have been eligible for AFDC under the AFDC requirements in effect on July 16, 1996 are generally still eligible for Medicaid. Although most persons covered by TANF receive Medicaid, it is not required by law.

Medicaid coverage may begin as early as the third month prior to application—if the person would have been eligible for Medicaid had he or she applied during that time. Medicaid coverage generally stops at the end of the month in which a person no longer meets the criteria of any Medicaid eligibility group. The BBA allows states to provide 12 months of continuous Medicaid coverage (without reevaluation) for eligible children under age 19.

The Ticket to Work and Work Incentives Improvement Act of 1999 (Public Law 106-170) provides or continues Medicaid coverage to certain disabled beneficiaries who work despite their disability. Beneficiaries with higher incomes may pay a sliding scale premium based on income.

The Deficit Reduction Act (DRA) of 2005 (Public Law 109-171) refined eligibility requirements for Medicaid beneficiaries by tightening standards for citizenship and immigration documentation and by changing the rules concerning long-term care eligibility—specifically, the look-back period for determining community spouse income and assets was lengthened from 36 months to 60 months, individuals whose homes exceed $500,000 in value are disqualified, and the states are required to impose partial months of ineligibility.

Beginning in 2014, the Affordable Care Act will give states the option to extend Medicaid eligibility to all individuals under age 65 in families with income below 138 percent of the FPL. (Technically, the income limit is 133 percent of the FPL, but the Act also provides for a 5-percent income disregard.) In addition to the higher level of allowable income, the new legislation expands eligibility to people under age 65 who have no other qualifying factors that would have made them eligible for Medicaid under prior law, such as being under age 18, disabled, pregnant, or parents of eligible children. Because individuals are not required to be parents of eligible children under the new law, nondisabled nonaged adults comprise the category expected to have the greatest increase in Medicaid enrollment. In *National Federation of Independent Businesses v. Sebelius (2012),* the U.S. Supreme Court ruled that states could not be required to expand Medicaid eligibility to 138 percent of the FPL as a condition of continuing to operate the existing Medicaid program and receiving Federal financial participation. This ruling has made the eligibility expansion effectively optional for each state's Medicaid program. Thus, it is possible that some states would choose not to expand Medicaid eligibility in 2014 and that the individuals who would potentially be newly eligible would remain ineligible in those states.

Scope of Medicaid Services

Title XIX of the Social Security Act allows considerable flexibility within the states' Medicaid plans. However, some federal requirements are mandatory if federal matching funds are to be received. A state's Medicaid program must offer medical assistance for certain basic services to most categorically needy populations. These services generally include:

- Inpatient hospital services;
- Outpatient hospital services;
- Pregnancy-related services, including prenatal care and 60 days postpartum pregnancy-related services;
- Vaccines for children;
- Physician services;
- Nursing facility services for persons aged 21 or older;
- Family planning services and supplies;
- Rural health clinic services;
- Home health care for persons eligible for skilled nursing services;
- Laboratory and x-ray services;
- Pediatric and family nurse practitioner services;
- Nurse-midwife services;
- Federally qualified health center (FQHC) services, and ambulatory services of an FQHC that would be available in other settings; and
- Early and periodic screening, diagnostic, and treatment (EPSDT) services for children under age 21.

States may also receive federal matching funds to provide certain optional services. Some of the most common currently approved optional Medicaid services are:

- Diagnostic services;
- Clinic services;
- Intermediate care facility services;
- Prescribed drugs and prosthetic devices;
- Optometrist services and eyeglasses;
- Nursing facility services for children under age 21;
- Transportation services;
- Rehabilitation and physical therapy services;
- Hospice care;
- Home and community-based care to certain persons with chronic impairments; and
- Targeted case management services.

The BBA included a state option known as Programs of All-inclusive Care for the Elderly (PACE). PACE provides an alternative to institutional care for persons aged 55 and older who require a nursing-facility level of care. The PACE team offers and manages all health, medical, and social services and mobilizes other services as needed to provide preventive, rehabilitative, curative, and supportive care. This care, provided in day health centers, homes, hospitals, and nursing homes, helps the person maintain independence, dignity, and quality of life. PACE functions within the Medicare program as well. Regardless of source of payment, PACE providers receive payment only through the PACE agreement and must make available all items and services covered under both Titles XVIII and XIX, without amount, duration, or scope limitations and without application of any deductibles, copayments, or other cost sharing. The individuals enrolled in PACE receive benefits solely through the PACE program.

Amount and Duration of Medicaid Services

Within broad federal guidelines and certain limitations, states determine the amount and duration of services offered under their Medicaid programs. States may limit, for example, the number of days of hospital care or the number of physician visits covered. Two restrictions apply: (1) limits must result in a sufficient level of services to reasonably achieve the purpose of the benefits, and (2) limits on benefits may not discriminate among beneficiaries based on medical diagnosis or condition.

In general, states are required to provide comparable amounts, duration, and scope of services to all categorically needy and categorically related eligible persons. There are two important exceptions: (1) medically necessary health care services that are identified under the EPSDT program for eligible children, and that are within the scope of mandatory or optional services under federal law, must be covered even if those services are not included as part of the covered services in that state's plan, and (2) states may request waivers to pay for otherwise uncovered home and community-based services for Medicaid-eligible persons who might otherwise be institutionalized. As long as the services are cost effective, states have few limitations on the services that may be covered under these waivers (except that states may not provide room and board for the beneficiaries, other than as a part of respite care). With certain exceptions, a state's Medicaid program must allow beneficiaries to have some informed choices among participating providers of health care and to receive quality care that is appropriate and timely.

Payment for Medicaid Services

Medicaid operates as a vendor payment program. States may pay health care providers directly on a fee-for-service basis, or states may pay for Medicaid services through various prepayment arrangements, such as health maintenance organizations (HMOs). Within federally imposed upper limits and specific restrictions, each state for the most part has broad discretion in determining the payment methodology and payment rate for services. Generally, payment rates must be sufficient to enlist enough providers so that covered services are available at least to the extent that comparable care and services are available to the general population within that geographic area. Providers participating in Medicaid must accept Medicaid payment rates as payment in full. States must make additional payments to qualified hospitals that provide inpatient services to a disproportionate number of Medicaid beneficiaries and/or to other low-income or uninsured persons under what is known as the "disproportionate share hospital" (DSH) adjustment. From 1988 to 1991, excessive and inappropriate use of the DSH adjustment resulted in rapidly increasing federal expenditures for Medicaid. Legislation passed in 1991 and 1993, and amended in the BBA of 1997 and later legislation, capped the federal share of payments to DSH hospitals.

States may impose nominal deductibles, coinsurance, or copayments on some Medicaid beneficiaries for certain services. The following Medicaid beneficiaries, however, must be excluded from cost sharing: pregnant women, children under age 18, and hospital or nursing home patients who are expected to contribute most of their income to institutional care. In addition, all Medicaid beneficiaries must be exempt from copayments for emergency services and family planning services. Under the DRA, new cost sharing and benefit rules provided states the option of imposing new premiums and increased cost sharing on all Medicaid beneficiaries except for those mentioned above and for terminally ill patients in hospice care. The DRA also established special rules for cost sharing for prescription drugs and for nonemergency services furnished in emergency rooms.

The federal government pays a share of the medical assistance expenditures under each state's Medicaid program. That share, known as the Federal Medical Assistance Percentage (FMAP), is determined annually by a formula that compares the state's average per capita income level with the national income average. States with a higher per capita income level are reimbursed a smaller share of their costs. By law, the FMAP cannot be lower than 50 percent or higher than 83 percent. In fiscal year 2013, the FMAPs varied from 50 percent in 19 states and the territories to 73.4 percent in Mississippi and averaged 59.5 percent overall. The BBA permanently raised the FMAP for the District of Columbia from 50 percent to 70 percent. For children covered through the CHIP program, the federal government pays states a higher share, or "enhanced" FMAP, which averaged 71.4 percent in fiscal year 2013.

The American Recovery and Reinvestment Act (ARRA) of 2009 (Public Law 111-5) provided states with an increase in their Medicaid FMAPs of up to 14 percentage points, depending on state unemployment rates, for the first quarter of fiscal year 2009 through the first quarter of fiscal year 2011. Section 201 of Public Law 111-226 (referred to as the Education, Jobs, and Medicaid Assistance Act of 2010) extended these increases for the second and third quarters of fiscal year 2011, but at lower levels than those under ARRA.

The federal government also reimburses states for 100 percent of the cost of services provided to American Indians and Alaska Natives through facilities of the Indian Health Service, for 100 percent of the cost of the Qualifying Individuals (QI) program (described later), and for 90 percent of the cost of family planning services, and shares in each state's expenditures for the administration of the Medicaid program. Most administrative costs are matched at 50 percent, although higher percentages are paid for certain activities and functions, such as development of mechanized claims processing systems.

Except for the CHIP program, the QI program, DSH payments, and payments to territories, federal payments to states for medical assistance have no set limit (cap). Rather, the federal government matches (at FMAP rates) state expenditures for the mandatory services, as well as for the optional services that the individual state decides to cover for eligible beneficiaries, and matches (at the appropriate administrative rate) all necessary and proper administrative costs.

Summary and Trends

Medicaid was initially formulated as a medical care extension of federally funded programs providing cash income assistance for the poor, with an emphasis on dependent children and their mothers, the disabled, and the elderly. Over the years, however, Medicaid eligibility has been incrementally expanded beyond its original ties with eligibility for cash programs. Legislation in the late 1980s extended Medicaid coverage to a larger number of low-income pregnant women and poor children and to some Medicare beneficiaries who are not eligible for any cash assistance program. Legislative changes also focused on increased access, better quality of care, specific benefits, enhanced outreach programs, and fewer limits on services.

In most years since its inception, Medicaid has had very rapid growth in expenditures. This rapid growth has been due primarily to the following factors:

- The increase in size of the Medicaid-covered populations as a result of federal mandates, increased state coverage of optional groups, general population growth, and economic recessions;
- The expansion of coverage and utilization of services;
- The DSH payment program, coupled with its inappropriate use to increase federal payments to states;
- The increase in the number of very old and disabled persons requiring extensive acute and/or long-term health care and various related services;
- The results of technological advances to keep a greater number of very low birth-weight babies and other critically ill or severely injured persons alive and in need of continued extensive and very costly care;
- The increase in drug costs and the availability of new expensive drugs; and
- The increase in payment rates to providers of health care services, when compared with general inflation.

As with all health insurance programs, most Medicaid beneficiaries incur relatively small average expenditures per person each year, and a relatively small proportion incurs very large costs. Moreover, the average cost varies substantially by type of beneficiary. National data for 2012, for example, indicate that Medicaid payments for services for 28.3 million children, who constituted 49 percent of all Medicaid beneficiaries, averaged $2,623 per child. Similarly, for 14.6 million nondisabled adults, who represented 25 percent of beneficiaries, payments averaged $4,458 per person. However, other groups had much larger per-person expenditures. Medicaid payments for services for 5.1 million aged, who constituted 9 percent of all Medicaid beneficiaries, averaged $15,990 per person; for 9.7 million disabled, who represented 17 percent of beneficiaries, payments averaged $16,781 per person. When expenditures for these high- and lower-cost beneficiaries are combined, the 2012 payments to health care vendors for 57.6 million Medicaid beneficiaries averaged $6,641 per person.

Long-term care is an important provision of Medicaid that will be increasingly utilized as our nation's population ages. The Medicaid program paid for nearly 40 percent of the total cost of nursing facility care in 2010. National data for 2010 show that Medicaid payments for nursing facility services (excluding intermediate care facilities) totaled $49.7 billion for more than 1.5 million beneficiaries of these services—an average expenditure of $32,153 per nursing home beneficiary. The national data also show that Medicaid payments for home health services totaled $4.8 billion for 1.1 million beneficiaries—an average expenditure of $4,196 per home health care beneficiary. With the percentage of our population who are elderly or disabled increasing faster than that of the younger groups, the need for long-term care is expected to increase.

Another significant development in Medicaid is the growth in managed care as an alternative service delivery concept different from the traditional fee-for-service system. Under managed care systems, HMOs, prepaid health plans (PHPs), or comparable entities agree to provide a specific set of services to Medicaid enrollees, usually in return for a predetermined periodic payment per enrollee. Managed care programs seek to enhance access to quality care in a cost-effective manner. Waivers may provide the states with greater flexibility in the design and implementation of their Medicaid managed care programs. Waiver authority under sections 1915(b) and 1115 of the Social Security Act is an important part of the Medicaid program. Section 1915(b) waivers allow states to develop innovative health care delivery or reimbursement systems. Section 1115 waivers allow experimental statewide health care reform demonstrations to cover uninsured populations and to test new delivery systems without increasing costs. Finally, the BBA provided states a new option to use managed care without a waiver. According to the *Medicaid Managed Care Enrollment Report*, the share of Medicaid beneficiaries enrolled in some form of managed care program grew steadily from 48 percent of enrollees in 1997 to 74 percent in 2011.

In fiscal year 2012, net outlays for the Medicaid program (federal and state) were $431.9 billion, including direct payment to providers of $251.9 billion, payments for various premiums (for HMOs, Medicare, etc.) of $132.5 billion, payments to disproportionate share hospitals of $14.1 billion, administrative costs of $22.6 billion, and various adjustments totaling

$7.2 billion. In addition, there were $3.6 billion in expenditures for the Vaccines for Children Program under Title XIX. With no other changes to the Medicaid program except for those already prescribed by current law (including the Affordable Care Act), spending is projected to reach $667 billion by fiscal year 2018.

Expenditures under the CHIP program in fiscal year 2012 were $12.3 billion. CHIP is currently funded through fiscal year 2015.

The Medicaid–Medicare Relationship

Medicare beneficiaries who have low incomes and limited resources may also receive help from the Medicaid program. For such persons who are eligible for full Medicaid coverage, the Medicare health care coverage is supplemented by services that are available under their state's Medicaid program. These additional services may include, for example, nursing facility care beyond the 100-day limit covered by Medicare, eyeglasses, and hearing aids. For persons enrolled in both programs, any services that are covered by Medicare are paid for by the Medicare program before any payments are made by the Medicaid program, since Medicaid is always the "payer of last resort."

Certain other Medicare beneficiaries may receive help with Medicare premium and cost-sharing payments through their state Medicaid program. Qualified Medicare Beneficiaries (QMBs) and Specified Low-Income Medicare Beneficiaries (SLMBs) are the best-known categories and the largest in numbers. QMBs are those Medicare beneficiaries who have financial resources at or below twice the standard allowed under the SSI program and incomes at or below 100 percent of the FPL. For QMBs, Medicaid pays the Hospital Insurance (HI, or Part A) and Supplementary Medical Insurance (SMI) Part B premiums and the Medicare coinsurance and deductibles, subject to limits that states may impose on payment rates. SLMBs are Medicare beneficiaries with resources like the QMBs but with incomes that are higher, though still less than 120 percent of the FPL. For SLMBs, the Medicaid program pays only the Part B premiums. A third category of Medicare beneficiaries who may receive help consists of disabled-and-working individuals. According to Medicare law, disabled-and-working individuals who previously qualified for Medicare because of a disability, but who lost entitlement because of their return to work (despite the disability), are allowed to purchase Medicare Part A and Part B coverage. If these persons have incomes below 200 percent of the FPL but do not meet any other Medicaid assistance category, they may qualify to have Medicaid pay their Part A premiums as Qualified Disabled and Working Individuals (QDWIs).

For Medicare beneficiaries with incomes above 120 percent and less than 135 percent of the FPL, states receive a capped allotment of federal funds for payment of Medicare Part B premiums. These beneficiaries are known as Qualifying Individuals (QIs). Unlike the QMBs and SLMBs, who may be eligible for other Medicaid benefits in addition to their QMB/SLMB benefits, the QIs cannot be otherwise eligible for medical assistance under a state plan. The QI benefit is 100 percent federally funded, up to the state's allotment. The QI program was established by the BBA for fiscal years 1998 through 2002 and has been extended numerous times, most recently through the end of December 2013.

The Centers for Medicare & Medicaid Services (CMS) estimates that, in 2012, Medicaid provided some level of supplemental health coverage for 9.6 million Medicare beneficiaries.

In January 2006, a new Medicare prescription drug benefit began that provides drug coverage for Medicare beneficiaries, including those who also receive coverage from Medicaid. In addition, under this benefit, individuals eligible for both Medicare and Medicaid receive a low-income subsidy for the Medicare drug plan premium and assistance with cost sharing for prescriptions. Medicaid no longer provides drug benefits for Medicare beneficiaries.

Because the Medicare drug benefit and low-income subsidy replace a portion of state Medicaid expenditures for drugs, states see a reduction in Medicaid expenditures. To offset this reduction, the Medicare Prescription Drug, Improvement, and Modernization Act (MMA) of 2003 (Public Law 108-173) requires each state to make a monthly payment to Medicare representing a percentage of the projected reduction. For 2006, this payment was 90 percent of the projected 2006 reduction in state spending. The percentage has decreased by 1⅔ percent per year since 2006 and will continue decreasing to 75 percent for 2015 and beyond.

Source: Reprinted from Klees, B. S., and C. J. Wolfe. 2014. *Medicaid Program Description and Legislative History.* Office of the Actuary, Centers for Medicare and Medicaid Services, US Department of Health and Human Services. Accessed March 13, 2014. www.ssa.gov/policy/docs/statcomps/supplement/2013/medicaid.html.

For additional information on Medicaid, see:

Kaiser Family Foundation. 2013. *Medicaid: A Primer.* Accessed March 13, 2014. https://kaiserfamilyfoundation.files.wordpress.com/2010/06/7334-05.pdf.

BRIEFLY ANNOTATED CHRONOLOGICAL LIST OF SELECTED US FEDERAL LAWS PERTAINING TO HEALTH[1]

1798

An act of July 16, 1798, passed by the Fifth Congress of the United States, taxed the employers of merchant seamen to fund arrangements for their healthcare through the Marine Hospital Service. In the language of the act, "the master or owner of every ship or vessel of the United States arriving from a foreign port into any port in the United States shall . . . render to the collector a true account of the number of seamen that shall have been employed on board such vessel . . . and shall pay to the said collector, at the rate of twenty cents per month, for every seaman so employed." The act stipulated in Section 2 that "the President of the United States is hereby authorized, out of the same, to provide for the temporary relief and mainte- nance of sick or disabled seamen in the hospitals, or other proper institutions now established in the several ports."

1882

An act of August 3, 1882, was the nation's first general immigration law and included the first federal medical excludability provisions affecting those who wished to immigrate to the United States. The act authorized state officials to board arriving ships to examine the condition of passengers. In the language of the act, "if on such examination, there shall be found among such passengers any convict, lunatic, idiot, or any person unable to take care of himself or herself with- out becoming a public charge . . . such persons shall not be permitted to land."

1891

An act of March 3, 1891, added the phrase "persons suffering from a loath- some or a contagious disease" to the list of medical excludability criteria for people seeking to immigrate to the United States.

1902

P.L. 57-244,[2] the Biologics Control Act, was the first federal law regulating the interstate and foreign sale of biologics (viruses, serums, toxins, and analogous products). The law established a national board and gave its members authority to establish regulations for licensing producers of biologics.

1906

P.L. 59-384, the Pure Food and Drug Act (also known as the Wiley Act), defined adulterated and mislabeled foods and drugs and prohibited their transport in interstate commerce. Passage of this legislation followed several years of intense campaigning by reformers and extensive newspaper coverage of examples of unwholesome and adulterated foods and of the widespread use of ineffective patent medicines.

1920

P.L. 66-141, the Snyder Act, was the first federal legislation pertaining to healthcare for Native Americans. Prior to the passage of this legislation, there were some health-related provisions in treaties between the government and the Native Americans, but this was the first formal legislation on the subject. The act provided for general assistance, directing "the Bureau of Indian Affairs, under the supervision of the Secretary of the Interior, to direct, supervise, and expend such monies as Congress may from time to time appropriate, for the benefit, care, and assistance of the Indians throughout the United States."

1921

P.L. 67-97, the Maternity and Infancy Act (also known as the Sheppard-Towner Act), provided grants to states to help them develop health services for mothers and their children. The law was allowed to lapse in 1929, although it has served as a prototype for federal grants-in-aid to the states.

1935

P.L. 74-271, the Social Security Act, a landmark law developed and passed during the Great Depression, established the Social Security program of old-age benefits. The legislation also included provisions for other benefits such as federal financial assistance to the states for their public assistance programs for low-income elderly individuals, dependent children, and blind citizens. This legislation also provided incentives for the establishment of state unemployment funds and provided financial assistance for maternal and child health and child welfare services and significantly increased federal assistance for state and local public health programs.

1936

P.L. 74-846, the Walsh-Healy Act, authorized federal regulation of industrial safety in companies doing business with the US government.

1937

P.L. 75-244, the National Cancer Institute Act, established the first categorical institute within the National Institutes of Health (NIH), which had been created in 1930 to serve as the administrative home for the research conducted by the US Public Health Service.

1938

P.L. 75-540, the LaFollette-Bulwinkle Act, provided grants-in-aid to the states to support their investigation and control of venereal disease.

P.L. 75-717, the Food, Drug, and Cosmetic Act, extended federal authority to ban new drugs from the market until they were approved by the Food and Drug Administration (FDA). This law also gave the federal government more extensive power in dealing with adulterated or mislabeled food, drugs, and cosmetic products.

1939

P.L. 76-19, the Reorganization Act, transferred the Public Health Service from the Treasury Department to the new Federal Security Agency (FSA). In 1953 the FSA was transformed into the US Department of Health, Education, and Welfare (DHEW), which, with the subsequent establishment of a new cabinet-level Department of Education in 1980, was itself transformed into the US Department of Health and Human Services (HHS).

1941

P.L. 77-146, the Nurse Training Act, provided schools of nursing with support to permit them to increase enrollments and improve their physical facilities.

1944

P.L. 78-410, the Public Health Service Act, revised and consolidated in one place all existing legislation pertaining to the US Public Health Service. The legislation provided for the organization, staffing, and functions and activities of the Public Health Service. This law has subsequently been used as a vehicle, through amendments to the legislation, for a number of important federal grant-in-aid programs.

1945

P.L. 79-15, the McCarran-Ferguson Act, expressly exempted the "business of insurance" from federal antitrust legislation (the Sherman Antitrust Act of 1890, the Clayton Act of 1914, and the Federal Trade Commission Act of 1914) to the extent that insurance was regulated by state law and did not involve "acts of boycott, coercion, or intimidation." A significant part of the underlying reasoning Congress used in exempting insurance, including health insurance, was the view that the determination of underwriting risks would require the cooperation and sharing of information among competing insurance companies.

1946

P.L. 79-487, the National Mental Health Act, authorized extensive federal support for mental health research and treatment programs and established grants-in-aid to the states for their mental health activities. The legislation also transformed the Public Health Service's Division of Mental Health into the National Institute of Mental Health.

P.L. 79-725, the Hospital Survey and Construction Act (also known as the Hill-Burton Act), was "an Act to amend the Public Health Service Act [see the 1944 P.L. 78-410 above] to authorize grants to the States for surveying their hospital and public health centers and for planning construction of additional facilities, and to authorize grants to assist in such construction." The legislation was enacted because Congress recognized a widespread shortage of hospital facilities (few were built during the Great Depression and World War II). Under provisions of the act, the states were required to submit a state plan for the construction of hospital facilities based on a survey of need to receive federal funds, which could be dispersed for projects within states.

1948

P.L. 80-655, the National Health Act, pluralized NIH by establishing a second categorical institute, the National Heart Institute. Hereafter, NIH became the National Institutes of Health.

P.L. 80-845, the Water Pollution Control Act, was enacted in part "in consequence of the benefits to the public health and welfare by the abatement of stream pollution." The act left the primary responsibility for water pollution control with the states.

1952

P.L. 82-414, the Immigration and Nationality Act (also known as the McCarran-Walter Act), followed an extensive study by Congress of immigration policy and practice. Among the law's provisions were a number of modifications in the medical excludability scheme affecting people wishing to immigrate to the United States. The act contained extensive provisions for observation and examination of aliens for the purpose of determining if they should be excluded for any of a number of specified "diseases or mental or physical defects or disabilities."

1954

P.L. 83-482, the Medical Facilities Survey and Construction Act, amended the Hill-Burton Act (see the 1946 P.L. 79-725) to greatly expand the Hill-Burton program's scope. The legislation authorized grants for surveys and construction of diagnostic and treatment centers (including hospital outpatient departments), chronic disease hospitals, rehabilitation facilities, and nursing homes.

P.L. 83-703, the Atomic Energy Act, established the Atomic Energy Commission and authorized it to license the use of atomic material in medical care.

1955

P.L. 84-159, the Air Pollution Control Act, provided for a program of research and technical assistance related to air pollution control. The law was enacted in part "in recognition of the dangers to the public health and welfare . . . from air pollution."

P.L. 84-377, the Polio Vaccination Assistance Act, provided for federal assistance to states for the operation of their polio vaccination programs.

1956

P.L. 84-569, the Dependents Medical Care Act, established the Civilian Health and Medical Program of the Uniformed Services for the dependents of military personnel.

P.L. 84-652, the National Health Survey Act, provided for the first system of regularly collected health-related data by the Public Health Service. This continuing process is called the Health Interview Survey and provides a national US household interview study of illness, disability, and health services utilization.

P.L. 84-660, the Water Pollution Control Act Amendments of 1956, amended the Water Pollution Control Act (see the 1948 P.L. 80-845) and provided for federal technical services and financial aid to the states and to municipalities in their efforts to prevent and control water pollution.

P.L. 84-911, the Health Amendments Act, amended the Public Health Service Act (see the 1944 P.L. 78-410) by initiating federal assistance for the education and training of health personnel. Specifically, the law authorized traineeships for public health personnel and advanced training for nurses. This support has been gradually broadened and extended by subsequent legislation to include many categories of health personnel.

1958

P.L. 85-544, Grants-in-Aid to Schools of Public Health, established a program of formula grants to the nation's schools of public health.

P.L. 85-929, the Food Additive Amendment, amended the Food, Drug, and Cosmetic Act (see the 1938 P.L. 75-717) to require premarketing clearance from FDA for new food additives. The so-called Delaney clause, after Representative James Delaney, who sponsored the provision, stated that "no additive shall be deemed to be safe if it is found to induce cancer when ingested by man or animal."

1959

P.L. 86-121, the Indian Sanitation Facilities Act, provided for the surgeon general to "construct, improve, extend, or otherwise provide and maintain, by contract or otherwise, essential sanitation facilities for Indian homes, communities, and lands."

P.L. 86-352, the Federal Employees Health Benefits Act, permitted Blue Cross to negotiate a contract with the Civil Service Commission to provide health insurance coverage for federal employees. The contract served as a prototype for Blue Cross's subsequent involvement in the Medicare and Medicaid programs as a fiscal intermediary.

1960

P.L. 86-778, the Social Security Amendments (also known as the Kerr-Mills Act), amended the Social Security Act (see the 1935 P.L. 74-271) to establish a new program of medical assistance for the aging population. Through this program, the federal government provided aid to the states for payments for medical care for "medically indigent" persons who were 65 years of age or older. The Kerr-Mills program, as it was called, was the forerunner of the Medicaid program established in 1965 (see P.L. 89-97).

1962

P.L. 87-692, the Health Services for Agricultural Migratory Workers Act, authorized federal grants to clinics serving migrant farmworkers and their families.

P.L. 87-781, the Drug Amendments (also known as the Kefauver-Harris amendments), amended the Food, Drug, and Cosmetic Act (see the 1938 P.L. 75-717) to significantly strengthen the provisions related to the regulation of therapeutic drugs. The changes required improved manufacturing practices and procedures and evidence that new drugs proposed for marketing be effective as well as safe. These amendments followed widespread adverse publicity about the serious negative side effects of the drug thalidomide.

1963

P.L. 88-129, the Health Professions Educational Assistance Act, inaugurated construction grants for teaching facilities that trained physicians, dentists, pharmacists, podiatrists, nurses, or professional public health personnel. The grants were made contingent on schools increasing their first-year enrollments. The legislation also provided for student loans and scholarships.

P.L. 88-156, the Maternal and Child Health and Mental Retardation Planning Amendments, amended the Social Security Act (see the 1935 P.L. 74-271). The changes were intended to "assist states and communities in preventing and combating mental retardation through expansion and improvement of the maternal and child health and crippled children's programs, through provision of prenatal, maternity, and infant care for individuals with conditions associated with childbearing that may lead to mental retardation, and through planning for comprehensive action to combat mental retardation."

P.L. 88-164, the Mental Retardation Facilities and Community Mental Health Centers Construction Act, was intended to "provide assistance in combating mental retardation through grants for construction of research centers and grants for facilities for the mentally retarded and assistance in improving mental health through grants for construction of community mental health centers, and for other purposes."

P.L. 88-206, the Clean Air Act, authorized direct grants to states and local governments to assist in their air pollution control efforts. The law also established federal enforcement of interstate air pollution restrictions.

1964

P.L. 88-352, the Civil Rights Act, affected almost every aspect of American life. Among its numerous provisions were some directly affecting healthcare. Specifically, Title VI included the provision "No person in the United States shall, on the ground of race, color, or national origin, be excluded from participation in, be denied the benefits of, or be subjected to discrimination under any program or activity receiving federal financial assistance." These words became the key to moving the nation toward racial equality in healthcare, a journey that continues. The 1946 P.L. 79-725, the Hospital Survey and Construction Act (also known as the Hill-Burton Act), included a provision requiring equal treatment of all patients in hospitals receiving funds under this program. However, the Hill-Burton Act also included a "separate but equal" provision by which hospitals could obtain funds through the program by demonstrating that quality of care in segregated facilities was equal. Because this was not actually demonstrable, this provision permitted continued discrimination until the provision was struck down by a court in the *Simkin v. Moses H. Cone Memorial Hospital* case in 1964.

P.L. 88-443, the Hospital and Medical Facilities Amendments, amended the Hill-Burton Act (see the 1946 P.L. 79-725) to specifically earmark grants for modernizing or replacing existing hospitals.

P.L. 88-452, the Economic Opportunity Act, sometimes referred to as the Antipoverty Program, was intended to "mobilize the human and financial resources of the nation to combat poverty in the United States." This broad legislation affected health in a number of ways as it sought to improve the economic and social conditions under which many people lived.

P.L. 88-581, the Nurse Training Act, added a new title, Title VIII, to the Public Health Service Act (see the 1944 P.L. 78-410). The legislation authorized separate funding for construction grants to schools of nursing, including associate degree and diploma schools. The law also provided for project grants whereby schools of nursing could strengthen their academic programs and provided for the establishment of student loan funds at these schools.

1965

P.L. 89-4, the Appalachian Redevelopment Act, sought to promote the economic, physical, and social development of the Appalachian region. Provisions in the law facilitated a number of steps to achieve this purpose, including the establishment of community health centers and training programs for health personnel.

P.L. 89-73, the Older Americans Act, established an Administration on Aging to administer programs for elderly individuals through state agencies on aging. The agenda for the joint efforts of the federal agency and the state agencies was detailed in ten specific objectives for the nation's older citizens, including several that were related to their health.

P.L. 89-92, the Federal Cigarette Labeling and Advertising Act, required that all cigarette packages sold in the United States bear the label "Caution: Cigarette Smoking May Be Hazardous to Your Health."

P.L. 89-97, the Social Security Amendments, a landmark in the nation's health policy, established two new titles to the Social Security Act (see the 1935 P.L. 74-271): (1) Title XVIII, Health Insurance for the Aged, or Medicare, and (2) Title XIX, Grants to the States for Medical Assistance Programs, or Medicaid. Enactment of these amendments followed many years of often acrimonious congressional debate about government's role and responsibility regarding ensuring access to health services for the citizenry. This legislation was made possible by the landslide dimensions of Lyndon B. Johnson's 1964 election to the presidency and by the accompanying largest Democratic majority in Congress since 1934.

In addition to establishing Titles XVIII and XIX, the Social Security Act Amendments of 1965 also amended Title V to authorize grant funds for maternal and child health and services for children with disabilities. These amendments also authorized grants for training professional personnel for the care of children with disabilities.

P.L. 89-239, the Heart Disease, Cancer and Stroke Amendments, amended the Public Health Service Act (see the 1944 P.L. 78-410) to establish a nationwide network of Regional Medical Programs. This legislation was intended to "assist in combating heart disease, cancer, stroke, and related diseases." Through its provisions, regional cooperative programs were established among medical schools, hospitals, and research institutions to foster research, training, continuing education, and demonstrations of patient care practices related to heart disease, cancer, and stroke.

P.L. 89-272, the Clean Air Act Amendments, amended the original Clean Air Act (see the 1963 P.L. 88-206) to provide for federal regulation of motor vehicle exhaust and to establish a program of federal research support and grants-in-aid in the area of solid waste disposal.

P.L. 89-290, the Health Professions Educational Assistance Amendments, amended the original act (see the 1963 P.L. 88-129) to provide further support to "improve the quality of schools of medicine, dentistry, osteopathy, optometry, and podiatry." The law expanded the availability of student loans and introduced a provision whereby 50 percent of a professional's student loan could be forgiven in exchange for practice in a designated shortage area.

1966

P.L. 89-564, the Highway Safety Act, sought to improve the nation's system of highways to make them safer for users.

P.L. 89-642, the Child Nutrition Act, established a federal program of support, including research, for child nutrition. A key component of the legislation was its authorization of the school breakfast program.

P.L. 89-749, the Comprehensive Health Planning Act (also known as the Partnership for Health Act), which amended the Public Health Service Act (see the 1944 P.L. 78-410), was intended to "promote and assist in the extension and improvement of comprehensive health planning and public health services, [and] to provide for a more effective use of available Federal funds for such planning and services." This legislation sought to promote comprehensive planning for health facilities, services, and personnel within the framework of a federal/state/local partnership. It also gave states greater flexibility in the use of their grants-in-aid for public health services through block grants.

The law, in Section 314a, authorized grants to states for the development of comprehensive state health planning and, in Section 314b, authorized grants to public or not-for-profit organizations "for developing comprehensive regional, metropolitan area or other local area plans for coordination of existing and planned health services." State planning agencies created or designated under this legislation became known as "A" agencies or as "314a" agencies. Within states, the other planning agencies created or designated under this legislation became known as "B," "areawide," or "314b" agencies.

P.L. 89-751, the Allied Health Professions Personnel Training Act, provided grant support for the training of allied health professionals. The legislation was patterned after the 1963 Health Professions Educational Assistance Act (see P.L. 88-129).

P.L. 89-794, the Economic Opportunity Act Amendments, amended the Economic Opportunity Act (see the 1964 P.L. 88-452) to establish Office of Economic Opportunity neighborhood health centers. Located especially in impoverished sections of cities and rural areas, these centers provided poor people with a comprehensive range of ambulatory health services. By the early 1970s, approximately 100 centers were to have been established under this program.

1967

P.L. 90-31, the Mental Health Amendments, amended the Mental Retardation Facilities and Community Mental Health Centers Construction Act (see the 1963 P.L. 88-164) to extend the program of construction grants for community mental health centers. The legislation also amended the term *construction* so that it covered acquisition of existing buildings.

P.L. 90-148, the Air Quality Act, amended the Clean Air Act (see the 1963 P.L. 88-206) to "authorize planning grants to air pollution control agencies; expand research provisions relating to fuels and vehicles; provide for interstate air pollution control agencies or commissions; authorize the establishment of air quality standards; and for other purposes." The act provided for each state to establish air quality standards depending on local conditions, but a minimum air quality was to be ensured through federal review of the states' standards.

P.L. 90-170, the Mental Retardation Amendments, also amended the Mental Retardation Facilities and Community Mental Health Centers Construction Act (see the 1963 P.L. 88-164) to extend the program of construction grants for university-affiliated and community-based facilities for individuals with mental retardation. The legislation also authorized a new program of grants for the education of physical educators and recreation workers who work with people who are mentally retarded and other children with disabilities and for research in these areas.

P.L. 90-174, the Clinical Laboratory Improvement Act, amended the Public Health Service Act (see the 1944 P.L. 78-410) to provide for the regulation of laboratories in interstate commerce by the Center for Disease Control through processes of licensure, standards setting, and proficiency testing.

P.L. 90-189, the Flammable Fabrics Act, was part of government's early efforts to rid the environment of hazards to human health. The legislation sought to regulate the manufacture and marketing of flammable fabrics.

P.L. 90-248, the Social Security Amendments, represented the first of many modifications to the Medicare and Medicaid programs, which were established by the Social Security Amendments of 1965 (see P.L. 89-97). Coming two years after their establishment, this legislation provided expanded coverage for such things as durable medical equipment for use in the home, podiatrist services for nonroutine foot care, outpatient physical therapy, and the addition of a lifetime reserve of 60 days of coverage for inpatient hospital care over and above the original coverage for up to 90 days during any spell of illness. In addition, certain payment rules were modified in favor of providers. For example, payment of full reasonable charges for radiologist and pathologist services provided to inpatients were authorized under one modification.

This law also sought to raise the quality of care provided in nursing homes by establishing a number of conditions that had to be met by nursing homes wanting to participate in the Medicare and Medicaid programs. There was also a provision for limiting the federal participation in medical assistance payments to families whose income did not exceed 133 percent of the income limit for Aid to Families with Dependent Children (AFDC) payments in any state.

1968

P.L. 90-490, the Health Manpower Act, extended previous programs of support for the training of health professionals (see the 1963 P.L. 88-129 and the 1964 P.L. 88-581), in effect authorizing formula institutional grants for training all health professionals.

1969

P.L. 91-173, the Federal Coal Mine Health and Safety Act, was intended to help secure and improve the health and safety of coal miners.

P.L. 91-190, the National Environmental Policy Act, was enacted to "declare a national policy which will encourage productive and enjoyable harmony between man and his environment; to promote efforts which will prevent or eliminate damage to the environment and biosphere and stimulate the health and welfare of man." This law established the Council on Environmental Quality to advise the president on environmental matters. The legislation required that environmental impact statements be prepared prior to the initiation of major federal actions.

1970

P.L. 91-222, the Public Health Cigarette Smoking Act, banned cigarette advertising from radio and television.

P.L. 91-224, the Water Quality Improvement Act, a comprehensive water pollution law, included among its numerous provisions those relating to oil pollution by vessels and on- and offshore oil wells, hazardous polluting substances other than oil, and pollution from sewage from vessels. It also provided for training people to work in the operation and maintenance of water treatment facilities. Perhaps its most important provisions, however, pertain to the procedures whereby all federal agencies must deal with water pollution, including requirements for cooperation among the various agencies.

P.L. 91-296, the Medical Facilities Construction and Modernization Amendments, amended the Hill-Burton Act (see the 1946 P.L. 79-725) by extending the program and by initiating a new program of project grants for emergency rooms, communications networks, and medical transportation systems.

P.L. 91-464, the Communicable Disease Control Amendments, amended the Public Health Service Act (see the 1944 P.L. 78-410), which had established the Communicable Disease Center (CDC), by renaming the CDC the Center for Disease Control. The legislation also broadened the CDC's functions beyond its traditional focus on communicable or infectious diseases (e.g., tuberculosis, venereal disease, rubella, measles, Rh disease, poliomyelitis, diphtheria, tetanus, whooping cough) to include other preventable conditions, including malnutrition.

P.L. 91-513, the Comprehensive Drug Abuse Prevention and Control Act, provided for special project grants for drug abuse and drug dependence treatment programs and grants for programs and activities related to drug education.

P.L. 91-572, the Family Planning Services and Population Research Act, established the Office of Population Affairs and added Title X, Population Research and Voluntary Family Planning Programs, to the Public Health

Service Act (see the 1944 P.L. 78-410). The legislation authorized a range of projects, formulas, training, and research grants and contracts to support family planning programs and services, except for abortion.

P.L. 91-596, the Occupational Safety and Health Act, established an extensive federal program of standard-setting and enforcement activities that were intended to ensure healthful and safe workplaces.

P.L. 91-601, the Poison Prevention Packaging Act, required that most drugs be dispensed in containers designed to be difficult for children to open.

P.L. 91-604, the Clean Air Amendments, was enacted because Congress became dissatisfied with progress toward control and abatement of air pollution under the Air Quality Act of 1967 (see the 1967 P.L. 90-148). This law took away the power of the states to establish different air quality standards in different air quality control regions. Instead, this legislation required states to achieve national air quality standards within each of their regions.

P.L. 91-616, the Comprehensive Alcohol Abuse and Alcoholism Prevention, Treatment, and Rehabilitation Act, established the National Institute of Alcohol Abuse and Alcoholism. The law provided a separate statutory base for programs and activities related to alcohol abuse and alcoholism. The legislation also provided a comprehensive program of aid to states and localities in their efforts addressed to combating alcohol abuse and alcoholism.

P.L. 91-623, the Emergency Health Personnel Act, amended the Public Health Service Act (see the 1944 P.L. 78-410) to permit the secretary of DHEW (now HHS) to assign commissioned officers and other health personnel of the US Public Health Service to areas of the country experiencing critical shortages of health personnel. This legislation also established the National Health Service Corps.

P.L. 91-695, the Lead-Based Paint Poisoning Prevention Act, represented a specific attempt to address the problem of lead-based paint poisoning through a program of grants to the states to aid them in their efforts to combat this problem.

1971

P.L. 92-157, the Comprehensive Health Manpower Training Act, at the time of its enactment was the most comprehensive health personnel legislation yet enacted. The legislation replaced institutional formula grants with a new system of capitation grants through which health professions schools received fixed sums of money for each of their students (contingent on increasing first-year enrollments). Loan provisions were broadened so that health professionals who practiced in designated personnel shortage areas could cancel 85 percent of education loans. The legislation also established the National

Health Manpower Clearinghouse, and the secretary of DHEW (now HHS) was directed to make every effort to provide to counties without physicians at least one National Health Service Corps physician.

1972

P.L. 92-294, the National Sickle Cell Anemia Control Act, authorized grants and contracts to support screening, treatment, counseling, information and education programs, and research related to sickle-cell anemia.

P.L. 92-303, the Federal Coal Mine Health and Safety Amendments, amended the earlier Federal Coal Mine Health and Safety Act (see the 1969 P.L. 91-173) to provide financial benefits and other assistance to coal miners who were afflicted with black lung disease.

P.L. 92-426, the Uniformed Services Health Professions Revitalization Act, established the Uniformed Services University of the Health Sciences. The legislation provided for this educational institution to be operated under the auspices of the US Department of Defense in Bethesda, Maryland. The legislation also created the Armed Forces Health Professions Scholarship Program.

P.L. 92-433, the National School Lunch and Child Nutrition Amendments, amended the Child Nutrition Act (see the 1966 P.L. 89-642) to add support for the provision of nutritious diets for pregnant and lactating women and for infants and children (the WIC program).

P.L. 92-573, the Consumer Product Safety Act, established the Consumer Product Safety Commission to develop safety standards and regulations for consumer products. Under provisions of the legislation, the administration of existing related legislation, including the Flammable Fabrics Act, the Hazardous Substances Act, and the Poison Prevention Packaging Act, was transferred to the commission.

P.L. 92-574, the Noise Control Act, much like the earlier Clean Air Act (see the 1963 P.L. 88-206) and the Flammable Fabrics Act (see the 1967 P.L. 90-189), continued government's efforts to rid the environment of harmful influences on human health.

P.L. 92-603, the Social Security Amendments, amended the Social Security Act (see the 1935 P.L. 74-271) to make several significant changes in the Medicare program. These amendments marked an important shift in the operation of the Medicare program as efforts were undertaken to help control its growing costs. Over the bitter opposition of organized medicine, the legislation established professional standards review organizations (PSROs) that were to monitor both the quality of services provided to Medicare beneficiaries and the medical necessity for the services.

One provision limited payments for capital expenditures by hospitals that had been disapproved by state or local planning agencies. Another provision authorized a program of grants and contracts to conduct experiments and demonstrations related to achieving increased economy and efficiency in the provision of health services. Some of the specifically targeted areas of these studies were to be prospective reimbursement, the requirement that patients spend three days in the hospital prior to admission to a skilled nursing home, the potential benefits of ambulatory surgery centers, payment for the services of physician assistants and nurse practitioners, and the use of clinical psychologists.

Coincident with these and other cost-containment amendments, several cost-increasing changes were also made in the Medicare program by this legislation. Notably, persons who were eligible for cash benefits under the disability provisions of the Social Security Act for at least 24 months were made eligible for medical benefits under the program. In addition, persons who were insured under Social Security, as well as their dependents, who required hemodialysis or renal transplantation for chronic renal disease were defined as disabled for the purpose of having them covered under the Medicare program for the costs of treating their end-stage renal disease (ESRD). The inclusion of coverage for individuals with disabilities and ESRD patients in 1972 was an extraordinarily expensive change in the Medicare program. In addition, certain less costly but still expensive additional coverages were extended, including chiropractic services and speech pathology services.

P.L. 92-714, the National Cooley's Anemia Control Act, authorized grants and contracts to support screening, treatment, counseling, information and education programs, and research related to Cooley's anemia.

1973

P.L. 93-29, the Older Americans Act, established the National Clearinghouse for Information on Aging and created the Federal Council on Aging. The legislation also authorized funds to establish gerontology centers and provided grants for training and research related to the field of aging.

P.L. 93-154, the Emergency Medical Services Systems Act, provided aid to states and localities to assist them in developing coordinated emergency medical service systems.

P.L. 93-222, the Health Maintenance Organization Act, amended the Public Health Service Act (see the 1944 P.L. 78-410) to "provide assistance and encouragement for the establishment and expansion of health maintenance organizations." The legislation—which added a new title, Title XIII, Health Maintenance Organizations (HMOs), to the Public Health Service

Act—authorized a program of grants, loans, and loan guarantees to support the conduct of feasibility and development studies and initial operations for new HMOs.

1974

P.L. 93-247, the Child Abuse Prevention and Treatment Act, created the National Center on Child Abuse and Neglect. The legislation authorized grants for research and demonstrations related to child abuse and neglect.

P.L. 93-270, the Sudden Infant Death Syndrome Act, added Part C, Sudden Infant Death Syndrome, to Title XI of the Public Health Service Act (see the 1944 P.L. 78-410). The legislation provided for the development of informational programs related to this syndrome for both public and professional audiences.

P.L. 93-296, the Research in Aging Act, established the National Institute on Aging within the NIH.

P.L. 93-344, the Congressional Budget and Impoundment Control Act, and its subsequent amendments provided Congress with the procedures through which it establishes target levels for revenues, expenditures, and the overall deficit for the coming fiscal year (FY). The congressional budget procedures are designed to coordinate decisions on sources and levels of federal revenues and on the objectives and levels of federal expenditures. These decisions have substantial impact on health policy. The procedures formally begin each year with the initial decision as to the overall size of the budget pie for a given year, as well as the sizes of its various pieces. To accomplish this, each year Congress adopts a concurrent resolution that imposes overall constraints on spending, based in part on the size of the anticipated revenue budget for the year, and distributes the overall constraint on spending among groups of programs and activities. These constraints are implemented through the reconciliation process. The result of this process is the annual omnibus reconciliation bill, which is a packaging together of all legislative changes made in the various standing committees necessitated by reconciling existing law with the budgetary targets established earlier in the concurrent resolution on the budget.

This act also established the US Congressional Budget Office (CBO). The nonpartisan CBO conducts studies and analyses of the fiscal and budget implications of various decisions facing Congress, including those related to health.

P.L. 93-360, the Nonprofit Hospital Amendments, amended the 1947 Labor–Management Relations Act (or the Taft-Hartley Act) to end the exclusion of nongovernmental, nonprofit hospitals from the provisions of this act as well as from the earlier National Labor Relations Act of 1935 (or the Wagner Act). Both of these acts pertain to fair labor practices and collective bargaining.

P.L. 93-406, the Employee Retirement Income Security Act (also known as ERISA), provided for the regulation of almost all pension and benefit plans for employees, including pensions, medical or hospital benefits, disability, and death benefits. The legislation provides for the regulation of many features of these benefit plans.

P.L. 93-523, the Safe Drinking Water Act, required the Environmental Protection Agency (EPA) to establish national drinking water standards and to aid states and localities in the enforcement of these standards.

P.L. 93-641, the National Health Planning and Resources Development Act, amended the Public Health Service Act (see the 1944 P.L. 78-410) in an attempt to ensure "the development of a national health policy and of effective state and area health planning and resource development programs, and for other purposes." The legislation added two new titles, XV and XVI, to the Public Health Service Act. These titles superseded and significantly modified the programs established under Sections 314a and 314b of Title III of the 1966 P.L. 89-749, the Comprehensive Health Planning Act (or the Partnership for Health Act) as well as the programs established under the Hill-Burton Act (see the 1946 P.L. 79-725).

The legislation essentially folded existing health planning activities into a new framework created by the legislation. The secretary of DHEW (now HHS) was to enter into an agreement with each state's governor for the designation of a state health planning and development agency (SHPDA). The states were to also establish state health coordinating councils to serve as advisors in setting overall state policy.

A network of local health systems agencies (HSAs) covering the entire nation was established by the legislation. The HSAs were to (1) improve the health of area residents; (2) increase the accessibility, acceptability, continuity, and quality of health services; and (3) restrain healthcare cost increases and prevent duplication of healthcare services and facilities. An important feature of the planning framework created by P.L. 93-641 was a provision that permitted the HSAs in states that had established certificate-of-need (CON) programs to conduct CON reviews and to make recommendations developed at the local level to the SHPDA.

Congress repealed this law in 1986 (effective January 1, 1987), leaving responsibility for the CON programs entirely in the hands of the states.

P.L. 93-647, the Social Security Amendments (also known as the Social Services Amendments), amended the Social Security Act (see the 1935 P.L. 74-271) to consolidate existing federal–state social service programs into a block grant program that would permit a ceiling on federal matching funds while providing more flexibility to the states in providing certain social services. The legislation added a new title, Title XX, Grants to the States for Services, to the Social Security Act.

The goals of the legislation pertained to the prevention and remedy of neglect, abuse, or exploitation of children or adults, the preservation of families, and the avoidance of inappropriate institutional care by substituting community-based programs and services. Social services covered under this law included childcare service; protective, foster, and daycare services for children and adults; counseling; family planning services; homemaker services; and home-delivered meals.

1976

P.L. 94-295, the Medical Devices Amendments, amended the Food, Drug, and Cosmetic Act (see the 1938 P.L. 75-717) to strengthen the regulation of medical devices. This legislation was passed, after previous attempts had failed, amid growing public concern with the adverse effects of such medical devices as the Dalcon Shield intrauterine device.

P.L. 94-317, the National Consumer Health Information and Health Promotion Act, amended the Public Health Service Act (see the 1944 P.L. 78-410) to add Title XVII, Health Information and Promotion. The legislation authorized grants and contracts for research and community programs related to health information, health promotion, preventive health services, and education of the public in the appropriate use of healthcare services.

P.L. 94-437, the Indian Health Care Improvement Act, an extensive piece of legislation, was intended to fill existing gaps in the delivery of healthcare services to Native Americans.

P.L. 94-460, the Health Maintenance Organization Amendments, amended the Health Maintenance Organization Act (see the 1973 P.L. 93-222) to ease the requirements that had to be met for an HMO to become federally qualified. One provision, however, required that HMOs must be federally qualified if they were to receive reimbursement from the Medicare or Medicaid programs.

P.L. 94-469, the Toxic Substances Control Act (TSCA), sought to regulate chemical substances used in various production processes. The legislation defined chemical substances broadly. The purpose of TSCA was to identify potentially harmful chemical substances before they were produced and entered the marketplace and, subsequently, the environment.

P.L. 94-484, the Health Professions Educational Assistance Act, extended the program of capitation grants to professional schools that had been established under the Comprehensive Health Manpower Training Act (see the 1971 P.L. 92-157). However, this legislation dropped the requirement that schools increase their first-year enrollments as a condition for receiving grants. Under this legislation, medical schools were required to have 50 percent of their graduates enter residency programs in primary care by 1980. They were also required to reserve positions in their third-year classes for US citizens who were studying medicine in foreign medical schools. However, under intense protest from medical schools, this earlier provision was repealed in 1975.

1977

P.L. 95-142, the Medicare-Medicaid Antifraud and Abuse Amendments, amended the legislation governing the Medicare and Medicaid programs (see the 1965 P.L. 89-97) in an attempt to reduce fraud and abuse in the programs as a means to help contain their costs. Specific changes included strengthening criminal and civil penalties for fraud and abuse affecting the programs, modifying the operations of the PSROs, and promulgating uniform reporting systems and formats for hospitals and certain other healthcare organizations participating in the Medicare and Medicaid programs.

P.L. 95-210, the Rural Health Clinic Services Amendments, amended the legislation governing the Medicare and Medicaid programs (see the 1965 P.L. 89-97) to modify the categories of practitioners who could provide reimbursable services to Medicare and Medicaid beneficiaries, at least in rural settings. Under the provisions of this act, rural health clinics that did not routinely have physicians available on site could, if they met certain requirements regarding physician supervision of the clinic and review of services, be reimbursed for services provided by nurse practitioners and physician assistants through the Medicare and Medicaid programs. This act also authorized certain demonstration projects in underserved urban areas for reimbursement of these nonphysician practitioners.

1978

P.L. 95-292, the Medicare End-Stage Renal Disease Amendments, further amended the legislation governing the Medicare program (see the 1965 P.L. 89-97) in an attempt to help control the program's costs. Since the addition of coverage for ESRD under the Social Security Amendments of 1972 (P.L. 92-603), the costs to the Medicare program had risen steadily and quickly. This legislation added incentives to encourage the use of home dialysis and renal transplantation in ESRD.

The legislation also permitted the use of a variety of reimbursement methods for renal dialysis facilities, and it authorized funding for the conduct of studies of ESRD itself, especially studies incorporating possible cost reductions in treatment for this disease. It also directed the secretary of DHEW (now HHS) to establish areawide network coordinating councils to help plan for and review ESRD programs.

P.L. 95-559, the Health Maintenance Organization Amendments, further amended the Health Maintenance Organization Act (see the 1973 P.L. 93-222) to add a new program of loans and loan guarantees to support the acquisition of ambulatory care facilities and related equipment. The legislation also provided for support for a program of training for HMO administrators and medical directors and for providing technical assistance to HMOs in their developmental efforts.

1979

P.L. 96-79, the Health Planning and Resources Development Amendments, amended the National Health Planning and Resources Development Act (see the 1974 P.L. 93-641) to add provisions intended to foster competition within the health sector, to address the need to integrate mental health and alcoholism and drug abuse resources into health system plans, and to make several revisions in the CON requirements.

1980

P.L. 96-398, the Mental Health Systems Act, extensively amended the Community Mental Health Centers program (the 1970 P.L. 91-211) by including provisions for the development and support of comprehensive state mental health systems. Subsequently, however, this legislation was almost completely superseded by the block grants to the states for mental health and alcohol and drug abuse that were provided under the Omnibus Budget Reconciliation Act of 1981 (see P.L. 97-35).

P.L. 96-499, the Omnibus Budget Reconciliation Act (OBRA '80), was contained in Title IX of the Medicare and Medicaid Amendments of 1980. These amendments made extensive modifications in the Medicare and Medicaid programs, with 57 separate sections pertaining to one or both of the programs. Many of the changes reflected continuing concern with the growing costs of the programs and were intended to help control these costs.

Examples of the changes that were specific to Medicare included removal of the 100 visits per year limitation on home health services and the requirement that patients pay a deductible for home care visits under Part B of the program. These changes were intended to encourage home care over more expensive institutional care. Another provision permitted small rural hospitals to use their beds as "swing beds" (alternating their use as acute or long-term care beds as needed) and authorized swing-bed demonstration projects for large and urban hospitals. An important change in the Medicaid program required the programs to pay for the services that the states had authorized nurse-midwives to perform.

P.L. 96-510, the Comprehensive Environmental Response, Compensation and Liability Act, established the Superfund program that intended to provide resources for the cleanup of inactive hazardous waste dumps. The legislation assigned retroactive liability for the costs of cleaning up the dumps to their owners and operators as well as to the waste generators and transporters who had used the dump sites.

1981

P.L. 97-35, the Omnibus Budget Reconciliation Act (OBRA '81), in its Title XXI, Subtitles A, B, and C, contained further amendments to the Medicare and Medicaid programs. Just as in 1980, this legislation included extensive changes in the programs, with 46 sections pertaining to them. Enacted in the context of extensive efforts to reduce the federal budget, many of the provisions hit Medicare and Medicaid especially hard. For example, one provision eliminated the coverage of alcohol detoxification facility services, another removed the use of occupational therapy as a basis for initial entitlement to home health service, and yet another increased the Part B deductible.

In other provisions, OBRA '81 combined 20 existing categorical public health programs into four block grants. The block grants were (1) Preventive Health and Health Services, which combined such previously categorical programs as rodent control, fluoridation, hypertension control, and rape crisis centers among others into one block grant to be distributed among the states by a formula based on population and other factors; (2) Alcohol Abuse, Drug Abuse, and Mental Health Block Grant, which combined existing programs created under the Community Mental Health Centers Act, the Mental Health Systems Act, the Comprehensive Alcohol Abuse and Alcoholism Prevention, Treatment, and Rehabilitation Act, and the Drug Abuse, Prevention, Treatment, and Rehabilitation Act; (3) Primary Care Block Grant, which consisted of the Community Health Centers; and (4) Maternal and Child Health Block Grant, which consolidated seven previously categorical grant programs from Title V of the Social Security Act and from the Public Health Services Act, including the maternal and child health and children with disabilities programs, genetic disease service, adolescent pregnancy services, sudden infant death syndrome, hemophilia treatment, Supplemental Security Income payments to children with disabilities, and lead-based poisoning prevention.

1982

P.L. 97-248, the Tax Equity and Fiscal Responsibility Act (TEFRA), made a number of important changes in the Medicare program. One provision added coverage for hospice services provided to Medicare beneficiaries. These benefits were extended later and are now an integral part of the Medicare program. However, the most important provisions, in terms of impact on the Medicare program, were those that sought to control the program's costs by setting limits on how much Medicare would reimburse hospitals on a per-case basis and by limiting the annual rate of increase for Medicare's reasonable costs per discharge. These changes in reimbursement methodology represented fundamental changes in the Medicare program and reflected a dramatic shift in the nation's Medicare policy.

Another provision of TEFRA replaced PSROs, which had been established by the Social Security Amendments of 1972 (see P.L. 92-603), with a new utilization and quality control program called peer review organizations. The TEFRA changes regarding the operation of the Medicare program were extensive, but they were only the harbinger of the most sweeping legislative changes in the history of the Medicare program the following year.

P.L. 97-414, the Orphan Drug Act, provided financial incentives for the development and marketing of orphan drugs, defined by the legislation to be drugs for the treatment of diseases or conditions affecting so few people that revenues from sales of the drugs would not cover their development costs.

1983

P.L. 98-21, the Social Security Amendments, another landmark in the evolution of the Medicare program, amended the legislation governing the program (see the 1965 P.L. 89-97) to initiate the Medicare prospective payment system (PPS). The legislation included provisions to base payment for hospital inpatient services on predetermined rates per discharge for diagnosis-related groups (DRGs). PPS was a major departure from the cost-based system of reimbursement that had been used in the Medicare program since its inception in 1965. The legislation also directed the administration to study physician payment reform options, a feature that was to later have significant impact (see the 1989 P.L. 10-239).

1984

P.L. 98-369, the Deficit Reduction Act (DEFRA), among many provisions, temporarily froze increases in physicians' fees paid under the Medicare program. Another provision in the legislation placed a specific limitation on the rate of increase in the DRG payment rates that the secretary of HHS could permit in the two subsequent years.

The legislation also established the Medicare Participating Physician/Supplier (PARDOC) program and created two classes of physicians in regard to their relationships to the Medicare program and outlined different reimbursement approaches for them depending on whether they were classified as "participating" or "nonparticipating." As part of this legislation, Congress mandated that the Office of Technology Assessment study alternative methods of paying for physician services so that the information could guide the reform of the Medicare program.

P.L. 98-417, the Drug Price Competition and Patent Term Restoration Act, provided brand-name pharmaceutical manufacturers with patent term extensions. These extensions significantly increased manufacturers' opportunities for earning profits during the longer effective patent life of their affected products.

P.L. 98-457, the Child Abuse Amendments, amended the Child Abuse Prevention and Treatment Act (see the 1974 P.L. 93-247) to involve Infant Care Review Committees in the medical decisions regarding the treatment of handicapped newborns, at least in hospitals with tertiary-level neonatal care units.

The legislation established treatment and reporting guidelines for newborns who were severely disabled, making it illegal to withhold "medically indicated treatment" from newborns except when "in the treating physician's reasonable medical judgment, (i) the infant is chronically and irreversibly comatose; (ii) the provision of such treatment would merely prolong dying, not be effective in ameliorating or correcting all of the infant's life-threatening conditions, or otherwise be futile in terms of survival of the infant; or (iii) the provision of such treatment would be virtually futile in terms of the survival of the infant and the treatment itself under such circumstances would be inhumane."

P.L. 98-507, the National Organ Transplant Act, made it illegal to "knowingly acquire, receive, or otherwise transfer any human organ for valuable consideration for use in human transplantation if the transfer affects interstate commerce."

1985

P.L. 99-177, the Emergency Deficit Reduction and Balanced Budget Act (also known as the Gramm-Rudman-Hollings Act), established mandatory deficit reduction targets for the five subsequent fiscal years. Under provisions of the legislation, the required budget cuts would come equally from defense spending and from domestic programs that were not exempted. The Gramm-Rudman-Hollings Act had significant impact on the Medicare program throughout the last half of the 1980s, as well as on other health programs such as community and migrant health centers, veteran and Native American health, health professions education, and the NIH. Among other things, this legislation led to substantial cuts in Medicare payments to hospitals and physicians.

P.L. 99-272, the Consolidated Omnibus Budget Reconciliation Act (COBRA '85), contained a number of provisions that affected the Medicare program. Hospitals that served a disproportionate share of poor patients received an adjustment in their PPS payments; hospice care was made a permanent part of the Medicare program, and states were given the ability to provide hospice services under the Medicaid program; FY1986 PPS payment rates were frozen at 1985 levels through May 1, 1986, and increased 0.5 percent for the remainder of the year; payment to hospitals for the indirect costs of medical education was modified; and a schedule to phase out payment of a return on equity to proprietary hospitals was established.

This legislation established the Physician Payment Review Commission (PPRC) to advise Congress on physician payment policies for the Medicare program. The legislation also required that PPRC advise Congress and the secretary of HHS regarding the development of a resource-based relative value scale for physician services.

Under another of COBRA's important provisions, employers were required to continue health insurance for employees and their dependents who would otherwise lose their eligibility for the coverage because of reduced hours of work or termination of their employment.

1986

P.L. 99-509, the Omnibus Budget Reconciliation Act (OBRA '86), altered the PPS payment rate for hospitals once again and reduced payment amounts for capital-related costs by 3.5 percent for part of FY1987, by 7 percent for FY1988, and by 10 percent for FY1989. In addition, certain adjustments were made in the manner in which "outlier" or atypical cases were reimbursed.

The legislation established further limits to balance billing by physicians providing services to Medicare clients by setting "maximum allowable actual charges" for physicians who did not participate in the PARDOC program (see the Deficit Reduction Act of 1984, P.L. 98-369). In another provision intended to realize savings for the Medicare program, OBRA '86 directed HHS to use the concept of "inherent reasonableness" to reduce payments for cataract surgery as well as for anesthesia during the surgery.

P.L. 99-660, the Omnibus Health Act, contained provisions to significantly liberalize coverage under the Medicaid program. Using family income up to the federal poverty line as a criterion, this change permitted states to offer coverage to all pregnant women, infants up to one year of age, and, by using a phase-in schedule, children up to five years of age.

One part of this omnibus health legislation was the National Childhood Vaccine Injury Act. This law established a federal vaccine injury compensation system. Under provisions of the legislation, parties injured by vaccines would be limited to awards of income losses plus $250,000 for pain and suffering or death.

Another important part of the omnibus health legislation of 1986 was the Health Care Quality Improvement Act. This law provided immunity from private damage lawsuits under federal or state law for "any professional review action" so long as that action followed standards set out in the legislation. This afforded members of peer review committees protection from most damage suits filed by physicians whom they disciplined. The law also mandated creation of a national data bank through which information on physician licensure actions, sanctions by boards of medical examiners, malpractice claims paid, and professional review actions that adversely affect the clinical privileges of physicians could be provided to authorized persons and organizations.

1987

P.L. 100-177, the National Health Service Corps Amendments, reauthorized the National Health Service Corps (NHSC), which had been created under a provision of the Emergency Health Personnel Act of 1970 (see P.L. 91-623).

P.L. 100-203, the Omnibus Budget Reconciliation Act (OBRA '87), contained a number of provisions that directly affected the Medicare program. It required the secretary of HHS to update the wage index used in calculating hospital PPS payments by October 1, 1990, and to do so at least every three years thereafter. It also required the secretary to study and report to Congress on the criteria being used by the Medicare program to identify referral hospitals. Deepening the reductions established by OBRA '86, one provision of the act reduced payment amounts for capital-related costs by 12 percent for FY1988 and by 15 percent for FY1989.

Regarding payments to physicians for services provided to Medicare clients, the legislation reduced fees for 12 sets of "overvalued" procedures. It also allowed higher fee increases for primary care than for other physician services and increased the fee differential between participating and nonparticipating physicians (see the 1984 P.L. 98-369).

The legislation also contained a number of provisions that affected the Medicaid program. Key among these, the law provided additional options for children and pregnant women and required states to cover eligible children up to age six with an option for allowing coverage up to age eight. The distinction between skilled nursing facilities (SNFs) and intermediate care facilities was eliminated. The legislation contained a number of provisions intended to enhance the quality of services provided in nursing homes, including requirements that nursing homes enhance the quality of life of each resident and operate quality assurance programs.

1988

P.L. 100-360, the Medicare Catastrophic Coverage Act, provided the largest expansion of the benefits covered under the Medicare program since its establishment in 1965 (see P.L. 89-97). Among other things, provisions of this legislation added coverage for outpatient prescription drugs and respite care and placed a cap on out-of-pocket spending by elderly individuals for copayment costs for covered services.

The legislation included provisions that would have the new benefits phased in over a four-year period and paid for by premiums charged to Medicare program enrollees. Thirty-seven percent of the costs were to be covered by a fixed monthly premium paid by all enrollees, and the remainder of the costs were to be covered by an income-related supplemental premium that was, in effect, an income surtax that would apply to fewer than half of the enrollees. Under intense pressure from many of their older constituents and their interest groups who objected to having to pay additional premiums or the income surtax, Congress repealed P.L. 100-360 in 1989 without implementing most of its provisions.

P.L. 100-578, the Clinical Laboratory Improvement Amendments, amended the Clinical Laboratory Improvement Act (see the 1967 P.L. 90-174) to extend and modify government's ability to regulate clinical laboratories.

P.L. 100-582, the Medical Waste Tracking Act, was enacted in response to the highly publicized incidents of used and discarded syringes and needles washing up on the shores of a number of states in the eastern United States in the summer of 1988. The legislation itself was rather limited in that it focused on the tracking of medical wastes from their origin to their disposal rather than on the broader regulation of transportation and disposal of these wastes.

P.L. 100-607, the National Organ Transplant Amendments, amended the National Organ Transplant Act (see the 1984 P.L. 98-507) to extend the prohibition against the sale of human organs to the organs and other body parts of human fetuses.

P.L. 100-647, the Technical and Miscellaneous Revenue Act, directed the PPRC (see the 1985 P.L. 99-272) to consider policies for moderating the rate of increase in expenditures for physician services in the Medicare program and for reducing the utilization of these services.

1989

P.L. 101-239, the Omnibus Budget Reconciliation Act (OBRA '89), included provisions for minor, primarily technical, changes in PPS and a provision to extend coverage for mental health benefits and add coverage for Pap smears. Small adjustments were made in the disproportionate share regulations, and the 15 percent capital-related payment reduction established in OBRA '87 was continued in OBRA '89. Another provision required the secretary of HHS to update the wage index annually in a budget-neutral manner beginning in FY1993.

As part of the OBRA '89 legislation, the Health Care Financing Administration was directed to begin implementing a resource-based relative value scale for reimbursing physicians under the Medicare program on January 1, 1992. The new system was to be phased in over a four-year period beginning in 1992.

Another important provision in this legislation initiated the establishment of the Agency for Health Care Policy and Research (now the Agency for Healthcare Research and Quality). This agency succeeded the National Center for Health Services Research and Technology Assessment. The new agency was created to conduct or foster the conduct of studies of healthcare quality, effectiveness, and efficiency. In particular, the agency was to conduct or foster the conduct of studies on the outcomes of medical treatments and provide technical assistance to groups seeking to develop practice guidelines.

1990

P.L. 101-336, the Americans with Disabilities Act, provided a broad range of protections for people with disabilities, in effect combining protections contained in the Civil Rights Act of 1964, the Rehabilitation Act of 1973, and the Civil Rights Restoration Act of 1988. The central goal of the legislation was independence for those individuals, to assist them in being self-supporting and able to lead independent lives.

P.L. 101-381, the Ryan White Comprehensive AIDS Resources Emergency Act, provided resources to 16 epicenters, including San Francisco and New York City, and to states hardest hit by acquired immunodeficiency syndrome (AIDS) to assist them in coping with the skyrocketing cost of care and treatment.

P.L. 101-508, the Omnibus Budget Reconciliation Act (OBRA '90), contained the Patient Self-Determination Act, which required healthcare institutions participating in the Medicare and Medicaid programs to provide all of their patients with written information on policies regarding self-determination and living wills. The institutions were also required under this legislation to inquire whether patients had advance medical directives and to document the replies in the patients' medical records.

The legislation made additional minor changes in PPS, including further adjustments in the wage index calculation and in the disproportionate share regulations. Regarding the wage index, one provision required the Prospective Payment Assessment Commission, which was established by the 1983 Social Security Amendments (see P.L. 98-21) to help guide Congress and the secretary of HHS on implementing PPS to further study the available data on wages by occupational category and to develop recommendations on modifying the wage index to account for occupational mix.

The legislation also included a provision that continued the 15 percent capital-related payment reduction that was established in OBRA '87 and continued in OBRA '89 and another provision that made the reduced teaching adjustment payment established in OBRA '87 permanent. One of its more important provisions provided a five-year deficit reduction plan that was to reduce total Medicare outlays by more than $43 billion between FY1991 and FY1995.

P.L. 101-629, the Safe Medical Devices Act, further amended the Federal Food, Drug and Cosmetic Act (see the 1938 P.L. 75-717) and the subsequent Medical Devices Amendments of 1976 (see P.L. 94-295) to require institutions that use medical devices to report device-related problems to the manufacturers and/or to FDA. Reportable problems include any incident in which any medical device may have caused or contributed to any person's death, serious illness, or serious injury.

P.L. 101-649, the Immigration and Nationality Act of 1990, restructured with minor modifications the medical exclusion scheme for screening people who desired to immigrate to the United States that had been in use since the enactment of the Immigration and Nationality Act of 1952 (see P.L. 82-414).

1992

P.L. 102-585, the Veterans Health Care Act, required the Department of Veterans Affairs to establish in each of its hospitals suitable indoor and outdoor smoking areas. This law ran counter to the department's 1991 internal policy of running its hospitals on a smoke-free basis and was out of step with the private-sector movement to establishing smoke-free hospitals.

1993

P.L. 103-43, the National Institutes of Health Revitalization Act, contained provisions for a number of structural and budgetary changes in the operation of NIH. It also set forth guidelines for the conduct of research on transplantation of human fetal tissue and added human immunodeficiency virus (HIV) infection to the list of excludable conditions covered by the Immigration and Nationality Act (see the 1990 P.L. 101-649).

P.L. 103-66, the Omnibus Budget Reconciliation Act (OBRA '93), established an all-time-record five-year cut in Medicare funding and included a number of other changes affecting the Medicare program. For example, the legislation included provisions to end return on equity payments for capital to proprietary SNFs and reduced the previously established rate of increase in payment rates for care provided in hospices. In addition, the legislation cut laboratory fees drastically by changing the reimbursement formula and froze payments for durable medical equipment, parenteral and enteral services, and orthotics and prosthetics in FY1994 and FY1995.

OBRA '93 contained the Comprehensive Childhood Immunization Act, which provided $585 million to support the provision of vaccines for children eligible for Medicaid, children who do not have health insurance, and Native American children.

Note on 1994 and 1995

Chronologies of American health policy will always show these years as a period in which health policymaking appeared dormant because almost no important new federal laws pertaining to health, nor amendments to existing laws, were enacted. This apparent dearth of health policy, however, is misleading. This was a period of extraordinary consideration of health legislation, although little was enacted. President Clinton attempted a fundamental reform of the American healthcare system through the introduction of his Health Security proposal in late 1993. The proposed legislation died with the 1994 Congress. The debate consumed almost all of the health-related legislation development energy expended during 1994. Then, following this bill's demise, the 1995 attempt to enact unprecedented cutbacks in the Medicare and Medicaid programs as part of a far-reaching budget reconciliation bill that sought a balanced federal budget ended in a veto by President Clinton. The political wrangling over the budget grew even worse in 1996. Proposed changes in the Medicare and Medicaid programs, changes that were linked to the development of a plan to balance the federal budget over a seven-year span, would have meant massive cuts in these programs. The differences over these plans between the Republican-controlled Congress and President Clinton, a Democrat, were so fundamental that they led to a complete impasse in the budget negotiations in 1996, including a brief shutdown of the federal government in the absence of budget authority to operate.

1995

P.L. 104-65, the Lobbying Disclosure Act, contained provisions requiring registration with the secretary of the Senate and the clerk of the House of Representatives by any individual lobbyist (or the individual's employer if it employs one or more lobbyists) within 45 days after the individual first makes, or is employed or retained to make, a lobbying contact with either the president, the vice president, a member of Congress, or any of a number of specified federal officers. This law defines a lobbyist as any individual employed or retained by a client for financial or other compensation for services that include more than one lobbying contact, unless the individual's lobbying activities constitute less than 20 percent of the time engaged in the services provided to that client over a six-month period.

1996

P.L. 104-134, the Departments of Veterans Affairs, Housing and Urban Development, and Independent Agencies Appropriations Act, contained several provisions that offered certain protections for enrollees in managed care plans. One provision prohibited plans from restricting hospital stays for mothers and newborns to less than 48 hours for vaginal deliveries and 96 hours following a cesarean section. Another provision required that group health plans that offer both medical and surgical benefits and mental health benefits not impose a more restrictive lifetime or annual limit on mental health benefits than is imposed on medical or surgical benefits.

P.L. 104-191, the Health Insurance Portability and Accountability Act (HIPAA; also known as the Kassebaum-Kennedy Act), provided employees who work for companies that offer health insurance to their employees with guaranteed access to health insurance in the event that they change jobs or become unemployed. In addition, the legislation guaranteed renewability of health insurance coverage so long as premiums are paid. It also provided for increased tax deductions for the self-employed who purchase health insurance and allowed tax deductions for medical expenses related to long-term care insurance coverage. The legislation also established a limited "medical savings accounts" demonstration project.

P.L. 104-193, the Personal Responsibility and Work Opportunity Reconciliation Act (also known as the Welfare Reform Act), made significant changes in the nation's welfare policy, with implications for such health determinants as the social and economic environments faced by affected people, and affected eligibility for the Medicaid program in a fundamental way. Since the establishment of the Medicaid program in 1965 (see P.L. 89-97), eligibility for a key welfare benefit, AFDC, and eligibility for Medicaid benefits have been linked. Families receiving AFDC have been automatically eligible for Medicaid and enrolled in the Medicaid program. The Personal Responsibility and Work Opportunity Reconciliation Act, however, replaced AFDC with the Temporary Assistance to Needy Families (TANF) block grant. Under the provisions of the TANF block grant, states are given broad flexibility to design income support and work programs for low-income families with children and are required to impose federally mandated restrictions, such as time limits, on federally funded assistance. The welfare reform law does provide that children and parents who would have qualified for Medicaid based on their eligibility for AFDC continue to be eligible for Medicaid, but, in the absence of AFDC, states must use different mechanisms to identify and enroll former AFDC recipients in their Medicaid programs.

1997

P.L. 105-33, the Balanced Budget Act of 1997 (BBA), contained the most significant changes in the Medicare program since the program's inception in 1965. Overall, this legislation required a five-year reduction of $115 billion in the Medicare program's expenditure growth and a $13 billion reduction in growth of the Medicaid program. A new "Medicare+Choice" program was created, which gives Medicare beneficiaries the opportunity to choose from a variety of health plan options the plan that best suits their needs and preferences. Significant changes were also made in the traditional Medicare program. Among them, hospital annual inflation updates were reduced, as were hospital payments for inpatient capital expenses and for bad debts. Other provisions established a cap on the number of medical residents supported by Medicare graduate medical education payments and provided incentives for reductions in the number of residents.

An important provision of this act established the State Children's Health Insurance Program (SCHIP) and provided states with $24 billion in federal funds for 1998 until 2002 to increase health insurance for children.

Other provisions established two new commissions. One of these, the Medicare Payment Review Commission (MedPAC), replaced the Physician Payment Review Commission and the Prospective Payment Review Commission. MedPAC was required to submit an annual report to Congress on the status of Medicare reforms and to make recommendations on Medicare payment issues. The second new commission established by this legislation, the National Bipartisan Commission on the Future of Medicare, was charged with developing recommendations for Congress on actions necessary to ensure the long-term fiscal health of the Medicare program. This commission was to consider several specific issues that were debated in the development of the BBA of 1997, but rejected. These issues included raising the eligibility age for Medicare, increasing the Part B premiums, and developing alternative approaches to financing graduate medical education.

P.L. 105-115, the Food and Drug Administration Modernization and Accountability Act, directs the secretary of HHS, at the request of a new drug's sponsor, to identify the drug as a "fast track product" and to facilitate development and expedite review if the new drug is intended for serious conditions and demonstrates the potential to address unmet medical needs for those conditions. The law also mandates development, prioritization, publication, and annual updating of a list of approved drugs for which additional pediatric information may produce health benefits in the pediatric population. It also mandates development of guidance on the inclusion of women and minorities in clinical trials. Among numerous other provisions, the law also authorizes the secretary of HHS to permit the shipment of investigational drugs or investigational devices for the diagnosis, monitoring, or treatment of a serious disease or condition in emergency situations. It permits any person through a licensed physician to request, and any manufacturer or distributor to provide to the physician, such a drug or device if specified requirements are met.

1998

P.L. 105-357, the Controlled Substances Trafficking Prohibition Act, amends the Controlled Substances Import and Export Act to prohibit US residents from importing into the United States a non-Schedule I controlled substance exceeding 50 dosage units if they (1) enter the United States through an international land border and (2) do not possess a valid prescription or documentation verifying such a prescription. This law has a provision that declares that the federal requirements under the law not limit states from imposing additional requirements.

P.L. 105-369, the Ricky Ray Hemophilia Relief Fund Act, establishes in the US Treasury the Ricky Ray Hemophilia Relief Fund. The law mandates a single payment of $100,000 from the fund to any individual infected with HIV if the individual has any blood-clotting disorder and was treated with blood-clotting agents between July 1, 1982, and December 31, 1987; is the lawful current or former spouse of such an individual; or acquired the HIV infection from a parent who is such an individual. The law declares that it does not create or admit any claim of the individual against the United States or its agents regarding HIV and anti-hemophilic factor treatment and that acceptance of a payment under this act is in full satisfaction of all such claims of the individual.

1999

P.L. 106-113, the Medicare, Medicaid and SCHIP Balanced Budget Refinement Act of 1999 (BBRA), changed the provisions in the BBA of 1997 in a number of ways. One change, for example, pertained to the way that hospitals treating a disproportionate share (DSH) of low-income Medicare and Medicaid patients receive additional payments from Medicare. BBRA froze DSH adjustments at 3 percent (the FY2000 level) through FY2001 and reduced the formula to 4 percent from the BBA-established 5 percent in FY2002 and then to 0 percent for subsequent years. The law increased hospice payment by 0.5 percent for FY2001 and by 0.75 percent for FY2002. Medicare reimburses teaching hospitals for their role in providing graduate medical education (GME). Prior to BBA, Medicare's indirect medical education adjustment (IME) payments increased 7.7 percent for each 10 percent increase in a hospital's ratio of interns and residents to beds. BBA decreased the adjustment to 6.5 percent in FY1999, 6.0 percent in FY 2000, and 5.5 percent in FY2001 and subsequent years. BBRA froze the IME adjustment at 6.5 percent through FY2000, reduced it to 6.25 percent in FY2001, and reduced it to 5.5 percent in FY2002 and subsequent years.

P.L. 106-117, the Veterans Millennium Health Care and Benefits Act, directs the secretary of Veterans Affairs to provide nursing home care to any veteran in need of such care through December 31, 2003, (1) for a service-connected disability or (2) who has a service-connected disability rated at 70 percent or more. The law prohibits a veteran receiving such care from being transferred from the providing facility without the consent of the veteran or his or her representative. It also directs the secretary to operate and maintain a program to provide the following extended care services to eligible veterans: (1) geriatric evaluation; (2) nursing home care, either in facilities of the Department of Veterans Affairs or in community-based facilities; (3) domiciliary services; (4) adult day healthcare; (5) noninstitutional alternatives to nursing home care; and (6) respite care. The law has a provision that prohibits the secretary from furnishing such services for a nonservice-connected disability unless the veteran agrees to make a copayment for services of more than 21 days in a year and requires the secretary to establish a methodology for establishing the copayment amount.

2000

P.L. 106-354, the Breast and Cervical Cancer Prevention and Treatment Act, amends Title XIX (Medicaid) of the Social Security Act to give states the option of making medical assistance for breast and cervical cancer–related treatment services available during a presumptive eligibility period to certain low-income women who have already been screened for such cancers under the Centers for Disease Control and Prevention breast and cervical cancer early detection program. The law also provides for an enhanced match of federal funds to help states pay for these treatment services through their Medicaid programs.

P.L. 106-430, the Needlestick Safety and Prevention Act, revised the blood-borne pathogens standard in effect under the Occupational Safety and Health Act of 1970 (see P.L. 91-596) to include safer medical devices, such as sharps with engineered sharps injury protections and needleless systems, as examples of engineering controls designed to eliminate or minimize occupational exposure to blood-borne pathogens through needlestick injuries. Other provisions require certain employers to (1) review and update exposure control plans to reflect changes in technology that eliminate or reduce such exposure and document their consideration and implementation of appropriate commercially available and effective safer medical devices for such purpose; (2) maintain a sharps injury log, noting the type and brand of device used, where the injury occurred, and an explanation of the incident (exempting employers who are not required to maintain specified OSHA logs); and (3) seek input on such engineering and work practice controls from the affected healthcare workers.

P.L. 106-525, the Minority Health and Health Disparities Research and Education Act, amends the Public Health Service Act to establish within the NIH the National Center on Minority and Health Disparities to conduct and support research, training, dissemination of information, and other programs with respect to minority health conditions and other populations with health disparities. This law requires the center director, in expending funds, to give priority to conducting and supporting minority health disparities research (research on minority health conditions, including research to prevent, diagnose, and treat such conditions). It also requires coordination of center research with other health disparities research conducted or supported by NIH and requires the center director, the NIH director, and the directors of all other agencies of NIH to, among other things, establish a comprehensive plan and budget for the conduct and support of all minority health and other health disparities research activities of the agencies of NIH. The law also has a provision requiring the directors to work together to carry out provisions of the act relating to participation by minority groups in clinical research.

P.L. 106-554, the Medicare, Medicaid, and SCHIP Benefits Improvement and Protection Act of 2000, changed numerous provisions previously enacted in BBA and BBRA. Among the important changes were

- an increase of 3.4 percent for Medicare inpatient payments in FY2001 and an estimated 3.5 percent in FY2002,
- an increase of 4.4 percent in Medicare outpatient payments in 2001,
- IME payments at 6.5 percent in FY2001 and FY2002,
- elimination of the additional 1 percent cut in Medicare DSH hospital payments in FY2001 and FY2002,
- an increase from 55 to 70 percent in Medicare payments for bad debt,
- an increase for the direct GME payment floor to 85 percent of the national average,
- elimination of BBA's FY2001 and FY2002 Medicaid DSH cut,
- removal of the 2 percent payment reduction for rehabilitation hospitals in FY2001,
- a 3.2 percent increase in skilled nursing service payments in FY2001,
- a one-year delay of the 15 percent reduction for home health and the full market basket in FY2001,
- an increase of 2 percent in incentive payments for psychiatric hospitals/ units, and
- expansion of Medicare payment for telehealth services to rural areas.

P.L. 106-580, the National Institute of Biomedical Imaging and Bioengineering Establishment Act, amends the Public Health Service Act to provide for the establishment of the National Institute of Biomedical Imaging and Bioengineering. The law requires the director of the institute to establish a national biomedical imaging and bioengineering program, which includes research and related technology assessments and development in biomedical imaging and bioengineering. It also requires the director to prepare and transmit to the secretary of HHS and the director of NIH a plan to initiate, expand, intensify, and coordinate institute biomedical imaging and bioengineering activities. It requires (1) the consolidation and coordination of institute biomedical imaging and bioengineering research and related activities with those of NIH and other federal agencies and (2) the establishment of an institute advisory council.

2001

P.L. 107-9, the Animal Disease Risk Assessment, Prevention, and Control Act, directs the Secretary of Agriculture to submit a preliminary report to specified congressional committees concerning (1) interagency measures to assess, prevent, and control the spread of foot and mouth disease and bovine spongiform encephalopathy ("mad cow disease") in the United States; (2) related federal information sources available to the public; and (3) the need for any additional legislative authority or product bans. The law directs the secretary, in consultation with governmental and private-sector parties, to submit a final report to such committees that discusses such diseases' economic impacts; public and animal health risks; and related legislative, federal agency, and product recommendations.

P.L. 107-38, the Emergency Supplemental Appropriations Act for Recovery from and Response to Terrorist Attacks on the United States, makes emergency supplemental appropriations for FY2001 for emergency expenses to respond to the terrorist attacks on the United States on September 11, 2001, to provide assistance to the victims, and to deal with other consequences of the attacks. The law makes $40 billion available to the Executive Office of the President and Funds Appropriated to the President for the Emergency Response Fund for such expenses as (1) providing federal, state, and local preparedness for mitigating and responding to the attacks; (2) providing support to counter, investigate, or prosecute domestic or international terrorism; (3) providing increased transportation security; (4) repairing damaged public facilities and transportation systems; and (5) supporting national security.

P.L. 107-109, Best Pharmaceuticals for Children Act, amends the Public Health Service Act to direct the secretary of HHS, through the NIH, to develop an annual list of approved drugs for which (1) there is a referral, an approved or pending new drug application, or no patent or market exclusivity protection and (2) additional pediatric safety and effectiveness studies are needed. The act also directs the secretary to award contracts to entities with appropriate experience for pediatric clinical trials of such drugs; requires the results of such trials to be reported to the commissioner of food and drugs, who shall then determine and request any necessary labeling changes; authorizes the commissioner to deem a drug misbranded if the holder of an approved application refuses to make the requested change; requires the secretary to send a nonbinding letter of recommendation to an approved application holder if such studies indicate a reformulation is necessary; and sets forth reporting, label change, and dispute resolution requirements.

P.L. 107-121, the Native American Breast and Cervical Cancer Treatment Technical Amendment Act of 2001, amends Title XIX of the Social Security Act to clarify that Indian women with breast or cervical cancer who are eligible for health services provided under a medical care program of the Indian Health Service or of a tribal organization are included in the optional Medicaid eligibility category of breast or cervical cancer patients added by the Breast and Cervical Prevention and Treatment Act of 2000.

P.L. 107-205, the Nurse Reinvestment Act, amends the Public Health Service Act to direct the secretary of HHS to promote the nursing profession through public service announcements and to make grants to support state and local advertising campaigns, excluding particular employment opportunities.

The legislation expands eligibility for the nursing loan repayment program to include service at any healthcare facility with a critical shortage of nurses. The legislation also authorizes the secretary to award grants or contracts to schools of nursing or healthcare facilities to expand nursing opportunities (1) in education, through increased enrollment in four-year degree programs, internship and residency programs, or new technologies such as distance learning; and (2) in practice, through care to underserved populations, care in noninstitutional settings or organized healthcare systems, and through developing cultural competencies.

2002

P.L. 107-250, the Medical Device User Fee and Modernization Act, amends the Federal Food, Drug, and Cosmetic Act to establish a new program that, beginning on October 1, 2002, subjects each medical device manufacturer to a medical device fee for certain applications, reports, application supplements, and submissions sent to the FDA for evaluation. The legislation grants exceptions, including for humanitarian devices and certain devices sponsored by state governments or the federal government, and directs the secretary of HHS to waive one premarket application, or one premarket report where the applicant is a small business submitting its first premarket application or its first premarket report, respectively, for review.

P.L. 107-251, the Health Care Safety Net Amendments of 2002, amends the Public Health Service Act to reauthorize and strengthen the health centers program and the National Health Service Corps and to establish the Healthy Communities Access Program to help coordinate services for the uninsured and underinsured.

P.L. 107-280, the Rare Diseases Act, amends the Public Health Service Act to (1) establish the Office of Rare Diseases at the NIH and (2) provide for rare disease regional centers of excellence. The legislation sets forth the duties of such an office and such regional centers, including research and educational duties. It also defines *rare disease* as any disease or condition affecting fewer than 200,000 persons in the United States.

P.L. 107-296, the Homeland Security Act, establishes the Department of Homeland Security (DHS) as an executive department of the United States, headed by the secretary of Homeland Security appointed by the president with the advice and consent of the Senate, to (1) prevent terrorist attacks within the United States; (2) reduce the vulnerability of the United States to terrorism; (3) minimize the damage, and assist in the recovery, from terrorist attacks that occur within the United States; (4) carry out all functions of entities transferred to DHS; (5) ensure that the functions of the agencies and subdivisions within DHS that are not related directly to securing the homeland are not diminished or neglected except by a specific act of Congress; (6) ensure that the overall economic security of the United States is not diminished by efforts, activities, and programs aimed at securing the homeland; and (7) monitor connections between illegal drug trafficking and terrorism, coordinate efforts to sever such connections, and otherwise contribute to efforts to interdict illegal drug trafficking.

P.L. 107-313, the Mental Health Parity Reauthorization Act, amends the Employee Retirement Income Security Act of 1974 (ERISA) and the Public Health Service Act to extend the mental health benefits parity provisions through 2003.

2003

P.L. 108-74, the State Children's Health Insurance Program Allotments Extension, amends Title XXI (State Children's Health Insurance

Program, or SCHIP) of the Social Security Act to revise the special rule for the redistribution and availability of unexpended FY1998 and FY1999 SCHIP allotments, including to (1) extend the availability of FY1998 and FY1999 reallocated funds through FY2004 and (2) permit 50 percent of the total amount of unexpended FY2000 and FY2001 SCHIP allotments that remain available to a state through the end of FY2002 and FY2003 to remain available for expenditure by the state through the end of FY2004 and FY2005, respectively.

P.L. 108-155, the Pediatric Research Equity Act, amends the Federal Food, Drug, and Cosmetic Act to authorize the FDA to require license applications for new drugs and biological products to assess such drugs' or products' safety and effectiveness, including dosage, for relevant pediatric subpopulations. The legislation permits deferral of such assessments under specified circumstances, including if the secretary of HHS finds that the drug or biological product is ready for approval for use in adults before pediatric studies are complete. It also permits full waiver of such assessments under certain conditions, including if (1) studies are highly impractical or impossible or (2) there is no meaningful therapeutic advantage or benefit in the pediatric population and the drug or biological product is not likely to be used in a substantial number of pediatric patients.

P.L. 108-170, the Veterans Health Care, Capital Asset, and Business Improvement Act, amends Title 38, *United States Code,* to improve and enhance the provision of healthcare for veterans, to authorize major construction projects and other facilities matters for the Department of Veterans Affairs, to enhance and improve authorities relating to the administration of personnel of the Department of Veterans Affairs, and for other purposes.

P.L. 108-173, the Medicare Prescription Drug, Improvement, and Modernization Act (MMA), created a new drug benefit as Part D of Medicare. The new benefit is to begin in 2006, with an interim Medicare-endorsed drug discount card available to beneficiaries. In addition, this law adds certain preventive benefits, including an initial routine physical examination for new beneficiaries, as well as cardiovascular blood screening tests and diabetes screening and services. MMA also renamed Medicare+Choice to Medicare Advantage (MA) and changed some of the enrollment and disenrollment rules for beneficiaries.

Another fundamental change in the Medicare program resulting from MMA is the Part B premium determination, which has been uniform for all beneficiaries since the program's inception. Beginning in 2007, this premium will be higher for those with incomes over $80,000 for a single beneficiary or $160,000 for a couple. In addition, the Part B deductible, set at $100 since 1991, is increased to $110 and thereafter will increase by the annual percentage increase in Part B expenditures.

2004

P.L. 108-216, the Organ Donation and Recovery Improvement Act, amends the Public Health Service Act to authorize the secretary of HHS to award grants to states, transplant centers, qualified organ procurement organizations, or other public or private entities to reimburse travel, subsistence, and incidental nonmedical expenses incurred by individuals toward making living organ donations. The legislation also directs the secretary to establish a public education program to increase awareness about organ donation and the need to provide for an adequate rate of donations. It authorizes the secretary to (1) make peer-reviewed grants to or contracts with public and not-for-profit private entities for studies and demonstration projects to increase organ donation and recovery rates, including living donations; (2) make grants to states for organ donor awareness, public education, and outreach activities and programs designed to increase the number of organ donors within the state; and (3) support the development and dissemination of educational materials to inform healthcare professionals about organ, tissue, and eye donation issues.

P.L. 108-276, the Project BioShield Act, amends the Public Health Service Act to provide protections and countermeasures against chemical, radiological, or nuclear agents that may be used in a terrorist attack against the United States by giving the NIH contracting flexibility to make infrastructure improvements and expedite the scientific peer review process and by streamlining the FDA approval process of countermeasures.

P.L. 108-355, the Garrett Lee Smith Memorial Act, amends the Public Health Service Act to support the planning, implementation, and evaluation of organized activities involving statewide youth suicide early intervention and prevention strategies and to authorize grants to institutions of higher education to reduce student mental and behavioral health problems.

P.L. 108-358, the Anabolic Steroid Control Act, amends the Controlled Substances Act to clarify the definition of anabolic steroids and to provide for research and education activities relating to steroids and steroid precursors. The legislation defines *anabolic steroid* as any drug or hormonal substance chemically and pharmacologically related to testosterone (other than estrogens, progestins, corticosteroids, and dehydroepiandrosterone).

2005

P.L. 109-18, the Patient Navigator Outreach and Chronic Disease Prevention Act, amends the Public Health Service Act to authorize a demonstration grant program to provide patient navigator services to reduce barriers and improve healthcare outcomes. This act permits the secretary of HHS, acting through the administrator of the Health Resources and Services Administration, to make grants to eligible entities for the development and operation of demonstration programs to provide patient navigator services to improve healthcare outcomes. The act requires the secretary to coordinate with and ensure the participation of the Indian Health Service, the National Cancer Institute, the Office of Rural Health Policy, and such other offices and agencies as deemed appropriate by the secretary regarding the design and evaluation of the demonstration programs.

P.L. 109-41, the Patient Safety and Quality Improvement Act, amends the Public Health Service Act to designate patient safety data as privileged and confidential. The act defines a patient safety organization (PSO) as an organization certified by the secretary of HHS that conducts efforts to improve patient safety and the quality of healthcare delivery through the collection and analysis of patient safety data. The act requires the secretary to (1) maintain a patient safety network of databases that has the capacity to accept, aggregate, and analyze nonidentifiable patient safety data voluntarily reported and that provides an interactive resource for providers and PSOs; (2) develop or adopt voluntary national standards to promote the electronic exchange of healthcare information; and (3) contract with a research organization to study the impact of medical technologies and therapies on healthcare.

P.L. 109-171, the Deficit Reduction Act (DRA) of 2005, established and funded the Medicare–Medicaid Data Match Program, which is designed to identify improper billing and utilization patterns by matching Medicare and Medicaid claims information. The funds also can be used (1) to coordinate actions by CMS, the states, the attorney general, and the HHS Office of Inspector General to prevent improper Medicaid and Medicare expenditures and (2) to increase the effectiveness and efficiency of both Medicare and Medicaid through cost avoidance, savings, and the recoupment of fraudulent, wasteful, or abusive expenditures.

2006

P.L. 109-307, the Children's Hospital GME Support Reauthorization Act of 2006, amends the Public Health Service Act to (1) require the secretary of HHS to make payments for FY2007–FY2011 to children's hospitals for expenses associated with operating approved graduate medical residency training programs; and (2) decrease from 26 to 12 the number of interim payments to hospitals per fiscal year. The act also requires the secretary, acting through the administrator of the Health Resources and Services Administration (HRSA), to report to Congress on the residency training programs.

P.L. 109-415, the Ryan White HIV/AIDS Treatment Modernization Act of 2006, amends provisions of Title XXVI of the Public Health Service Act (popularly known as the Ryan White Care Act [RWCA]) concerning emergency relief grants for metropolitan areas to assist in delivering and enhancing HIV-related services. The act reauthorizes for three years the RWCA, providing $2.1 billion annually for HIV/AIDS programs in the United States. These amendments have the effect of shifting additional funds to rural areas and the South, where the disease is a newer phenomenon.

P.L. 109-417, the Pandemic and All-Hazards Preparedness Act, amends the Public Health Service Act with respect to public health security and all-hazards preparedness and response. This act improves the public health and medical preparedness and response capabilities for emergencies, whether deliberate, accidental, or natural. The act enhances the nation's capacity to handle a major medical surge during an emergency by establishing a national infrastructure for registering health professional volunteers, improving core training, strengthening logistical support, and developing a clear organizational framework for healthcare providers.

The act establishes overarching preparedness goals for essential federal, state, and local public health and medical capabilities to increase accountability and incentivize regional coordination, including

1. integrating public health and public and private medical capabilities with other first responder systems;
2. developing and maintaining federal, state, local, and tribal essential public health security capabilities;
3. increasing the preparedness and response capabilities, and the surge capacity of hospitals and healthcare facilities;
4. taking into account the needs of at-risk individuals during a public health emergency;
5. ensuring coordination of federal, state, local, and tribal planning, preparedness, and response activities; and
6. maintaining continuity of operations of vital public health and medical services in the event of a public health emergency.

2007

P.L. 110-18, the National Breast and Cervical Cancer Early Detection Program Reauthorization Act of 2007, amends the Public Health Service Act to change from 2000 to 2020 the target year for the committee coordinating Public Health Service activities to achieve the objectives established by the secretary of HHS for reductions in the rate of mortality from breast and cervical cancers in the United States. The act also directs the secretary to establish a demonstration project that allows the secretary to waive certain requirements for awarding breast and cervical cancer grants for preventive health measures with respect to breast and cervical cancers.

P.L. 110-23, the Trauma Care Systems Planning and Development Act of 2007, amends the Public Health Service Act to direct the secretary of HHS to (1) collect, compile, and disseminate information on achievements and problems in providing trauma care and emergency medical services; and (2) promote the collection and categorization of trauma data in a consistent and standardized manner.

The act authorizes the secretary, acting through the administrator of the Health Resources and Services Administration, to make grants to states, political subdivisions, or consortia thereof to improve access to and enhance the development of trauma care systems. It requires grant funds be used to (1) integrate and broaden the reach of such a system; (2) strengthen, develop, and improve an existing system; (3) expand communications between the system and emergency medical services through improved equipment or a telemedicine system; (4) improve data collection and retention; or (5) increase education, training, and technical assistance opportunities. The act requires the secretary to give priority to applicants who will use the grants to focus on improving access to trauma care systems and to give special consideration to projects that demonstrate strong state or local support.

P.L. 110-26, the American National Red Cross Governance Modernization Act of 2007, amends the congressional charter of the American National Red Cross (ANRC) to modernize its governance structure, to enhance the ability of its board of governors to support the critical mission of ANRC in the twenty-first century. The act requires the corporation to submit a report to the secretary of defense on the activities of the corporation during the preceding fiscal year, including a complete, itemized report of all receipts and expenditures.

P.L. 110-85, the Food and Drug Administration Amendments Act of 2007, amends the Federal Food, Drug, and Cosmetic Act (FFDCA) to revise and extend the user-fee programs for prescription drugs and for medical devices. The act also amends FFDCA to include postmarket safety activities within the process for the review of human drug applications or supplements, including (1) developing and using improved adverse event data collection systems and improved analytical tools to assess potential safety problems; (2) implementing and enforcing provisions relating to postapproval studies, clinical trials, labeling changes, and risk evaluation and mitigation strategies; and (3) conducting screenings of the Adverse Event Reporting System database and reporting on new safety concerns.

P.L. 110-173, the Medicare, Medicaid, and SCHIP Extension Act of 2007, prevented a 10.1 percent reduction in Medicare payments to physicians that was scheduled to take effect in 2008 and instead gave physicians a 0.5 percent increase through June 30, 2008.

2008

P.L. 110-233, the Genetic Information Nondiscrimination Act of 2008, amends the Employee Retirement Income Security Act of 1974 (ERISA), the Public Health Service Act, and the Internal Revenue Code to prohibit a group health plan from adjusting premium or contribution amounts for a group on the basis of genetic information. The act also prohibits a group health plan from requesting or requiring an individual or family member of an individual from undergoing a genetic test and requires the plan to request only the minimum amount of information necessary to accomplish the intended purpose. The act prohibits an issuer of a Medicare supplemental policy from (1) requesting or requiring an individual or a family member to undergo a genetic test, or (2) requesting, requiring, or purchasing genetic information for underwriting purposes or for any individual prior to enrollment.

P.L. 110-275, the Medicare Improvements for Patients and Providers Act of 2008, extended the planned reduction in Medicare payments to physicians through the end of 2008 and increased payment of their fees for all of 2009 by 1.1 percent. Benefit improvements for Medicare beneficiaries included reduced coinsurance payments for mental health visits and elimination of the deductibles for Welcome to Medicare physical examinations.

P.L. 110-314, the Consumer Product Safety Improvement Act of 2008, treats as a banned hazardous substance under the Federal Hazardous Substances Act any children's product (a consumer product designed or intended primarily for children 12 years of age or younger) containing more than specified amounts of lead. The act establishes a more stringent limit on the amount of lead allowed in paint. It also requires the Consumer Product Safety Commission to (1) evaluate the effectiveness, precision, and reliability of X-ray fluorescence technology and other alternative methods for measuring lead in paint or other surface coatings when used on a children's product or furniture article to determine compliance with specified regulations; and (2) conduct an ongoing effort to study and encourage the further development of alternative methods for measuring lead in paint and other surface coatings.

The act requires a manufacturer of a children's product, before importing any children's product that is subject to a safety rule, to have the product tested by an accredited third party for compliance with such rule and to certify that such product complies.

P.L. 110-335, the Health Care Safety Net Act of 2008, amends the Public Health Service Act to reauthorize appropriations for FY2008–FY2012 for health centers to meet the healthcare needs of medically underserved populations. The act requires the comptroller general to study the economic costs and benefits of school-based health centers and their impact on the health of students, including an analysis of (1) the impact that federal funding could have on the operation of such centers, (2) any cost savings to other federal programs derived from providing health services in such centers, and (3) the impact of such centers in rural or underserved areas.

The act also requires the secretary of HHS, acting through the administrator of HRSA, to submit a report to the relevant congressional committees that describes efforts to expand and accelerate quality improvement activities in community health centers. It also requires the administrator to establish a mechanism for the dissemination of initiatives, best practices, and other information that may assist healthcare quality improvement efforts in community health centers.

P.L. 110-354, the Breast Cancer and Environmental Research Act of 2008, amends the Public Health Service Act to require the secretary of HHS to establish the Interagency Breast Cancer and Environmental Research Coordinating Committee to (1) share and coordinate information on existing breast cancer research activities and make recommendations for the improvement of research programs; (2) develop a comprehensive strategy and advise the NIH and other federal agencies in the solicitation of proposals for collaborative, multidisciplinary research, including proposals to evaluate environmental and genomic factors that may be related to the etiology of breast cancer; (3) develop a summary of advances in federal breast cancer research relevant to the diagnosis, prevention, and treatment of cancer and other diseases and disorders; and (4) make recommendations to the secretary regarding changes to research activities, avoiding unnecessary duplication of effort among federal agencies, public participation in decisions relating to breast cancer research, how best to disseminate information on breast cancer research progress, and how to expand partnerships between public and private entities to expand collaborative, crosscutting research. The act authorizes appropriations for FY2009–FY2012.

P.L. 110-374, the Emergency Economic Stabilization Act of 2008, contains in Title V, Subtitle B, the Paul Wellstone and Pete Domenici Mental Health Parity and Addiction Equity Act of 2008, which amends the Employee Retirement Income Security Act of 1974 (ERISA), the Public Health Service Act, and the Internal Revenue Code to require a group health plan that provides both medical and surgical benefits and mental health or substance use disorder benefits to ensure that (1) the financial requirements, such as deductibles and copayments, applicable to such mental health or substance use disorder benefits are no more restrictive than the predominant financial requirements applied to substantially all medical and surgical benefits covered by the plan; (2) there are no separate cost-sharing requirements that are applicable only with respect to mental health or substance use disorder benefits; (3) the treatment limitations applicable to such mental health or substance use disorder benefits are no more restrictive than the predominant treatment limitations applied to substantially all medical and surgical benefits covered by the plan; and (4) there are no separate treatment limitations that are applicable only with respect to mental health or substance use disorder benefits.

P.L. 110-377, the Poison Center Support, Enhancement, and Awareness Act of 2008, amends the Public Health Service Act to require the secretary of HHS to provide coordination and assistance for the maintenance of the nationwide toll-free phone number to access poison control centers.

The act requires the secretary to carry out and expand on a national media campaign to educate the public and healthcare providers about poison prevention and the availability of poison control center resources in local communities. The secretary is authorized to enter into contracts with nationally recognized organizations in the field of poison control and national media firms for the development and implementation of a nationwide poison prevention and poison control center awareness campaign.

This act also expands the poison control center grant program to allow the secretary to award grants for poison control centers to comply with the operational requirements needed to sustain certification. The act authorizes appropriations for FY2009–FY2014.

2009

P.L. 111-3, the Children's Health Insurance Program Reauthorization Act of 2009, amends Title XXI of the Social Security Act to extend and improve the Children's Health Insurance Program (CHIP). The act reauthorizes CHIP through 2013 at increased levels of funding by providing an additional $35 billion over five years. Among other things, the act lowers the rate of uninsured low-income children, in part by providing states with incentives and tools for outreach and enrollment to accomplish this. Other provisions improve the quality of care for low-income children and reduce racial and ethnic disparities in coverage and quality. The legislation also reduces administrative barriers, maintains state flexibility, and enhances premium assistance options for low-income families.

P.L. 111-5, the American Recovery and Reinvestment Act of 2009, was enacted in response to the global financial crisis that emerged in 2008. The purposes of the act are

- to preserve and create jobs and promote economic recovery;
- to assist those most affected by the recession;
- to provide investments needed to increase economic efficiency by spurring technological advances in science and health;
- to invest in transportation, environmental protection, and other infrastructure that will provide long-term economic benefits; and
- to stabilize state and local government budgets, in order to minimize and avoid reductions in essential services and counterproductive state and local tax increases.

Within this massive economic stimulus package ($787 billion), a significant amount of the resources (about $150 billion in new funds) are directed to healthcare. The specific allocations to healthcare are shown in the table on page 427.

P.L. 111-31, the Family Smoking Prevention and Tobacco Control Act, amends the FFDCA to provide for the regulation of tobacco products by the secretary of HHS through the FDA. The act directs the secretary to establish within the FDA (1) the Center for Tobacco Products to implement this act; and (2) an identifiable office to provide technical and other nonfinancial assistance to assist small tobacco product manufacturers in complying with this act. The act also requires tobacco product manufacturers or importers to submit to the secretary (1) a listing of all ingredients, including ingredients added by the manufacturer to the tobacco, paper, or filter, by brand and quantity; (2) a description of the content, delivery, and form of nicotine in each tobacco product; (3) a listing of all constituents, including smoke constituents, identified by the secretary as harmful or potentially harmful to health in each tobacco product; and (4) all documents developed that relate to the health, toxicological, behavioral, or physiologic effects of tobacco products and their constituents, ingredients, components, and additives.

The act directs the secretary to prescribe regulations to protect the public health and ensure that tobacco products are in compliance with this act by requiring good manufacturing practices or hazard analysis and critical control point methodology. It also requires the secretary to (1) provide a reasonable period for manufacturers to conform to good manufacturing practices, and (2) not require any small tobacco product manufacturer to comply with such regulations for at least four years.

P.L. 111-87, Ryan White HIV/AIDS Treatment Extension Act of 2009, amends provisions of Title XXVI of the Public Health Service Act (popularly known as the Ryan White Care Act [RWCA]) to extend the RWCA and revive any expired programs retroactively to September 30, 2009. The act reauthorizes appropriations for RWCA provisions, including provisions concerning (1) emergency relief grants for metropolitan areas to

Program or Investment Area	Amount and Purpose of Funding
Comparative effectiveness research	$1.1 billion, of which $300 million will be administered by the Agency for Healthcare Research and Quality, $400 million by the NIH, and $400 million by the secretary of health and human services.
Continuation of health insurance coverage for unemployed workers	$24.7 billion to provide a 65% federal subsidy for up to 9 months of premiums under the Consolidated Omnibus Budget Reconciliation Act. The subsidy will help workers who lose their jobs to continue coverage for themselves and their families.
Departments of Defense and Veterans Affairs	More than $1.4 billion for the construction and renovation of healthcare facilities.
Health information technology	$19.2 billion, including $17.2 billion for financial incentives to physicians and hospitals through Medicare and Medicaid to promote the use of electronic health records and other health information technology and $2 billion for affiliated grants and loans to be administered by the Office of the National Coordinator for Health Information Technology. Physicians may be eligible for grants of $40,000 to $65,000 over multiple years, and hospitals for up to $11 million.
Health Resources and Services Administration	$2.5 billion, including $1.5 billion for construction, equipment, and health information technology at community health centers; $500 million for services at these centers; $300 million for the NHSC; and $200 million for other health professions training programs.
Medicare	$338 million for payments to teaching hospitals, hospice programs, and long-term care hospitals.
Medicaid and other state health programs	$87 billion for additional federal matching payments for state Medicaid programs for a 27-month period that began October 1, 2008, and $3.2 billion for additional state fiscal relief related to Medicaid and other health programs.
National Institutes of Health	$10 billion, including $8.2 billion for new grants and related activities and $1.8 billion for construction and renovation of NIH buildings and facilities, extramural research facilities, and research equipment.
Prevention and wellness	$1 billion, including $650 million for clinical and community-based prevention activities that will address rates of chronic diseases, as determined by the secretary of health and human services; $300 million to the Centers for Disease Control and Prevention for immunizations for low-income children and adults; and $50 million to states to reduce healthcare–associated infections.
Public Health and Social Services Emergency Fund	$50 million to the HHS to improve the security of information technology.

assist in delivering and enhancing HIV-related services; (2) grants to enable states to improve healthcare and support services for individuals and families with HIV/AIDS (Care grants); (3) early intervention grants to public and nonprofit private entities to provide early intervention services; (4) programs to provide coordinated services for women, infants, children, and youth with HIV/AIDS; (5) grants for HIV/AIDS education and training for healthcare personnel; (6) grants to dental schools and programs for providing oral healthcare to patients with HIV/AIDS; and (7) the Minority AIDS Initiative.

2010

P.L. 111-148, the Patient Protection and Affordable Care Act of 2010 (ACA), is a major health reform law, culminating a centurylong effort to expand health insurance coverage to nearly all Americans. It is a massive law, more fully described in Appendix 1 of this book. Only its main provisions are summarized here. Most of the description of the provisions of the ACA provided here are abstracted from Redhead, C. S., H. Chaikind, B. Fernandez, and J. Staman. 2012. *ACA: A Brief Overview of the Law, Implementation, and Legal Challenges.* Washington, DC: Congressional Research Service Report R41664.

The primary goal of the ACA is to increase access to affordable health insurance for the millions of Americans without coverage and make health insurance more affordable for those already covered. In addition, the ACA makes numerous changes in the way healthcare is financed, organized, and delivered. Among its many provisions, the ACA restructures the private health insurance market, sets minimum standards for health coverage, creates a mandate for most US residents to obtain health insurance coverage, and provides for the establishment of state-based insurance marketplaces (previously called exchanges) for the purchase of private health insurance. Certain individuals and families will be able to receive federal subsidies to reduce the cost of purchasing coverage through the insurance marketplaces. The new law also expands eligibility for Medicaid; amends the Medicare program in ways that are intended to reduce the growth in Medicare spending; imposes an excise tax on insurance plans found to have high premiums; and makes numerous other changes to the tax code, Medicare, Medicaid, CHIP, and many other federal programs.

The major expansion and reform provisions in the ACA took effect beginning in 2014. States are expected to establish health insurance marketplaces that provide access to private health insurance plans with standardized benefit and cost-sharing packages for eligible individuals and small employers. In 2017, states may allow larger employers to purchase health insurance through the marketplaces, but are not required to do so. The secretary of HHS will establish marketplaces in states that do not create their own approved marketplace. Premium credits and cost-sharing subsidies will be available to individuals who enroll in marketplace plans, provided their income is generally at or above 100 percent and does not exceed 400 percent of the federal poverty level (FPL) and they meet certain other requirements.

Also beginning in 2014, most individuals are required to have insurance or pay a penalty (an individual mandate). Certain employers with more than 50 employees who do not offer health insurance may be subject to penalties. While most of these employers who offer health insurance will meet the law's requirements, some also may be required to pay a penalty if any of their full-time workers enroll in marketplace plans and receive premium tax credits.

In addition to the expanding private health insurance coverage, the ACA, as enacted, requires state Medicaid programs to expand coverage to all eligible nonpregnant, nonelderly legal residents with incomes up to 133 percent of the FPL, or risk losing their federal Medicaid matching funds. The federal government will initially cover all the costs for this group, with the federal matching percentage phased down to 90 percent of the costs by 2020. The law also requires states to maintain the current CHIP structure through FY2019, and provides federal CHIP appropriations through FY2015 (thus providing a two-year extension on CHIP funding).

The ACA incorporates numerous Medicare payment provisions intended to reduce the rate of growth in spending. They include reductions in Medicare Advantage plan payments and a lowering of the annual payment update for hospitals and certain other providers. The ACA established an Independent Payment Advisory Board (IPAB) to make recommendations for achieving specific Medicare spending reductions if costs exceed a target growth rate. IPAB's recommendations will take effect unless Congress overrides them, in which case Congress would be responsible for achieving the same level of savings. Also, the ACA provides tools to help reduce fraud, waste, and abuse in both Medicare and Medicaid.

Other provisions establish pilot, demonstration, and grant programs to test integrated models of care, including accountable care organizations, medical homes that provide coordinated care for high-need individuals, and bundled payments for acute-care episodes (including hospitalization and follow-up care). The ACA creates the Center for Medicare and Medicaid Innovation to pilot payment and service delivery models, primarily for Medicare and Medicaid beneficiaries. The law also establishes new pay-for-reporting and pay-for-performance programs within Medicare that will pay providers based on the reporting of, or performance on, selected quality measures.

Additionally, the ACA creates incentives for promoting primary care and prevention; for example, by increasing primary care payment rates under

Medicare and Medicaid, covering some preventive services without cost-sharing, and funding community-based prevention and employer wellness programs, among other things. The law increases funding for community health centers and the National Health Service Corps to expand access to primary care services in rural and medically underserved areas and reduce health disparities. Finally, the ACA requires the HHS secretary to develop a national strategy for healthcare quality to improve care delivery, patient outcomes, and population health.

P.L. 111-152, the Health Care and Education Reconciliation Act of 2010, amends a number of aspects of the ACA and other laws. These are details necessary to implement the ACA for the most part. For example, Internal Revenue Code provisions are added to revise the formula for calculating the refundable tax credit for premium assistance for coverage under a qualified health plan by establishing a sliding scale from the initial to the final premium percentage for individuals and families with household incomes up to 400 percent of the federal poverty line. The act required an adjustment after 2014 and another after 2018 of the initial and final premium percentages to reflect the excess (if any) of the rate of premium growth over the rate of growth of income and the consumer price index.

The act revises the provisions setting forth penalties to be imposed on individuals who decline to purchase healthcare coverage by (1) lowering the maximum penalty amount from $495 to $325 in 2015 and from $750 to $695 in 2016; and (2) increasing the penalty rates based on taxpayer household income for taxable years beginning in 2014 and 2015 and for taxable years beginning after 2015. It also revises the provisions setting forth penalties to be imposed on employers with 50 or more employees who decline to offer employees healthcare coverage to allow an exemption for the first 30 employees (including part-time employees) when calculating the penalty, and it increases the applicable penalty amount per employee to $2,000.

The act requires exchanges (now called health insurance marketplaces) that offer healthcare plans to provide the secretary of the Treasury and taxpayers with specified information, including information about the level of coverage, the total premium for coverage, and the aggregate amount of any advance payment of the premium assistance tax credit.

The act establishes a Health Insurance Reform Implementation Fund within HHS and makes appropriations to the fund for the administrative costs of carrying out this act. It also makes numerous changes in Medicare and Medicaid required by the ACA.

P.L. 111-163, the Caregivers and Veterans Omnibus Health Services Act of 2010, directs the secretary of veterans affairs to establish a program of comprehensive assistance for family caregivers of any veteran who (1) is undergoing medical discharge from the armed forces; (2) has a serious injury incurred or aggravated in the line of duty on or after September 11, 2001; and (3) is in need of personal care services.

Title II of this act, Women Veterans Health Care Matters, requires the secretary to study, and report to the veterans committees on, barriers to the receipt of comprehensive VA healthcare encountered by women veterans. Title III of the act, Rural Health Improvements, authorizes the secretary to carry out demonstration projects to examine the feasibility and advisability of alternatives for expanding care for veterans in rural areas.

P.L. 111-264, the Stem Cell Therapeutic and Research Reauthorization Act of 2010, amends the Stem Cell Therapeutic and Research Act of 2005 to revise provisions related to the National Cord Blood Inventory, including to establish an inventory goal of at least 150,000 new units of cord blood to be made available under the C.W. Bill Young Cell Transplantation Program. (Currently, the number of units of cord blood is capped at 150,000.) The act revises application requirements for cord blood banks participating in the Inventory and authorizes appropriations for FY2011–FY2015 for the Inventory.

P.L. 111-268, the Combat Methamphetamine Enhancement Act of 2010, amends the Controlled Substances Act to require each regulated retail seller of any scheduled listed chemical product at retail (i.e., a product used to make methamphetamine) to submit a self-certification of compliance with the requirements of such act to the attorney general. The act requires the attorney general to (1) establish criteria for certifications of mail-order distributors that are consistent with the criteria for the certifications of regulated sellers; and (2) develop a list of all self-certified individuals and make it publicly available on the website of the Drug Enforcement Administration.

P.L. 111-309, the Medicare and Medicaid Extenders Act of 2010, amends Title XVIII (Medicare) of the Social Security Act to set the 2011 update to the single conversion factor in the formula for the physicians' fee schedule at zero (thus freezing the physician payment update for 2011). The act requires the conversion factor for 2012 and subsequent years to be computed as if the zero update for 2011 had never applied. It also amends the Tax Relief and Health Care Act of 2006, as modified by other federal law, to extend Section 508 hospital reclassifications through FY2011. ("Section 508" refers to Section 508 of the MMA of 2003, which allows the temporary reclassification of a hospital with a low Medicare area wage index, for reimbursement purposes, to a nearby location with a higher Medicare area wage index, so that the "Section 508 hospital" will receive the higher Medicare reimbursement rate.)

P.L. 111-332, the National Foundation on Fitness, Sports, and Nutrition Establishment Act, establishes the National Foundation on Fitness,

Sports and Nutrition as a charitable, nonprofit corporation (1) to develop, in conjunction with the Office of the President's Council on Fitness, Sports and Nutrition, a list and description of activities that would further the purposes and functions outlined in Executive Order 13265 (established by the President's Council on Physical Fitness and Sports) and with respect to which combined private and governmental efforts would be beneficial; (2) to promote private organization participation in, and private gifts to support, those activities; and (3) in consultation with such office, to undertake and support activities to further the purposes and functions of such executive order. The act prohibits the foundation from accepting any federal funds.

P.L. 111-347, the James Zadroga 9/11 Health and Compensation Act of 2010, amends the Public Health Service Act to establish the World Trade Center Health Program (WTC Program) within HHS to provide (1) medical monitoring and treatment benefits to eligible emergency responders and recovery and cleanup workers (including those who are federal employees) who responded to the September 11, 2001, terrorist attacks; and (2) initial health evaluation, monitoring, and treatment benefits to residents and other building occupants and area workers in New York City who were directly and adversely affected by such attacks.

Included within the WTC Program are (1) medical monitoring, including clinical examinations and long-term health monitoring and analysis for enrolled WTC responders who were likely to have been exposed to airborne toxins that were released, or to other hazards, as a result of the September 11, 2001, terrorist attacks; (2) initial health evaluation, including an evaluation to determine eligibility for follow-up monitoring and treatment; (3) follow-up monitoring and treatment and payment for all medically necessary health and mental healthcare expenses of an individual with respect to a WTC-related health condition, including necessary prescription drugs; (4) establishment of an education and outreach program to potentially eligible individuals concerning the benefits under this act; (5) collection and analysis of health and mental health data relating to individuals receiving monitoring or treatment benefits in a uniform manner in collaboration with the collection of epidemiological data; and (6) establishment of a research program on health conditions resulting from the terrorist attacks.

P.L. 111-351, the Predisaster Hazard Mitigation Act of 2010, amends the Robert T. Stafford Disaster Relief and Emergency Assistance Act to (1) increase the amount guaranteed to each state under the predisaster hazard mitigation program to $575,000; (2) require the president to award financial assistance under the program on a competitive basis; (3) eliminate the current termination date for such program (September 30, 2010); and (4) authorize appropriations for the program through FY2013. It also directs the administrator of the Federal Emergency Management Agency to submit to Congress a certification regarding whether all financial assistance under the program was awarded in accordance with such act.

P.L. 111-353, the FDA Food Safety Modernization Act, amends the FFDCA to expand the food safety activities of the secretary of HHS, including authorizing the secretary to inspect records related to food. The act requires each owner, operator, or agent in charge of a food facility to identify and implement preventive controls to significantly minimize or prevent hazards that could affect food manufactured, processed, packed, or held by such facility, and it sets forth provisions governing exemptions from such requirements for certain facilities. It directs the secretary to develop voluntary food allergy and anaphylaxis management guidelines for schools and early childhood education programs. It also requires the secretary, acting through the director of the CDC, to enhance foodborne illness surveillance systems to improve the collection, analysis, reporting, and usefulness of data on foodborne illnesses. Provisions related to the safety of imported food require US importers to perform risk-based foreign supplier verification activities to verify that imported food is produced in compliance with applicable requirements related to hazard analysis and standards for produce safety and is not adulterated or misbranded.

The act also requires the secretary to establish a program to expedite review and importation of food offered for importation by US importers who have voluntarily agreed to participate in such program. It authorizes the secretary to (1) require a certification that an article of food imported or offered for import complies with applicable requirements of this act, and (2) enter into arrangements and agreements with foreign governments to facilitate the inspection of registered foreign facilities.

P.L. 111-373, the Pedestrian Safety Enhancement Act of 2010, directs the secretary of transportation to initiate a rulemaking to promulgate a phased-in motor vehicle safety standard (1) establishing performance requirements for an alert sound that allows blind and other pedestrians to detect a nearby electric or hybrid vehicle operating below the cross-over speed, if any; and (2) requiring such vehicles to provide an alert sound conforming to established standard requirements. The act prescribes requirements for such standards and prohibits requiring either driver or pedestrian activation of the alert sound. It also directs the secretary to study and report to Congress on whether there is a safety need to apply such standard to conventional motor vehicles. In addition it requires the allocation of funds to the administrator of the National Highway Transportation Safety Administration to carry out this rulemaking.

P.L. 111-375, the National Alzheimer's Project Act, requires the secretary of HHS to (1) be responsible for the creation and maintenance of an integrated national plan to overcome Alzheimer's; (2) provide information and coordination of Alzheimer's research and services across all federal agencies; (3) accelerate the development of treatments that would prevent, halt, or reverse the course of Alzheimer's; (4) improve the early diagnosis of Alzheimer's disease and coordination of the care and treatment of citizens with Alzheimer's; (5) ensure the inclusion of ethnic and racial populations at higher risk for Alzheimer's, or least likely to receive care for Alzheimer's, in clinical, research, and service efforts with the purpose of decreasing health disparities in Alzheimer's; and (6) coordinate with international bodies to integrate and inform the fight against Alzheimer's globally.

P.L. 111-380, the Reduction of Lead in Drinking Water Act, amends the Safe Drinking Water Act to exempt from prohibitions on the use or sale of lead pipes, solder, and flux (1) pipes or pipe or plumbing fittings or fixtures, including backflow preventers, that are used exclusively for nonpotable services such as manufacturing, industrial processing, irrigation, outdoor watering, or any other uses where the water is not anticipated to be used for human consumption; or (2) toilets, bidets, urinals, fill valves, flushometer valves, tub fillers, shower valves, service saddles, or water distribution main gate valves that are two inches in diameter or larger.

The act redefines *lead free* to mean (1) not containing more than 0.2 percent lead when used with respect to solder and flux (current law); and (2) not more than a weighted average of 0.25 percent lead when used with respect to the wetted surfaces of pipes and pipe and plumbing fittings and fixtures. It also establishes a formula to calculate the weighted average lead content of a pipe or pipe or plumbing fitting or fixture.

2011

P.L. 112-32, the Combating Autism Reauthorization Act of 2011, amends the Public Health Service Act to extend and reauthorize through FY2014 (1) the surveillance and research program for autism spectrum disorder and other developmental disabilities; (2) the education, early detection, and intervention program for autism spectrum disorder and other developmental disabilities; and (3) the Interagency Autism Coordinating Committee.

P.L. 112-144, the Food and Drug Administration Safety and Innovation Act, amends the FFDCA to reauthorize and establish new FDA prescription drug user-fee programs and revise and impose new requirements relating to (1) prescription, pediatric, and generic drugs; (2) medical devices; (3) biosimilar biological products; (4) new infectious disease drugs; and (5) drug manufacturer reporting.

The act extends through FY2017 the authority of the secretary of HHS to assess and collect human drug application and supplement fees, prescription drug establishment fees, and prescription drug product fees to support the FDA drug development process and the process for the review of human drug applications. It also increases for FY2013–FY2017 the level of required prescription drug user fee revenues and provides for an inflation adjustment and a workload adjustment for FY2013 and for FY2014 and subsequent fiscal years for the required level of user fee revenue amounts.

The act directs the secretary, beginning FY2013, to assess and collect the following fees related to biosimilar biological products: (1) biosimilar program development fees, encompassing an initial biosimilar biological development fee, an annual biosimilar biological product development fee, and a reactivation fee; (2) a biosimilar biological product application and supplement fee; (3) a biosimilar biological product establishment fee; and (4) a biosimilar biological product fee. It waives such fees for a small business's first biosimilar biological product application and terminates such authority on October 1, 2017.

2012

P.L. 112-242, the Medicare IVIG Access and Strengthening Medicare and Repaying Taxpayers Act of 2012, directs the secretary of HHS to establish a three-year demonstration project under Part B (supplementary medical insurance) of Title XVIII (Medicare) of the Social Security Act to evaluate the benefits of providing payment for items and services needed for the in-home administration of intravenous immune globulin (IVIG) for the treatment of primary immune deficiency diseases. The act authorizes the secretary to waive such Medicare requirements as may be necessary to carry out the demonstration project.

2013

P.L. 113-5, the Pandemic and All-Hazards Preparedness Act Reauthorization of 2013, amends the Public Health Service Act to require the secretary of HHS to submit the National Health Security Strategy to the relevant congressional committees in 2014. The act revises the strategy's preparedness goals, in part to specify that the drills and exercises included in periodic evaluations of federal, state, local, and tribal preparedness and response capabilities also include drills and exercises to ensure medical surge capacity for events without notice.

The act requires the strategy to include (1) provisions for increasing the preparedness, response capabilities, and surge capacity of ambulatory care facilities, dental health facilities, and critical care service systems; (2) plans for optimizing a coordinated and flexible approach to the medical surge capacity of hospitals, other healthcare facilities, critical care, and trauma care and emergency medical systems; (3) provisions taking into account the unique needs of individuals with disabilities in a public health emergency; and (4) strategic initiatives to advance countermeasures to diagnose, mitigate, prevent, or treat harm from any biological agent or toxin or any chemical, radiological, or nuclear agent or agents, whether naturally occurring, unintentional, or deliberate.

The act also requires the secretary to (1) monitor emerging issues and concerns as they relate to medical and public health preparedness and response for at-risk individuals in the event of a public health emergency; (2) disseminate and update novel and best practices of outreach to and care of at-risk individuals before, during, and following public health emergencies in as timely a manner as is practicable, including from the time a public health threat is identified; and (3) ensure that public health and medical information distributed by HHS during a public health emergency is delivered in a manner that takes into account the range of communication needs of the intended recipients, including at-risk individuals.

P.L. 113-51, the HIV Organ Policy Equity Act, amends the Public Health Service Act to repeal the requirement that the Organ Procurement and Transplantation Network adopt and use standards of quality for the acquisition and transportation of donated organs that include standards for preventing the acquisition of organs infected with the etiologic agent for AIDS. The act replaces this requirement with authorization for the network to adopt and use such standards with respect to organs infected with HIV, provided that any such standards ensure that organs infected with HIV may be transplanted only into individuals who are (1) infected with such virus before receiving such an organ; and (2) participating in clinical research approved by an institutional review board under the criteria, standards, and regulations regarding organs infected with HIV developed under this act or, if participation in such research is no longer warranted, receiving a transplant under such standards and regulations.

P.L. 113-55, the Prematurity Research Expansion and Education for Mothers Who Deliver Infants Early Reauthorization Act (or the PREEMIE Reauthorization Act), amends the Prematurity Research Expansion and Education for Mothers Who Deliver Infants Early Act to revise and reauthorize requirements for research on prematurity and preterm births.

The act authorizes the director of the CDC to (1) conduct epidemiological studies (as currently required) on the clinical, biological, social, environmental, genetic, and behavioral factors related to prematurity, as appropriate; (2) conduct activities to improve national data to facilitate tracking preterm births; and (3) continue efforts to prevent preterm birth through the identification of opportunities for prevention and the assessment of their impact.

Title II of this act, known as the National Pediatric Research Network Act of 2013, amends the Public Health Service Act to authorize the director of the NIH, in carrying out the Pediatric Research Initiative, to consult with the director of the Eunice Kennedy Shriver National Institute of Child Health and Human Development to provide for the establishment of a national pediatric research network.

The act authorizes the director of the institute to award funding to public or private nonprofit entities for providing support for pediatric research consortia, including with respect to basic, clinical, behavioral, or translational research and the training of researchers in pediatric research techniques. It also requires consortia to (1) be formed from a collaboration of cooperating institutions; (2) be coordinated by a lead institution or institutions; (3) agree to disseminate scientific findings rapidly and efficiently to other consortia, NIH, FDA, and other relevant agencies; and (4) meet requirements prescribed by the director of NIH. The act allows such support to be for a period of five years, with additional extensions at the discretion of the director of NIH.

2014

P.L. 113-77, the Poison Center Network Act, amends the Public Health Service Act to reauthorize through FY2019 (1) a poison control nationwide toll-free phone number; and (2) a national media campaign to educate the public and healthcare providers about poison prevention and the availability of poison control center resources in local communities and to conduct advertising campaigns about the nationwide toll-free number.

The act revises and reauthorizes through FY2019 a grant program for accredited (currently, certified) poison control centers. It allows grant funds to be used to research, improve, and enhance the communications and response capability and capacity of the poison control centers to facilitate increased access to such centers through the integration and modernization of communications and data systems.

P.L. 113-146, the Veterans' Access to Care through Choice, Accountability, and Transparency Act, approved overwhelmingly in the House and Senate, was in response to significant access problems in which veterans experienced long wait times to see physicians and other healthcare providers in Veterans Health Administration (VHA) facilities. An important provision requires hospital care and medical services to be furnished to veterans through contracts with specified non-VA facilities if the veterans (1) have been unable to schedule an appointment at a VA medical facility within the VHA's wait-time goals for hospital care or medical services, and (2) opt for non-VA care or services. The act provides for such care through contracts with any healthcare provider participating in the Medicare program, any federally qualified health center, the Department of Defense, and the Indian Health Service.

Other important provisions of the act expand the hiring and training of VA staff in the healthcare occupations and expand the use of telemedicine to serve veterans. Another provision establishes the Commission on Access to Care to examine veterans' access to VA healthcare and to strategically examine how best to organize the VHA, locate healthcare resources, and deliver healthcare to veterans over the next 10 to 20 years. The act directs the commission to submit an interim and final report to the president on its findings and recommendations for improving access to healthcare through the VHA.

Notes

1. The Library of Congress maintains a website (www.congress.gov), on which extensive information on federal legislation is provided. This is an excellent source of additional information on public laws that pertain to health.
2. Reflecting the convention adopted by Congress, acts began to be referred to by their public law numbers. These numbers reflect both the number of the enacting Congress and the sequence in which the laws are enacted. For example, Public Law (P.L.) 57-244 means the two hundred forty-fourth law passed by the Fifty-Seventh Congress. Hereafter, the public law numbers of health-related federal laws in this chronology are provided.

NATIONAL INSTITUTE OF BIOMEDICAL IMAGING AND BIOENGINEERING ESTABLISHMENT ACT

P.L. 106-580
106th Congress

To amend the Public Health Service Act to establish the National Institute of Biomedical Imaging and Bioengineering.

Be it enacted by the Senate and House of Representatives of the United States of America in Congress assembled,

SECTION 1. SHORT TITLE.

This Act may be cited as the "National Institute of Biomedical Imaging and Bioengineering Establishment Act."

SEC. 2. FINDINGS.

The Congress makes the following findings:

(1) Basic research in imaging, bioengineering, computer science, informatics, and related fields is critical to improving health care but is fundamentally different from the research in molecular biology on which the current national research institutes at the National Institutes of Health (NIH; www.nih.gov) are based. To ensure the development of new techniques and technologies for the 21st century, these disciplines therefore require an identity and research home at the NIH that is independent of the existing institute structure.

(2) Advances based on medical research promise new, more effective treatments for a wide variety of diseases, but the development of new, non-invasive imaging techniques for earlier detection and diagnosis of disease is essential to take full advantage of such new treatments and to promote the general improvement of health care.

(3) The development of advanced genetic and molecular imaging techniques is necessary to continue the current rapid pace of discovery in molecular biology.

(4) Advances in telemedicine, and teleradiology in particular, are increasingly important in the delivery of high-quality, reliable medical care to rural citizens and other underserved populations. To fulfill the promise of telemedicine and related technologies fully, a structure is needed at the NIH to support basic research focused on the acquisition, transmission, processing, and optimal display of images.

(5) A number of Federal departments and agencies support imaging and engineering research with potential medical applications, but a central coordinating body, preferably housed at the NIH, is needed to coordinate these disparate efforts and facilitate the transfer of technologies with medical applications.

(6) Several breakthrough imaging technologies, including magnetic resonance imaging (MRI) and computed tomography (CT), have been developed primarily abroad, in large part because of the absence of a home at the NIH for basic research in imaging and related fields. The establishment of a central focus for imaging and bioengineering research at the NIH would promote both scientific advance[s] and United States economic development.

(7) At a time when a consensus exists to add significant resources to the NIH in coming years, it is appropriate to modernize the structure of the NIH to ensure that research dollars are expended more effectively and efficiently and that the fields of medical science that have contributed the most to the detection, diagnosis, and treatment of disease in recent years receive appropriate emphasis.

(8) The establishment of a National Institute of Biomedical Imaging and Bioengineering at the NIH would accelerate the development of new technologies with clinical and research applications, improve coordination and efficiency at the NIH and throughout the Federal Government, reduce duplication and waste, lay the foundation for a new medical information age, promote economic development, and provide a structure to train the young researchers who will make the path-breaking discoveries of the next century.

SEC. 3. ESTABLISHMENT OF NATIONAL INSTITUTE OF BIOMEDICAL IMAGING AND BIOENGINEERING.

(a) In General.—Part C of Title IV of the Public Health Service Act (42 U.S.C. 285 et seq.) is amended by adding at the end the following subpart:

Subpart 18—National Institute of Biomedical Imaging and Bioengineering

PURPOSE OF THE INSTITUTE

Sec. 464z. (a) The general purpose of the National Institute of Biomedical Imaging and Bioengineering (in this section referred to as the "Institute") is the conduct and support of research, training, the dissemination of health information, and other programs with respect to biomedical imaging, biomedical engineering, and associated technologies and modalities with biomedical applications (in this section referred to as "biomedical imaging and bioengineering").

(b)(1) The Director of the Institute, with the advice of the Institute's advisory council, shall establish a National Biomedical Imaging and Bioengineering Program (in this section referred to as the "Program").

(2) Activities under the Program shall include the following with respect to biomedical imaging and bioengineering:

(A) Research into the development of new techniques and devices.

(B) Related research in physics, engineering, mathematics, computer science, and other disciplines.

(C) Technology assessments and outcomes studies to evaluate the effectiveness of biologics, materials, processes, devices, procedures, and informatics.

(D) Research in screening for diseases and disorders.

(E) The advancement of existing imaging and bioengineering modalities, including imaging, biomaterials, and informatics.

(F) The development of target-specific agents to enhance images and to identify and delineate disease.

(G) The development of advanced engineering and imaging technologies and techniques for research from the molecular and genetic to the whole organ and body levels.

(H) The development of new techniques and devices for more effective interventional procedures (such as image-guided interventions).

(3)(A) With respect to the Program, the Director of the Institute shall prepare and transmit to the Secretary and the Director of NIH a plan to initiate, expand, intensify, and coordinate activities of the Institute with respect to biomedical imaging and bioengineering. The plan shall include such comments and recommendations as the Director of the Institute determines appropriate. The Director of the Institute shall periodically review and revise the plan and shall transmit any revisions of the plan to the Secretary and the Director of NIH.

(B) The plan under subparagraph (A) shall include the recommendations of the Director of the Institute with respect to the following:

(i) Where appropriate, the consolidation of programs of the National Institutes of Health for the express purpose of enhancing support of activities regarding basic biomedical imaging and bioengineering research.

(ii) The coordination of the activities of the Institute with related activities of the other agencies of the National Institutes of Health and with related activities of other Federal agencies.

(c) The establishment under section 406 of an advisory council for the Institute is subject to the following:

(1) The number of members appointed by the Secretary shall be 12.

(2) Of such members—

(A) six members shall be scientists, engineers, physicians, and other health professionals who represent disciplines in biomedical imaging and bioengineering and who are not officers or employees of the United States; and

(B) six members shall be scientists, engineers, physicians, and other health professionals who represent other disciplines and are knowledgeable about the applications of biomedical imaging and bioengineering in medicine, and who are not officers or employees of the United States.

(3) In addition to the ex officio members specified in section 406(b)(2), the ex officio members of the advisory council shall include the Director of the Centers for Disease Control and Prevention, the Director of the National Science Foundation, and the Director of the National Institute of Standards and Technology (or the designees of such officers).

(d)(1) Subject to paragraph (2), for the purpose of carrying out this section:

(A) For fiscal year 2001, there is authorized to be appropriated an amount equal to the amount obligated by the National Institutes of Health during fiscal year 2000 for biomedical imaging and bioengineering, except that such amount shall be adjusted to offset any inflation occurring after October 1, 1999.

(B) For each of the fiscal years 2002 and 2003, there is authorized to be appropriated an amount equal to the amount appropriated under subparagraph (A) for fiscal year 2001, except that such amount shall be adjusted for the fiscal year involved to offset any inflation occurring after October 1, 2000.

(2) The authorization of appropriations for a fiscal year under paragraph (1) is hereby reduced by the amount of any appropriation made for such year for the conduct or support by any other national research institute of any program with respect to biomedical imaging and bioengineering.

(b) USE OF EXISTING RESOURCES.—In providing for the establishment of the National Institute of Biomedical Imaging and Bioengineering pursuant to the amendment made by subsection (a), the Director of the National Institutes of Health (referred to in this subsection as "NIH")—

(1) may transfer to the National Institute of Biomedical Imaging and Bioengineering such personnel of NIH as the Director determines to be appropriate;

(2) may, for quarters for such Institute, utilize such facilities of NIH as the Director determines to be appropriate; and

(3) may obtain administrative support for the Institute from the other agencies of NIH, including the other national research institutes.

(c) CONSTRUCTION OF FACILITIES.—None of the provisions of this Act or the amendments made by the Act may be construed as authorizing the construction of facilities, or the acquisition of land, for purposes of the establishment or operation of the National Institute of Biomedical Imaging and Bioengineering.

(d) DATE CERTAIN FOR ESTABLISHMENT OF ADVISORY COUNCIL.—Not later than 90 days after the effective date of this Act under section 4, the Secretary of Health and Human Services shall complete the establishment of an advisory council for the National Institute of Biomedical Imaging and Bioengineering in accordance with section 406 of the Public Health Service Act and in accordance with section 464z of such Act (as added by subsection (a) of this section).

(e) CONFORMING AMENDMENT.—Section 401(b)(1) of the Public Health Service Act (42 U.S.C. 281(b)(1)) is amended by adding at the end the following subparagraph:

(R) The National Institute of Biomedical Imaging and Bioengineering.

SEC. 4. EFFECTIVE DATE.

This Act takes effect October 1, 2000, or upon the date of the enactment of this Act, whichever occurs later.

Approved December 29, 2000.

Source: National Institute of Biomedical Imaging and Bioengineering Establishment Act of 2000, Pub. L. No. 106-580, 114 Stat. 3088 (2000). Accessed January 16, 2014. www.gpo .gov/fdsys/pkg/PLAW-106publ580/pdf/PLAW-106publ580.pdf.

6

SUMMARIES OF A PROPOSED AND A FINAL RULE

A Proposed Rule

DEPARTMENT OF HEALTH AND HUMAN SERVICES

Centers for Medicare & Medicaid Services

42 CFR Parts 403, 411, 417, and 423

[CMS-4068-P]

RIN 0938-AN08

Medicare Program; Medicare Prescription Drug Benefit

AGENCY: Centers for Medicare & Medicaid Services (CMS), HHS.

ACTION: Proposed rule.

SUMMARY: This proposed rule would implement the new Medicare Prescription Drug Benefit. This new voluntary prescription drug benefit program was enacted into law on December 8, 2003, in section 101 of the Medicare Prescription Drug, Improvement, and Modernization Act of 2003 (MMA). The addition of a prescription drug benefit to Medicare represents a landmark change to the Medicare program that will significantly improve the healthcare coverage available to millions of Medicare beneficiaries. The MMA specifies that the prescription drug benefit program will become available to beneficiaries beginning on January 1, 2006. Please see the executive summary in the SUPPLEMENTARY INFORMATION section for further synopsis of this rule.

DATES: To be assured consideration, comments must be received at one of the addresses provided below, no later than 5:00 p.m. on October 4, 2004.

ADDRESSES: In commenting, please refer to file code CMS-4068-P. Because of staff and resource limitations, we cannot accept comments by facsimile (FAX) transmission.

You may submit comments in one of three ways (no duplicates, please):

1. Electronically. You may submit electronic comments to http://www
   .cms.hhs.gov/regulations/ecomments (attachments should be in
   Microsoft Word, WordPerfect, or Excel; however, we prefer Microsoft
   Word).
2. By mail. You may mail written comments (one original and two copies)
   to the following address only: Centers for Medicare & Medicaid
   Services, Department of Health and Human Services, Attention: CMS-
   4068-P, P.O. Box 8014, Baltimore, MD 21244-8014.

   Please allow sufficient time for mailed comments to be received
   before the close of the comment period.
3. By hand or courier. If you prefer, you may deliver (by hand or courier)
   your written comments (one original and two copies) before the
   close of the comment period to one of the following addresses. If you
   intend to deliver your comments to the Baltimore address, please call
   telephone number (410) 786-7197 in advance to schedule your arrival
   with one of our staff members.

(Because access to the interior of the HHH Building is not readily
available to persons without Federal Government identification, commenters
are encouraged to leave their comments in the CMS drop slots located in the
main lobby of the building. A stamp-in clock is available for persons wishing
to retain a proof of filing by stamping in and retaining an extra copy of the
comments being filed.)

Comments mailed to the addresses indicated as appropriate for hand
or courier delivery may be delayed and received after the comment period.

Submission of comments on paperwork requirements. You may submit
comments on this document's paperwork requirements by mailing your
comments to the addresses provided at the end of the "Collection of Information Requirements" section in this document.

For information on viewing public comments, see the beginning of
the SUPPLEMENTARY INFORMATION section.

FOR FURTHER INFORMATION CONTACT: Lynn Orlosky (410) 786-
9064 or Randy Brauer (410) 786-1618 (for issues related to eligibility, elections, enrollment, including auto-enrollment of dual eligible beneficiaries,
and creditable coverage).

Wendy Burger (410) 786-1566 (for issues related to marketing and
user fees).

Vanessa DuranScirri (214) 767-6435 (for issues related to benefits and beneficiary protections, including Part D benefit packages, Part D covered drugs, coordination of benefits in claims processing and tracking of out-of-pocket costs, pharmacy network access standards, plan information dissemination requirements, and privacy of records).

Craig Miner, RPh. (410) 786-1889 or Tony Hausner (410) 786-1093 (for issues of pharmacy benefit cost and utilization management, formulary development, quality assurance, medication therapy management, and electronic prescribing).

Mark Newsom (410) 786-3198 (for issues of submission, review, negotiation, and approval of risk and limited risk bids for PDPs [prescription drug plans] and MA-PD [Medicare Advantage prescription drug] plans; the calculation of the national average bid amount; determination and collection of enrollee premiums; calculation and payment of direct and reinsurance subsidies and risksharing; and retroactive adjustments and reconciliations).

Jim Owens (410) 786-1582 (for issues of licensing and waiver of licensure, the assumption of financial risk for unsubsidized coverage, and solvency requirements for unlicensed sponsors or sponsors who are not licensed in all States in the region in which it wants to offer a PDP).

Terese Klitenic (410) 786-5942 (for issues of coordination of Part D plans with providers of other prescription drug coverage including Medicare Advantage plans, state pharmaceutical assistance programs (SPAPs), Medicaid, and other retiree prescription drug plans; also for issues related to eligibility for and payment of subsidies for assistance with premium and cost-sharing amounts for Part D eligible individuals with lower income and resources; for rules for states on eligibility determinations for low-income subsidies and general state payment provisions including the phased-down state contribution to drug benefit costs assumed by Medicare).

Frank Szeflinski (303) 844-7119 (for issues related to conditions necessary to contract with Medicare as a PDP sponsor, as well as contract requirements, intermediate sanctions, termination procedures and change of ownership requirements; employer group waivers and options; also for issues related to cost-based HMOs and CMPs offering Part D coverage).

John Scott (410) 786-3636 (for issues related to the procedures PDP sponsors must follow with regard to grievances, coverage determinations, and appeals).

Tracey McCutcheon (410) 786-6715 (for issues related to solicitation, review and approval of fallback prescription drug plan proposals; fallback contract requirements; and enrollee premiums and plan payments specific to fallback plans).

Jim Mayhew (410) 786-9244 (for issues related to the alternative retiree drug subsidy).

Joanne Sinsheimer (410) 786-4620 (for issues related to physician self-referral prohibitions).

Brenda Hudson (410) 786-4085 (for issues related to PACE organizations offering Part D coverage).

Julie Walton (410) 786-4622 or Kathryn McCann (410) 786-7623 (for issues related to provisions on Medicare supplemental (Medigap) policies).

For general questions: Please call (410) 786-1296.

Supplementary Information

EXECUTIVE SUMMARY. Generally, coverage for the prescription drug benefit will be provided under private prescription drug plans (PDPs), which will offer only prescription drug coverage, or through Medicare Advantage prescription drug plans (MA-PDs), which will offer prescription drug coverage that is integrated with the healthcare coverage they provide to Medicare beneficiaries under Part C of Medicare. PDPs must offer a basic prescription drug benefit. MA-PDs must offer either a basic benefit or broader coverage for no additional cost. If this required level of coverage is offered, the PDP or MA-PD plan may also offer supplemental benefits through enhanced alternative coverage for an additional premium. All organizations offering drug plans will have flexibility in the design of the prescription drug benefit. Consistent with the MMA, this proposed rule provides for subsidy payments to sponsors of qualified retiree prescription drug plans.

We intend to implement the drug benefit to permit and encourage a range of options for Medicare beneficiaries to augment the standard Medicare coverage for drug costs above the initial coverage limit ($2250 in 2006) and below the annual out-of-pocket threshold ($5100 in 2006). In addition to the coverage established by the statute for low-income beneficiaries, we seek comments on the best way to support options for expanding beneficiaries' drug coverage. Potential options include facilitating coverage through employer plans, MAPD plans and/or high-option PDPs, as well as through charity organizations and State pharmaceutical assistance programs. We specifically seek comments on ways to maximize the continued use of non-Medicare resources (private contributions, employer/union contributions, state contributions, health plan contributions, and other sources) that currently provide at least partial coverage for three-fourths of Medicare beneficiaries. See sections II.C, II.J, and II.P, and II R of this preamble for further details on these issues. We are also considering establishing a CMS demonstration to evaluate possible ways of achieving such extended coverage, and we welcome all suggestions in this regard.

Throughout the preamble, we identify options and alternatives to the provisions we propose. We strongly encourage comments and ideas on our approach and on alternatives to help us design the Medicare Prescription Drug Benefit Program to operate as effectively and efficiently as possible in meeting the needs of Medicare beneficiaries.

Although this proposed rule specifies most of the requirements for implementing the new prescription drug program, readers should note that we are also issuing a closely related proposed rule that concerns Medicare Advantage plans, which will usually combine medical and prescription drug coverage. In addition, although this proposed rule specifies requirements related to PDP regions it does not designate those regions. Regional boundary decisions will be made through a separate process. Additional non-regulatory guidance on this and other topics will also be forthcoming.

We have considered and, in some places, have identified how this proposed rule intersects with other Federal laws, such as the Health Insurance Portability and Accountability Act (HIPAA) of 1996 Certification of Creditable Coverage and the HIPAA Privacy Rule. We are interested in learning how this proposed rule may interact with other legal obligations to which the PDP sponsors and MA-PD plans may be subject and intend to make appropriate changes in the final rule to address such issues.

SUBMITTING COMMENTS: We welcome comments from the public on all issues set forth in this rule to assist us in fully considering issues and developing policies. Comments will be most useful if they are organized by the section of the proposed rule to which they apply. You can assist us by referencing the file code [CMS-4068-P] and the specific "issue identifier" that precedes the section on which you choose to comment.

INSPECTION OF PUBLIC COMMENTS: All comments received before the close of the comment period are available for viewing by the public, including any personally identifiable or confidential business information that is included in a comment. After the close of the comment period, CMS posts all electronic comments received before the close of the comment period on its public website. Comments received timely will be available for public inspection as they are received, generally beginning approximately 3 weeks after publication of a document, at the headquarters of the Centers for

Medicare & Medicaid Services, 7500 Security Boulevard, Baltimore, Maryland 21244, Monday through Friday of each week from 8:30 a.m. to 4:00 p.m. To schedule an appointment to view public comments, phone (410) 786-7197.

COPIES: To order copies of the Federal Register containing this document, send your request to: New Orders, Superintendent of Documents, P.O. Box 371954, Pittsburgh, PA 15250-7954. Specify the date of the issue requested and enclose a check or money order payable to the Superintendent of Documents, or enclose your Visa or Master Card number and expiration date. Credit card orders can also be placed by calling the order desk at (202) 512-1800 (or toll-free at 1-888-293-6498) or by faxing to (202) 512-2250. The cost for each copy is $10. As an alternative, you can view and photocopy the Federal Register document at most libraries designated as Federal Depository Libraries and at many other public and academic libraries throughout the country that receive the Federal Register. This Federal Register document is also available from the Federal Register online database through GPO Access, a service of the U.S. Government Printing Office. The Web site address is: *http://www.access.gpo.gov/fr/index.html.*

Source: Reprinted from "Medicare Program; Medicare Prescription Drug Benefit." 69 Fed. Reg. 148 (August 3, 2004), 46631–33. Accessed January 16, 2014. www.cms.gov /Regulations-and-Guidance/Regulations-and-Policies/QuarterlyProviderUpdates /Downloads/cms4068p.pdf.

A Final Rule

DEPARTMENT OF HEALTH AND HUMAN SERVICES

Centers for Medicare & Medicaid Services

42 CFR Parts 400, 403, 411, 417, and 423

[CMS-4068-F]

RIN 0938-AN08

Medicare Program; Medicare Prescription Drug Benefit

AGENCY: Centers for Medicare & Medicaid Services (CMS), HHS.

ACTION: Final rule.

SUMMARY: This final rule implements the provisions of the Social Security Act (the Act) establishing and regulating the Medicare Prescription Drug

Benefit. The new voluntary prescription drug benefit program was enacted into law on December 8, 2003 in section 101 of Title I of the Medicare Prescription Drug, Improvement, and Modernization Act of 2003 (MMA; Pub. L. 108-173). Although this final rule specifies most of the requirements for implementing the new prescription drug program, readers should note that we are also issuing a closely related rule that concerns Medicare Advantage organizations, which, if they offer coordinated care plans, must offer at least one plan that combines medical coverage under Parts A and B with prescription drug coverage. Readers should also note that separate CMS guidance on many operational details appears or will soon appear on the CMS website, such as materials on formulary review criteria, risk plan and fallback plan solicitations, bid instructions, solvency standards and pricing tools, and plan benefit packages.

The addition of a prescription drug benefit to Medicare represents a landmark change to the Medicare program that will significantly improve the healthcare coverage available to millions of Medicare beneficiaries. The MMA specifies that the prescription drug benefit program will become available to beneficiaries beginning on January 1, 2006.

Generally, coverage for the prescription drug benefit will be provided under private prescription drug plans (PDPs), which will offer only prescription drug coverage, or through Medicare Advantage prescription drug plans (MA-PDs), which will offer prescription drug coverage that is integrated with the healthcare coverage they provide to Medicare beneficiaries under Part C of Medicare. PDPs must offer a basic prescription drug benefit. MA-PDs must offer either a basic benefit or broader coverage for no additional cost. If this required level of coverage is offered, MA-PDs or PDPs, but not fallback PDPs, may also offer supplemental benefits through enhanced alternative coverage for an additional premium. All organizations offering drug plans will have flexibility in the design of the prescription drug benefit. Consistent with the MMA, this final rule also provides for subsidy payments to sponsors of qualified retiree prescription drug plans to encourage retention of employer-sponsored benefits.

We are implementing the drug benefit in a way that permits and encourages a range of options for Medicare beneficiaries to augment the standard Medicare coverage. These options include facilitating additional coverage through employer plans, MA-PD plans and high-option PDPs, and through charity organizations and State pharmaceutical assistance programs. See sections II.C, II.J, and II.P, and II.R of this preamble for further details on these issues.

The proposed rule identified options and alternatives to the provisions we proposed and we strongly encouraged comments and ideas on our approach and on alternatives to help us design the Medicare Prescription Drug Benefit Program to operate as effectively and efficiently as possible in meeting the needs of Medicare beneficiaries.

DATES: These regulations are effective on March 22, 2005.

FOR FURTHER INFORMATION CONTACT: [*This Final Rule contains a long list of contacts similar to the one shown above for the Proposed Rule; the list is omitted here.*]

Table of Contents [*Condensed*]

I.   Background
     A. Medicare Prescription Drug, Improvement, and Modernization Act of 2003
     B. Codification of Regulations
     C. Organizational Overview of Part 423

II. Discussion of the Provisions of the Final Rule
     A. General Provisions
     B. Eligibility and Enrollment
     C. Voluntary Prescription Benefits and Beneficiary Protections
     D. Cost Control and Quality Improvement Requirements for Part D Plans
     E. RESERVED
     F. Submission of Bids and Monthly Beneficiary Premiums: Plan Approval
     G. Payments to Part D Plan Sponsors for Qualified Prescription Drug Coverage
     H. RESERVED
     I. Organization Compliance with State Law and Preemption by Federal Law
     J. Coordination Under Part D Plans with Other Prescription Drug Coverage
     K. Application Procedures and Contracts with PDP Sponsors
     L. Effect of Change of Ownership or Leasing of Facilities During the Term of Contract
     M. Grievances, Coverage Determinations, and Appeals
     N. Medicare Contract Determinations and Appeals
     O. Intermediate Sanctions
     P. Premiums and Cost-Sharing Subsidies for Low-Income Individuals
     Q. Guaranteeing Access to a Choice of Coverage (Fallback Prescription Drug Plans)
     R. Payments to Sponsors of Retiree Prescription Drug Plans

S. Special Rules for States-Eligibility Determinations for Low-Income Subsidies, and General Payment Provisions

T. Part D Provisions Affecting Physician Self-Referral, Cost-Based HMO, PACE, and Medigap Requirements

III. Provisions of the Final Rule

IV. Collection of Information Requirements

V. Regulatory Impact Analysis

Source: Reprinted from "Medicare Program; Medicare Prescription Drug Benefit." 70 Fed. Reg. 18 (January 28, 2005), 4194–96. Accessed January 16, 2015. www.gpo.gov/fdsys /pkg/FR-2005-01-28/pdf/05-1321.pdf.

NEWS RELEASE: FDA ALLOWS MARKETING OF FIRST MEDICAL DEVICE TO PREVENT MIGRAINE HEADACHES

Today, the U.S. Food and Drug Administration allowed marketing of the first device as a preventative treatment for migraine headaches. This is also the first transcutaneous electrical nerve stimulation (TENS) device specifically authorized for use prior to the onset of pain.

"Cefaly provides an alternative to medication for migraine prevention," said Christy Foreman, director of the Office of Device Evaluation at the FDA's Center for Devices and Radiological Health. "This may help patients who cannot tolerate current migraine medications for preventing migraines or treating attacks."

Migraine headaches are characterized by intense pulsing or throbbing pain in one area of the head, accompanied by nausea or vomiting and sensitivity to light and sound. A migraine can last from four to 72 hours when left untreated. According to the National Institutes of Health, these debilitating headaches affect approximately 10 percent of people worldwide and are three times more common in women than men.

Cefaly is a small, portable, battery-powered, prescription device that resembles a plastic headband worn across the forehead and atop the ears. The user positions the device in the center of the forehead, just above the eyes, using a self-adhesive electrode. The device applies an electric current to the skin and underlying body tissues to stimulate branches of the trigeminal nerve, which has been associated with migraine headaches. The user may feel a tingling or massaging sensation where the electrode is applied. Cefaly is indicated for patients 18 years of age and older and should only be used once per day for 20 minutes.

The FDA reviewed the data for Cefaly through the de novo premarket review pathway, a regulatory pathway for generally low- to moderate-risk medical devices that are not substantially equivalent to an already legally marketed device.

The agency evaluated the safety and effectiveness of the device based on data from a clinical study conducted in Belgium involving 67 individuals who experienced more than two migraine headache attacks a month and who had not taken any medications to prevent migraines for three months prior to using Cefaly, as well as a patient satisfaction study of 2,313 Cefaly users in France and Belgium.

The 67-person study showed that those who used Cefaly experienced significantly fewer days with migraines per month and used less migraine attack medication than those who used a placebo device. The device did not completely prevent migraines and did not reduce the intensity of migraines that did occur.

The patient satisfaction study showed that a little more than 53 percent of patients were satisfied with Cefaly treatment and willing to buy the device for continued use. The most commonly reported complaints were dislike of the feeling and not wanting to continue using the device, sleepiness during the treatment session, and headache after the treatment session.

No serious adverse events occurred during either study.

Cefaly is manufactured by STX-Med in Herstal, Liege, Belgium.

Source: Reprinted from US Food and Drug Administration. 2014. "FDA Allows Marketing of First Medical Device to Prevent Migraine Headaches." News release. Issued March 11. www.fda.gov/NewsEvents/Newsroom/PressAnnouncements/ucm388765.htm.

SMOKEFREE LAWS

Since the 1970s, the nonsmokers' rights movement has made significant progress toward clean indoor air. As of January 2, 2014, there were 4,019 states, commonwealths, territories, and municipalities with laws in effect that restrict where smoking is allowed as follows:

Local

- A total of 3,964 municipalities in the United States have laws in effect that restrict where smoking is allowed.
- Of these 3,964, a total of 1,087 municipalities have a 100 percent smokefree provision in effect—either in non-hospitality workplaces, and/or restaurants, and/or bars.
- There are 867 municipalities with laws in effect that require non-hospitality workplaces to be 100 percent smokefree.
- There are 901 municipalities with laws in effect that require restaurants to be 100 percent smokefree.
- There are 771 municipalities with laws in effect that require bars to be 100 percent smokefree.
- There are 598 municipalities with laws in effect that require non-hospitality workplaces, restaurants, and bars to be 100 percent smokefree.
- There are 685 municipalities with laws in effect that require both non-hospitality workplaces and restaurants to be 100 percent smokefree.
- There are 764 municipalities with laws in effect that require both restaurants and bars to be 100 percent smokefree.

State and Local

- Across the United States, 22,487 municipalities, representing 81.5 percent of the US population, are covered by a 100 percent smokefree provision in non-hospitality workplaces, and/or restaurants, and/or bars, by either a state, commonwealth, territorial, or local law.

- A total of 39 states and the District of Columbia have local laws in effect that require non-hospitality workplaces and/or restaurants and/or bars to be 100 percent smokefree.

- There are 2,695 states, commonwealths, territories, cities, and counties with a law that restricts smoking in one or more outdoor areas, including 1,238 that restrict smoking near entrances, windows, and ventilation systems of enclosed places; 2,034 that restrict smoking in public outdoor places such as parks, beaches, and service lines; 322 that prohibit smoking in all outdoor stadiums and other sports and entertainment venues, and 427 that restrict smoking in some areas within outdoor stadiums and other sports and entertainment venues.

State, Commonwealth, and Territory

- A total of 36 states, along with the District of Columbia, American Samoa, the Northern Mariana Islands, Puerto Rico, and the US Virgin Islands, have laws in effect that require non-hospitality workplaces and/or restaurants and/or bars and/or state-run gambling establishments to be100 percent smokefree:
  - American Samoa: Restaurants
  - Arizona: Workplaces, Restaurants, Bars, and State-Regulated Gambling
  - California: Restaurants, Bars, and State-Regulated Gambling
  - Colorado: Restaurants, Bars, and State-Regulated Gambling
  - Connecticut: Restaurants and Bars
  - Delaware: Workplaces, Restaurants, Bars, and State-Regulated Gambling
  - District of Columbia: Workplaces, Restaurants, and Bars
  - Florida: Workplaces, Restaurants, and State-Regulated Gambling
  - Hawaii: Workplaces, Restaurants, and Bars
  - Idaho: Restaurants
  - Illinois: Workplaces, Restaurants, Bars, and State-Regulated Gambling
  - Indiana: Workplaces and Restaurants
  - Iowa: Workplaces, Restaurants, and Bars
  - Kansas: Workplaces, Restaurants, and Bars
  - Louisiana: Workplaces and Restaurants

- Maine: Workplaces, Restaurants, Bars, and State-Regulated Gambling Facilities opened in July 2003 or later
- Maryland: Workplaces, Restaurants, Bars, and State-Regulated Gambling
- Massachusetts: Workplaces, Restaurants, Bars, and State-Regulated Gambling
- Michigan: Workplaces, Restaurants, and Bars
- Minnesota: Workplaces, Restaurants, Bars, and State-Regulated Gambling
- Montana: Workplaces, Restaurants, Bars, and State-Regulated Gambling
- Nebraska: Workplaces, Restaurants, Bars, and State-Regulated Gambling
- Nevada: Workplaces and Restaurants
- New Hampshire: Restaurants and Bars
- New Jersey: Workplaces, Restaurants, and Bars
- New Mexico: Restaurants and Bars
- New York: Workplaces, Restaurants, Bars, and State-Regulated Gambling
- North Carolina: Restaurants and Bars
- North Dakota: Workplaces, Restaurants, Bars, and State-Regulated Gambling
- Northern Mariana Islands: Workplaces
- Ohio: Workplaces, Restaurants, Bars, and State-Regulated Gambling
- Oregon: Workplaces, Restaurants, Bars, and State-Regulated Gambling
- Pennsylvania: Workplaces
- Puerto Rico: Workplaces, Restaurants, Bars, and State-Regulated Gambling
- Rhode Island: Workplaces, Restaurants, and Bars
- South Dakota: Workplaces, Restaurants, Bars, and State-Regulated Gambling
- US Virgin Islands: Workplaces, Restaurants, Bars, and State-Regulated Gambling
- Utah: Workplaces, Restaurants, and Bars
- Vermont: Workplaces, Restaurants, Bars, and State-Regulated Gambling
- Washington: Workplaces, Restaurants, Bars, and State-Regulated Gambling

- Wisconsin: Workplaces, Restaurants, Bars, and State-Regulated Gambling

• There are 24 states, along with the District of Columbia, Puerto Rico, and the US Virgin Islands, which have laws in effect that require non-hospitality workplaces, restaurants, and bars to be 100 percent smokefree. These laws, along with local laws in other states, protect 49.1 percent of the US population.

• There are 30 states, along with the District of Columbia, Puerto Rico, and the US Virgin Islands, which have laws in effect that require restaurants and bars to be 100 percent smokefree. These laws, along with local laws in other states, protect 65 percent of the US population.

• There are 20 states, along with Puerto Rico and the US Virgin Islands, which have laws in effect that require all state-regulated gambling to be 100 percent smokefree. (Note: Maine's smokefree gambling law is for those facilities opened July 2003 or later.)

Source: Reprinted with permission from American Nonsmokers' Rights Foundation. 2014. "Overview List—How Many Smokefree Laws?" Accessed February 18. www.no-smoke.org /pdf/mediaordlist.pdf.

LAWS IMPLEMENTED BY THE EPA

The mission of the Environmental Protection Agency (EPA; www.epa.gov) is to protect human health and the environment. Established in 1970, EPA develops and enforces regulations that implement environmental laws enacted by Congress. EPA's FY2014 budget was approximately $8.2 billion. The major pieces of legislation that EPA implements or partially implements include the following.

Atomic Energy Act (AEA; 1946)—The AEA established the Atomic Energy Commission to promote the use of atomic energy for peaceful purposes to the maximum extent consistent with the common defense and security and with the health and safety of the public.

Clean Air Act (CAA; 1970)—The CAA is the comprehensive federal law that regulates air emissions from area, stationary, and mobile sources. This law authorizes EPA to establish national ambient air quality standards (NAAQS) to protect public health and the environment.

Clean Water Act (CWA; 1977)—Growing public awareness of and concern for controlling water pollution led to enactment of the Federal Water Pollution Control Act Amendments of 1972. As amended in 1977, this law became commonly known as the Clean Water Act. The CWA established the basic structure for regulating discharges of pollutants into the waters of the United States. It gave EPA the authority to implement pollution control programs such as setting wastewater standards for industry.

Comprehensive Environmental Response, Compensation, and Liability Act (CERCLA or Superfund; 1980)—The CERCLA created a tax on the chemical and petroleum industries and provided broad federal authority to respond directly to releases or threatened releases of hazardous substances that may endanger public health or the environment. Over five years, $1.6 billion was collected, and the tax went to a trust fund (called the Superfund) for cleaning up abandoned or uncontrolled hazardous waste sites. The CERCLA established prohibitions and requirements concerning closed and abandoned hazardous waste sites, provided for liability of persons responsible for releases of hazardous waste at these sites, and established a trust fund to provide for cleanup when no responsible party could be identified.

Emergency Planning and Community Right-to-Know Act (EPCRA; 1986)—The EPCRA was enacted by Congress as the national legislation on community safety. This law was designated to help local communities protect public health, safety, and the environment from chemical hazards. To implement the EPCRA, Congress required each state to appoint a state emergency response commission (SERC). The SERCs were required to divide their states into emergency planning districts and to name a local emergency planning committee (LEPC) for each district.

Endangered Species Act (ESA; 1973)—The ESA provides a program for the conservation of threatened and endangered plants and animals and the habitats in which they are found. EPA's decision to register a pesticide is based on the risk of adverse effects on endangered species and on environmental fate (how a pesticide will affect habitats).

Energy Independence and Security Act (EISA; 2007)—The EISA aims to move the United States toward greater energy independence, increase the production of clean renewable fuels, and increase US energy security. It promotes research on and the deployment of greenhouse gas capture and storage options.

Energy Policy Act (EPA; 2005)—The EPA addresses energy production in the United States, including (1) energy efficiency; (2) renewable energy; (3) oil and gas; (4) coal; (5) Tribal energy; (6) nuclear matters and security; (7) vehicles and motor fuels, including ethanol; (8) hydrogen; (9) electricity; (10) energy tax incentives; (11) hydropower and geothermal energy; and (12) climate change technology.

Federal Food, Drug, and Cosmetic Act (FFDCA; 1938)—The FFDCA extended federal authority to ban new drugs from the market until they were approved by the Food and Drug Administration (FDA). The law also gave the federal government more extensive power in dealing with adulterated or mislabeled food, drugs, and cosmetic products.

Federal Insecticide, Fungicide, and Rodenticide Act (FIFRA; 1972)—The FIFRA provides for federal control of pesticide distribution, sale, and use. It gives EPA authority not only to study the consequences of pesticide usage but also to require users (farmers, utility companies, and others) to register when purchasing pesticides. Through later amendments to the law, users also must take exams for certification as applicators of pesticides. All pesticides used in the United States must be registered (licensed) by EPA.

Food Quality Protection Act (FQPA; 1996)—The FQPA amended the FIFRA and FFDCA. These amendments fundamentally changed the way EPA regulates pesticides. The requirements included a new safety standard—reasonable certainty of no harm—that must be applied to all pesticides used on foods.

Marine Protection, Research, and Sanctuaries Act (MPRSA; 1988)—The MPRSA, also referred to as the Ocean Dumping Act, generally prohibits (1) transportation of material from the United States for the purpose of ocean dumping; (2) transportation of material from anywhere for the purpose of ocean dumping by US agencies or US-flagged vessels; (3) dumping of material transported from outside the United States into the US territorial sea.

National Environmental Policy Act (NEPA; 1969)—The NEPA established a broad national framework for protecting the nation's environment. It is the basic national charter for protection of the environment. It seeks to ensure that all branches of government give proper consideration to the environment before undertaking any actions that significantly affect the environment. For example, NEPA requirements are invoked when airports, buildings, military complexes, and highways are proposed. Environmental Assessments (EAs) and Environmental Impact Statements (EISs), which are assessments of the likelihood of impacts from alternative courses of action, are the most visible NEPA requirements.

Noise Control Act (1972)—This act establishes a national policy to promote an environment free from noise that jeopardizes the health and welfare of people. The act also serves to (1) establish a means for effective coordination of federal research and activities in noise control; (2) authorize the establishment of federal noise emission standards for products distributed in commerce; and (3) provide information to the public regarding the noise emission and noise reduction characteristics of such products.

Nuclear Waste Policy Act (NWPA; 1982)—The NWPA supports the use of deep geologic repositories for the safe storage and/or disposal of radioactive waste. The act establishes procedures to evaluate and select sites for geologic repositories and for the interaction of state and federal governments. It also provides a timetable of key milestones the federal agencies must meet in carrying out the program.

Occupational Safety and Health Act (OSHA; 1970)—The OSHA was enacted to ensure worker and workplace safety. It requires employers to provide workers with a place of employment free from recognized hazards to safety and health, such as exposure to toxic chemicals, excessive noise levels, mechanical dangers, heat or cold stress, or unsanitary conditions.

Oil Pollution Act (OPA; 1990)—The OPA streamlined and strengthened EPA's ability to prevent and respond to catastrophic oil spills. It established a trust fund, financed by a tax on oil, to fund the cleanup of spills when the responsible party is incapable of doing so or unwilling to do so.

Pollution Prevention Act (PPA; 1990)—The PPA focused industry, government, and public attention on reducing the amount of pollution through cost-effective changes in production, operation, and raw materials use. Opportunities for source reduction are often not realized because existing regulations and the industrial resources required for compliance focus on treatment and disposal. Source reduction is fundamentally different than waste management or pollution control.

Resource Conservation and Recovery Act (RCRA; 1976)—The RCRA gave EPA the authority to control hazardous waste from the "cradle to the grave." This includes the generation, transportation, treatment, storage, and disposal of hazardous waste.

Safe Drinking Water Act (SDWA; 1974)—The SWDA was established to protect the quality of drinking water in the United States. This law focuses on all waters actually or potentially designed for drinking use, whether from aboveground or underground sources. It authorized EPA to establish safe standards of purity and required all owners or operators of public water systems to comply with primary (health-related) standards.

Shore Protection Act (SPA; 1988)—The *Marine Protection, Research, and Sanctuaries Act of 1988,* also known as the Ocean Dumping Act, created the Shore Protection Act, which prohibits the transportation of municipal or commercial waste within coastal waters by a vessel without a permit and number or other marking. The goal of the act is to minimize deposit of waste into coastal waters during vessel loading, transport, and unloading, and to ensure that any deposited waste is reported and cleaned up.

Superfund Amendments and Reauthorization Act (SARA; 1986)— The SARA amended the CERCLA to reflect EPA's experience in administering the complex Superfund program during its first six years and made several important changes and additions to the program. The SARA

- stressed the importance of permanent remedies and innovative treatment technologies in cleaning up hazardous waste sites,
- required Superfund actions to consider the standards and requirements found in other state and federal environmental laws and regulations,
- provided new enforcement authorities and settlement tools,
- increased state involvement in every phase of the Superfund program,
- increased the focus on human health problems posed by hazardous waste sites,
- encouraged greater citizen participation in making decisions on how sites should be cleaned up, and
- increased the size of the trust fund to $8.5 billion.

Toxic Substances Control Act (TSCA; 1976)—The TSCA gave EPA the ability to track the industrial chemicals produced or imported into the United States. EPA repeatedly screens these chemicals and can require reporting or testing of those that may pose an environmental or human-health hazard. EPA can ban the manufacture and import of those chemicals that pose an unreasonable risk.

Source: Adapted from Environmental Protection Agency. 2014. "Laws and Executive Orders." Accessed March 20. www2.epa.gov/laws-regulations/laws-and-executive -orders#influence.

MEDICARE REVISITED—AGAIN AND AGAIN **10**

This chronological list contains some of the key legislative changes that have been made in the Medicare program since its enactment. The list reflects how frequently and substantively the program has been modified.

- **1965.** Medicare was enacted as Title XVIII of the Social Security Act, extending health coverage to almost all Americans aged 65 or older. Medicare was implemented and more than 19 million individuals enrolled on July 1, 1966.
- **1972.** Medicare eligibility was extended to individuals under age 65 with long-term disabilities and to individuals with end-stage renal disease (ESRD). Medicare was given the authority to conduct demonstration programs.
- **1977.** The Health Care Financing Administration (HCFA) was established to administer the Medicare program. On July 1, 2001, HCFA became the Centers for Medicare & Medicaid Services (CMS).
- **1980.** Coverage of Medicare home health services was broadened. Medicare supplemental insurance, also called "Medigap," was brought under federal oversight.
- **1982.** The Tax Equity and Fiscal Responsibility Act made it easier and more attractive for health maintenance organizations to contract with the Medicare program. In addition, the act expanded CMS's quality oversight efforts through peer review organizations (PROs).
- **1983.** An inpatient acute hospital prospective payment system (PPS) for the Medicare program, based on patients' diagnoses, was adopted to replace cost-based payments.
- **1985.** The Emergency Medical Treatment and Labor Act (EMTALA) required hospitals participating in Medicare that operated active emergency rooms to provide appropriate medical screenings and stabilizing treatments.
- **1988.** The Medicare Catastrophic Coverage Act, which included the most significant changes since enactment of the Medicare program, improved hospital and skilled nursing facility benefits for beneficiaries, covered mammography, and included an outpatient prescription drug

benefit (the Medicare Catastrophic Coverage Act) and a cap on patient liability.

The Qualified Medicare Beneficiary (QMB) program was established to pay Medicare premiums and cost-sharing charges for beneficiaries with incomes and resources below established thresholds.

- **1989.** The Medicare Catastrophic Coverage Act of 1988 was repealed after higher-income older adults protested new premiums. A new Medicare fee schedule was established for physician and other professional services, and a resource-based relative value scale replaced charge-based payments. Limits were placed on physician balance billing above the new fee schedule. Physicians were prohibited from referring Medicare patients to clinical laboratories in which the physicians, or physicians' family members, have a financial interest.

- **1990.** Specified Low-Income Medicare Beneficiary (SLMB) eligibility group was established for Medicaid programs to pay Medicare premiums for beneficiaries with incomes at least 100 percent but not more than 120 percent of the FPL (federal poverty level) and limited financial resources. Additional federal standards for Medicare supplemental insurance were enacted.

- **1996.** The Health Insurance Portability and Accountability Act of 1996 (HIPAA) had implications for the Medicare program. The act created the Medicare Integrity Program, which dedicated funding to program integrity activities and allowed CMS to competitively contract for program integrity work. HIPAA also created national administrative simplification standards for electronic healthcare transactions that applied to Medicare.

- **1997.** The Balanced Budget Act of 1997 (BBA) changed Medicare in a number of ways, including the following:

  - It established an array of new Medicare managed care and other private health plan choices for beneficiaries, offered through a coordinated open enrollment process.
  - It expanded education and information to help beneficiaries make informed choices about their healthcare.
  - It required CMS to develop and implement five new prospective payment systems for Medicare services (for inpatient rehabilitation hospital or unit services, skilled nursing facility services, home health services, hospital outpatient department services, and outpatient rehabilitation services).
  - It slowed the rate of growth in Medicare spending and extended the life of the trust fund for ten years.
  - It provided a broad range of beneficiary protections.

- It expanded preventive benefits.
- It called for testing other innovative approaches to payment and service delivery through research and demonstrations.

- **1998.** The Internet site www.medicare.gov was launched to provide updated information about Medicare.
- **1999.** The toll-free number 1-800-MEDICARE (1-800-633-4227) became available nationwide. The first annual *Medicare & You* handbook was mailed to all Medicare beneficiary households.

    The Ticket to Work and Work Incentives Improvements Act of 1999 (TWWIIA) expanded the availability of Medicare and Medicaid for certain beneficiaries with disabilities who return to work. The Balanced Budget Refinement Act of 1999 (BBRA) increased payments for some Medicare providers.

- **2000.** The Benefits Improvement and Protection Act (BIPA) further increased Medicare payments to providers and managed healthcare organizations, reduced certain Medicare beneficiary copayments, and improved Medicare's coverage of preventive services.

- **2003.** The Medicare Prescription Drug, Improvement, and Modernization Act (MMA) made the most significant changes to Medicare since the program began. The MMA created a prescription drug discount card until 2006, allowed for competition among health plans to foster innovation and flexibility in coverage, covered new preventive benefits, and made numerous other changes. As of 2006, the voluntary Part D outpatient prescription drug benefit became available to beneficiaries from private drug plans as well as Medicare Advantage plans. Employers who provide retiree drug coverage comparable to Medicare's are eligible for a federal subsidy. Medicare considered beneficiary income for the first time: beneficiaries with incomes less than 150 percent of the federal poverty limit became eligible for subsidies for the Part D prescription drug program. As of 2007, beneficiaries with higher incomes paid a greater share of the Part B premium.

- **2004.** The Medicare-Approved Drug Discount Card Program began. It was accompanied by the transitional assistance program, which provided annual credits of $600 to low-income Medicare beneficiaries who did not have prescription drug coverage in 2004–2005.

- **2005.** The "Welcome to Medicare" physical examination began to be covered. Several preventive services, including cardiovascular screening blood tests and diabetes screening tests, began to be covered for Medicare beneficiaries. Beginning on November 15, 2005, Medicare conducted the first open enrollment period for the new Part D prescription drug benefit. This permitted beneficiaries to enroll in a Medicare Prescription Drug Plan (PDP) or a Medicare Advantage Prescription Drug Plan (MAPD).

- **2006.** The Medicare Drug Benefit, which was established by the Medicare Prescription Drug, Improvement, and Modernization Act of 2003, took effect on January 1. By June 11, 2006, 22.5 million Medicare beneficiaries were enrolled in Part D plans.

- **2007.** Higher-income Medicare beneficiaries (above $80,000 for individuals or $160,000 for couples) paid higher monthly Part B premiums. The payments ranged from $105.80 to $161.40 per month and were based on income.

  The Medicare, Medicaid, and SCHIP Extension Act of 2007 prevented a 10.1 percent reduction in Medicare payments to physicians that was scheduled to take effect in 2008 and, instead, gave physicians a 0.5 percent increase through June 30, 2008.

- **2008.** The Medicare Improvements for Patients and Providers Act of 2008 (MIPPA) extended the planned reduction in Medicare payments to physicians through the end of 2008 and increased payment of their fees for all of 2009 by 1.1 percent. Benefit improvements for Medicare beneficiaries included reduced coinsurance payments for mental health visits and elimination of the deductibles for "Welcome to Medicare" physical examinations.

- **2009.** Although the American Recovery and Reinvestment Act of 2009, which was enacted in response to the global financial crisis that emerged in 2008, was a massive and far-reaching economic stimulus package ($787 billion), a significant amount of the resources (about $150 billion in new funds) was directed to healthcare. Of this, Medicare received a new allocation of $338 million for payments to teaching hospitals, hospice programs, and long-term care hospitals.

- **2010.** The Patient Protection and Affordable Care Act (ACA) amended the Medicare program by incorporating numerous Medicare payment provisions intended to reduce the rate of growth in spending. They include reductions in Medicare Advantage (MA) plan payments and a lowering of the annual payment update for hospitals and certain other providers. The ACA established an Independent Payment Advisory Board (IPAB) to make recommendations for achieving specific Medicare spending reductions if costs exceed a target growth rate. IPAB's recommendations will take effect unless Congress overrides them, in which case Congress would be responsible for achieving the same level of savings. Also, the ACA provided tools to help reduce fraud, waste, and abuse in both Medicare and Medicaid.

The ACA created the Center for Medicare and Medicaid Innovation (CMI) to pilot payment and service delivery models, primarily for Medicare and Medicaid beneficiaries. These include pilot, demonstration, and grant programs to test integrated models of care, including accountable care organizations (ACOs), medical homes that provide coordinated care for high-need individuals, and bundling payments for acute care episodes (including hospitalization and follow-up care). The law also established new pay-for-reporting and pay-for-performance programs within Medicare that will pay providers based on the reporting of, or performance on, selected quality measures. Additionally, the ACA created incentives for promoting primary care and prevention; for example, by increasing primary care payment rates under Medicare and Medicaid.

- **2012.** The Medicare IVIG Access and Strengthening Medicare and Repaying Taxpayers Act directed the secretary of the Department of Health and Human Services (HHS) to establish a three-year demonstration project under Part B (Supplementary Medical Insurance) of Title XVIII (Medicare) of the Social Security Act (SSA) to evaluate the benefits of providing payment for items and services needed for the in-home administration of intravenous immune globulin (IVIG) for the treatment of primary immune deficiency diseases. The act authorized the secretary to waive such Medicare requirements as may be necessary to carry out the demonstration project.

- **2014.** The Protecting Access to Medicare Act of 2014 amended Title XVIII (Medicare) of the Social Security Act (SSA) with respect to the physician payment update to (1) extend the update currently scheduled for January through March of 2014 to the entire calendar year of 2014; (2) freeze the update to the single conversion factor at 0.00 percent for January 1, 2015, through March 31, 2015; and (3) require that the conversion factor for April 1, 2015, through December 31, 2015, and for 2016 and subsequent years be computed as if such freeze had never applied.

  This act also amended the Medicare Improvements for Patients and Providers Act of 2008, as amended by the Patient Protection and Affordable Care Act (ACA), the American Taxpayer Relief Act, and the Pathway for SGR Reform Act of 2013 to extend through March 31, 2015, the funding of various programs, including the area agencies on aging and the contract with the National Center for Benefits and Outreach Enrollment.

  The act also extended (1) the geographic practice cost index (GPCI) floor through April 1, 2015; (2) the therapy cap exceptions process through March 15, 2015; (3) add-on payments for ground ambulance and super rural ground ambulance services through April 1, 2015; (4) the increased inpatient hospital payment adjustment for certain low-volume hospitals starting on April 1, 2015, for FY2016, and subsequent fiscal years; (5) the Medicare-Dependent Hospital (MDH) program through March 31, 2015; (6) specialized Medicare Advantage (MA) plans for individuals with special needs through December 31, 2016; (7) through December 31, 2016, authority to renew a reasonable cost reimbursement contract with a health maintenance organization and competitive medical plan; and (8) through March 31, 2015, the funding for any contract with a consensus-based entity regarding performance measurement as well as multi-stakeholder group input into selection of quality and efficiency measures (endorsement, input, and selection).

Sources: Adapted from the following:

Congress.gov. 2014. "Legislation." Accessed December 1. www. congress.gov/legislation.

Kaiser Family Foundation. 2005. "Medicare: A Timeline of Key Developments." Accessed December 1, 2014. http://kff.org/search/?s=Medicare:+A+timeline+of+key+developments.

US Department of Health and Human Services. 2004. "Key Milestones in CMS Programs." Accessed April 3, 2014. www.cms.gov/About-CMS/Agency-Information/History/down loads/CMSProgramKeyMilestones.pdf.

THE UNITED STATES CONSTITUTION AND THE FEDERAL GOVERNMENT

11

The US Constitution, adopted in 1789 and amended only rarely since then, is the supreme law of the United States. It established a republic under which the individual states retain considerable sovereignty and authority. Each state, for example, has its own elected executive (governor), legislature, and court system. The federal, or national, government is one of strong, but limited, powers. It may exercise only the powers specified in the Constitution itself. All other powers are reserved by the Constitution to the states and the people. This system of divided powers between the national and state governments is known as *federalism.*

The Bill of Rights is set forth as the first ten amendments to the Constitution. It guarantees fundamental rights to the people and protects them against improper acts by the government. The rights protected include such matters as free speech, freedom of assembly, freedom to seek redress of grievances, freedom from unreasonable searches and seizures, due process of law, protection against compelled self-incrimination, protection against seizure of property without just compensation, a speedy and public trial in criminal cases, trial by jury in both criminal and civil cases, and assistance of counsel in criminal prosecutions.

The Constitution established three separate branches of government—legislative (Article I), executive (Article II), and judicial (Article III). The three branches of the federal government operate within a constitutional system known as *checks and balances.* Each branch is formally separate from the other two, and each has certain constitutional authority to check the actions of the others.

The Legislative Branch

Congress, the national legislature of the United States, is composed of two houses or chambers—the Senate and the House of Representatives. Each state has two senators who are elected for six-year terms. One-third of the Senate is elected every two years. Members of the House of Representatives are elected from local districts within states. Each state receives a number of representatives in proportion to its population. The entire House is elected every two years.

To become law, proposed legislation must be passed by both houses and approved by the president. If the president does not sign, or vetoes, a bill, it may still be enacted, but only by a two-thirds vote of each house of Congress.

The Constitution did not establish a parliamentary or cabinet system of government, as in the United Kingdom and many other democracies around the world. Under the US Constitution, the president is both the head of state and the head of the government. The president appoints a cabinet—consisting of the heads of major executive departments and agencies—but neither the president nor any member of the cabinet sits in Congress. The president's political party, moreover, does not need to hold a majority of the seats in Congress to stay in office. In fact, it is not unusual for one or both houses of Congress to be controlled by the opposition party.

Each house of Congress has committees of its members, organized by subject matter, that draft laws, exercise general oversight over government agencies and programs, enact appropriation bills to fund government operations, and monitor the operation of federal programs. The federal courts, for example, maintain regular communications with the judiciary committees and the appropriations committees of the Senate and the House of Representatives.

The Executive Branch

The president is elected every four years, and under the Constitution may serve no more than two terms in office. Once elected, the president selects a cabinet, each member of which must be confirmed by a majority vote in the Senate. Each cabinet member is the head of a department in the executive branch. The cabinet includes, for example, the secretary of state, the secretary of defense, the secretary of the treasury, the secretary of health and human services, and the attorney general.

The president, the cabinet, and other members of the president's administration are responsible for operating the executive branch of the federal government and for executing and enforcing the laws. The attorney general, who is head of the Department of Justice, is responsible for all criminal prosecutions, for representing the government's legal interests in civil cases, and for administration of the Bureau of Prisons, the Federal Bureau of Investigation, the Marshals Service, the Immigration and Naturalization Service, and certain other law enforcement organizations. At the local level, the chief prosecutor in each of the 94 federal judicial districts is the US attorney, who is appointed by the president and reports to the attorney general.

The Department of Justice plays no role in administration or budgeting for the federal courts. The judiciary communicates separately and directly to Congress on legislative and appropriations matters.

The Judicial Branch

The federal judiciary is a totally separate, self-governing branch of the government. The federal courts often are called the guardians of the Constitution because their rulings protect the rights and liberties guaranteed by the Constitution. Through fair and impartial judgments, they determine facts and interpret the law to resolve legal disputes.

The courts do not make the laws. That is the responsibility of Congress. Nor do the courts have the power to enforce the laws. That is the role of the president and the many executive branch departments and agencies. But the judicial branch has the authority to interpret and decide the constitutionality of federal laws and to resolve other disputes over federal laws.

The framers of the Constitution considered an independent federal judiciary essential to ensure fairness and equal justice to all citizens of the United States. The Constitution they drafted promotes judicial independence in two principal ways. First, federal judges appointed under Article III of the Constitution can serve for life, and they can be removed from office only through impeachment and conviction by Congress of "Treason, Bribery, or other high Crimes and Misdemeanors." Second, the Constitution provides that the compensation of Article III federal judges "shall not be diminished during their Continuance in Office," which means that neither the president nor Congress can reduce the salaries of most federal judges. These two protections help an independent judiciary decide cases free from popular passion and political influence.

Source: Adapted from Hogan, T. F. 2010. *The Federal Court System in the United States,* third edition. Accessed July 9, 2014. www.uscourts.gov/uscourts/FederalCourts/Publications /English.pdf.

12

STATE LEGALIZATION OF RECREATIONAL MARIJUANA: SELECTED LEGAL ISSUES

May a state authorize the use of marijuana for recreational purposes even if such use is forbidden by federal law? This novel and unresolved legal question has vexed judges, politicians, and legal scholars, and it has also generated considerable public debate among supporters and opponents of "legalizing" the recreational use of marijuana.

Under the federal Controlled Substances Act (CSA), the cultivation, distribution, and possession of marijuana are prohibited for any reason other than to engage in federally approved research. Yet 18 states and the District of Columbia currently exempt qualified users of medicinal marijuana from penalties imposed under state law. In addition, in November 2012 Colorado and Washington became the first states to legalize, regulate, and tax small amounts of marijuana for nonmedicinal (so-called recreational) use by individuals over the age of 21. Thus, the current legal status of marijuana appears to be both contradictory and in a state of flux: as a matter of federal law, activities related to marijuana are generally prohibited and punishable by criminal penalties, whereas at the state level certain marijuana usage is increasingly being permitted. Individuals and businesses engaging in marijuana-related activities that are authorized by state law nonetheless remain subject to federal criminal prosecution or other consequences under federal law.

The Colorado and Washington laws that legalize, regulate, and tax an activity the federal government expressly prohibits appear to be logically inconsistent with established federal policy toward marijuana, and are therefore potentially subject to a legal challenge under the constitutional doctrine of preemption. This doctrine generally prevents states from enacting laws that are inconsistent with federal law. Under the supremacy clause, state laws that conflict with federal law are generally preempted and therefore void and without effect. Yet Congress intended that the CSA would not displace all state laws associated with controlled substances, as it wanted to preserve a role for the states in regulating controlled substances. States thus remain free to pass laws relating to marijuana, or any other controlled substance, so long as they do not create a "positive conflict" with federal law, such that the two laws "cannot consistently stand together."

This report summarizes the Washington and Colorado marijuana legalization laws and evaluates whether, or the extent to which, they may be preempted by the CSA or by international agreements. It also describes and analyzes the US Department of Justice's (DOJ's) response to these legalization initiatives as set forth in a memorandum sent to all federal prosecutors in late August 2013. The report then identifies certain noncriminal consequences that marijuana users may face under federal law. Finally, the report closes with a description of selected legislative proposals introduced in the One Hundred Thirteenth Congress relating to the treatment of marijuana under federal law, including H.R. 499 (Ending Federal Marijuana Prohibition Act of 2013); H.R. 501 (Marijuana Tax Equity Act of 2013); H.R. 689 (States' Medical Marijuana Patient Protection Act); H.R. 710 (Truth in Trials Act); H.R. 784 (States' Medical Marijuana Property Rights Protection Act); H.R. 964 (Respect States' and Citizens' Rights Act of 2013); H.R. 1523 (Respect State Marijuana Laws Act of 2013); H.R. 1635 (National Commission on Federal Marijuana Policy Act of 2013); and H.R. 2652 (Marijuana Businesses Access to Banking Act of 2013).

Source: Garvey, T., and B. T. Yeh. 2014. "State Legalization of Recreational Marijuana: Selected Legal Issues." Congressional Research Service Report R43034. Published January 13. www.fas.org/sgp/crs/misc/R43034.pdf.

FINDING BETTER SOLUTIONS: CMS INNOVATION CENTER DEVELOPS NEW PAYMENT AND SERVICE DELIVERY MODELS

The CMS Innovation Center (http://innovation.cms.gov) has categorized its efforts to develop new payment and delivery models that might address cost and quality problems into seven categories as follows:

1. **Accountable Care:** Accountable Care Organizations and similar care models are designed to incentivize healthcare providers to become accountable for a patient population and to invest in infrastructure and redesigned care processes that provide for coordinated care, high quality, and efficient service delivery.

2. **Bundled Payments for Care Improvement:** Medicare currently makes separate payments to various providers for the services they furnish to the same beneficiary for a single illness or course of treatment (an episode of care). Offering these providers a single, bundled payment for an episode of care makes them jointly accountable for the patient's care. It also allows providers to achieve savings based on effectively managing resources as they provide treatment to the beneficiary throughout the episode.

3. **Primary Care Transformation:** Primary care providers are a key point of contact for patients' healthcare needs. Strengthening and increasing access to primary care is critical to promoting health and reducing overall healthcare costs. Advanced primary care practices—also called "medical homes"—utilize a team-based approach, while emphasizing prevention, health information technology, care coordination, and shared decision making among patients and their providers.

4. **Initiatives Focused on the Medicaid and CHIP Population:** Medicaid and the Children's Health Insurance Program (CHIP) are administered by the states but are jointly funded by the federal government and states. Initiatives in this category are administered by the participating states.

5. **Initiatives Focused on the Medicare–Medicaid Enrollees**: The Medicare and Medicaid programs were designed with distinct purposes. Individuals enrolled in both Medicare and Medicaid (the "dual eligibles") account for a disproportionate share of the programs' expenditures. A fully integrated, person-centered system of care that ensures that all their needs are met could better serve this population in a high-quality, cost-effective manner.

6. **Initiatives to Speed the Adoption of Best Practices:** Recent studies indicate that it takes nearly 17 years on average before best practices—backed by research—are incorporated into widespread clinical practice, and even then the application of the knowledge is very uneven. The Innovation Center is partnering with a broad range of healthcare providers, federal agencies, professional societies, and other experts and stakeholders to test new models for disseminating evidence-based best practices and significantly increasing the speed of adoption.

7. **Initiatives to Accelerate the Development and Testing of New Payment and Service Delivery Models:** Many innovations necessary to improve the healthcare system will come from local communities and healthcare leaders from across the entire country. By partnering with these local and regional stakeholders, CMS can help accelerate the testing of models today that may be the next breakthrough tomorrow.

Source: Centers for Medicare & Medicaid Services. 2014. "Innovation Models." Accessed March 21. http://innovation.cms.gov/initiatives/index.html#views=models.

COALITION LETTER REQUESTING CHANGES TO MEANINGFUL USE FOR GREATER SYSTEMS INTEROPERABILITY

October 15, 2014

The Honorable Sylvia M. Burwell
Secretary
U.S. Department of Health & Human Services
200 Independence Avenue, S.W.
Washington, D.C. 20201

Dear Secretary Burwell:

The undersigned organizations write to express our immediate concerns with the Meaningful Use (MU) program and the current state of interoperability and usability of health information technology (HIT), including electronic health records and electronic medical records (EHRs/EMRs). Our respective members believe that the MU program and greater adoption of HIT could promote improvements in patient safety, care quality, and efficiency. Yet, based on our collective member experience, we are facing growing barriers to achieving these goals. Without changes to the MU program and a new emphasis for interoperable EHRs/EMRs systems and HIT infrastructure, we believe that the opportunity to leverage these technologies will not be realized.

Currently, health information stored in most EHRs/EMRs and other HIT systems and devices do not facilitate data exchange but "lock-in" important patient data and other information that is needed to improve care. Recent data from the Office of the National Coordinator for Health Information Technology (ONC) shows that less than 14 percent of physicians are able to electronically transmit health information outside of their organization and other providers are facing similar challenges. These barriers to data exchange proliferated as a result of a variety of factors; include strict MU requirements and deadlines that do not provide sufficient time to focus on achieving interoperability. This dynamic is also in part due to the strict

EHR certification requirements that have forced all the stakeholders involved to focus on meeting MU measures as opposed to developing more innovative technological solutions that will enhance patient care and safety while growing the marketplace.

In addition to HIT interoperability challenges, existing systems also lack usability, complicating physician and provider workflows, and diverting resources away from patient care. For instance, many of the physicians have vocalized concerns that these challenges and greater administrative burdens are creating significant dissatisfaction with EHR/EMR usability; yet, their vendors are limited from addressing these concerns as they focus on meeting increasingly complex certification requirements.

Unfortunately, the recently released final rule that provided relief for unavailable technology did not address or improve the challenges of interoperability and usability. It also only limited its impact to 2014, despite the growing concern with future stages of the MU program. Our organizations remain concerned that without changes the forward trajectory of the MU program will be in jeopardy.

For these reasons, we collectively recommend a different approach to improve the MU program and HIT. Such an approach should emphasize the following:

- Streamline and focus the ONC certification requirements on interoperability, quality measure reporting, and privacy/security. Removing a heavy handed set of certification mandates and allowing instead for a flexible and scalable standard based on open system architectural features like application program interfaces (APIs) will promote the delivery of more innovative and usable solutions. This in turn will allow data to move more freely across the health care system, reducing data lock-in and promoting more usable systems.
- Foster collaboration among stakeholders to promote the development of new HIT that is focused on meeting clinical care needs.
- Remove restrictive MU policies that stifle HIT innovation.
- Recognize vendors and providers need adequate time to develop, implement, and use newly deployed technology and systems before continuing on with subsequent stages of the MU program. Testing and achievement of specific performance benchmarks should occur before providers are held accountable for any new MU requirements.

We believe that rather than stopping momentum, these changes will keep the MU program on track and advance new uses of HIT. We appreciate your leadership on this important issue and look forward to working with you to achieve these needed improvements.

Sincerely,

American Academy of Family Physicians
American Medical Association
Medical Group Management Association
National Rural Health Association
Memorial Healthcare System
Mountain States Health Alliance
Premier healthcare alliance
Summa Health System

Source: Reprinted with permission from Premier Inc. 2014. "Coalition Letter Requesting Changes to Meaningful Use for Greater Systems Interoperability." Published October 15. www.premierinc.com/coalition-letter-requesting-changes-meaningful-use-greater-systems -interoperability/.

TYPES OF GROUPS INVOLVED IN FINANCING POLITICAL CAMPAIGNS

501(c) groups. Nonprofit, tax-exempt groups organized under section 501(c) of the Internal Revenue Code that can engage in varying amounts of political activity, depending on the type of group. For example, 501(c)(3) groups operate for religious, charitable, scientific, or educational purposes. These groups are not supposed to engage in any political activities, though some voter registration activities are permitted. 501(c)(4) groups are commonly called "social welfare" organizations that may engage in political activities, as long as these activities do not become their primary purpose. Similar restrictions apply to Section 501(c)(5) labor and agricultural groups, and to Section 501(c)(6) business leagues, chambers of commerce, real estate boards, and boards of trade.

527 group. A tax-exempt group organized under section 527 of the Internal Revenue Code to raise money for political activities including voter mobilization efforts, issue advocacy, and the like. Currently, the FEC only requires a 527 group to file regular disclosure reports if it is a political party or political action committee (PAC) that engages in either activities expressly advocating the election or defeat of a federal candidate, or in electioneering communications. Otherwise, it must file either with the government of the state in which it is located or the Internal Revenue Service. Many 527s run by special interest groups raise unlimited "soft money," which they use for voter mobilization and certain types of issue advocacy, but not for efforts that expressly advocate the election or defeat of a federal candidate or amount to electioneering communications.

Nonfederal group. A group set up to raise unlimited contributions called "soft money," which it spends on voter mobilization efforts and so-called issue ads that often criticize or tout a candidate's record just before an election in a not-so-subtle effort to influence the election's outcome. 501(c) groups and 527 groups may raise nonfederal funds.

Political action committee (PAC). A political committee that raises and spends limited "hard" money contributions for the express purpose of electing or defeating candidates. Organizations that raise soft money for issue advocacy may also set up a PAC. Most PACs represent business, such as the Microsoft PAC; labor, such as the Teamsters PAC; or ideological interests, such as the EMILY's List PAC or the National Rifle Association PAC. An organization's PAC will collect money from the group's employees or members and make contributions in the name of the PAC to candidates and political parties. Individuals contributing to a PAC may also contribute directly to candidates and political parties, even those also supported by the PAC. A PAC can give $5,000 to a candidate per election (primary, general, or special) and up to $15,000 annually to a national political party. PACs may receive up to $5,000 each from individuals, other PACs and party committees per year. A PAC must register with the Federal Election Commission within 10 days of its formation, providing the name and address of the PAC, its treasurer, and any affiliated organizations.

Source: Reprinted with permission from Center for Responsive Politics. 2014. "Types of Advocacy Groups." Accessed March 21. www.opensecrets.org/527s/types.php.

TESTIMONY ON HEART DISEASE EDUCATION, ANALYSIS RESEARCH, AND TREATMENT FOR WOMEN ACT (OR "HEART FOR WOMEN ACT")

Statement of Susan K. Bennett, MD
Clinical Director, Women's Heart Program, The George Washington University Hospital, Before the House Subcommittee on Health of the Committee on Energy and Commerce

Legislative Hearing on H.R. 1014, the Heart Disease Education, Analysis Research, and Treatment for Women Act

May 1, 2007

My name is Susan Bennett, and I am a practicing cardiologist; and I think first and foremost, I am one of the doctors in the trenches. I see patients five days a week, and I see men and women. About 70 percent of my practice is women, and that is primarily what I do. I am a clinical assistant professor of medicine and director of the Women's Heart Program at George Washington University Medical Center. I am also a volunteer and national spokeswoman for the American Heart Association and president of the Association of Women's Heart Programs, and I also serve on the Advisory Board of WomenHeart, which is the national coalition for women with heart disease.

On behalf of the American Heart Association, or AHA, and its more than 22 million volunteers and supporters, I appreciate the opportunity to testify today on H.R. 1014, known as the HEART for Women Act. We wish to thank this House Committee on Energy and Commerce, Subcommittee on Health, for holding today's hearing on this Act, which we strongly support along with many other nonprofit health organizations.

Heart disease, stroke, and other forms of cardiovascular diseases are the number one killer of American women, claiming more than 460,000 lives each year or about a death a minute. That is more female lives than the next five causes of death combined, including deaths from lung and breast cancer. An estimated 42 million women, about one in three, are living with the chronic effects of heart disease, stroke, or some other form of cardiovascular disease.

In 1984, women achieved equality and then surpassed men in one area where they don't want it: heart disease mortality. Every year since then, more women than men have died of cardiovascular disease, or CVD. During that time, we have made good progress in reducing CVD mortality for men but the same cannot be said for women. Although mortality rates have gone down for women, the decline is not nearly as steep as it is for men.

The HEART for Women Act is intended to help close that gap by focusing on three strategies to improve diagnosis, treatment, and prevention of heart disease and stroke in women. Part of the problem is that there are not enough women or physicians who recognize heart disease as the serious health threat that it truly is. Efforts like the AHA's Go Red for Women movement and the NHLDI's Heart Truth campaign have helped to increase awareness among women about their risk of heart disease, but much more work remains.

The latest American Heart Association survey tracking women's awareness of heart disease found that 43 percent of women are still not aware that heart disease is the leading cause of death for women. Women of color are significantly less likely to know this important fact, despite being at greater risk for cardiovascular disease.

Even more alarming, especially to me, is the pervasive lack of awareness about women and heart disease among physicians. According to an American Heart Association–sponsored survey published in 2005, fewer than one in five physicians surveyed recognized that more women than men die of heart disease than other cardiovascular disease each year. Astoundingly, only 8 percent of primary care physicians knew this basic fact.

Healthcare professionals treat what they perceive to be a problem; and partially as a result of the above statistics, we see that women are often treated less aggressively. For instance, women are more likely to die within a year of their first heart attack, but are less likely to be referred for diagnostic testing ahead of time that could have caught the disease early in the preventive phase. And according to the Agency for Health Care Research and Quality's 2006 National Healthcare Disparities Report, female Medicare patients who suffer from a heart attack are less likely to receive the recommended care compared to their male counterparts.

The HEART for Women Act would help to increase awareness among populations for which there are still gaps, particularly older women and healthcare professionals. For healthcare professionals, the bill authorizes the Health Resources and Services Administration to conduct an education campaign to increase professionals' understanding about the prevalence and unique aspects of care for women in the prevention and treatment of forms of CVD.

The bill also authorizes the Secretary of Health and Human Services to develop and distribute educational materials to women 65 years and older to educate them about a woman's risk for heart attacks and strokes, risk factors, and symptoms.

Another problem that I struggle with every day in my practice is the lack of information available to us about the safety and efficacy of heart and stroke treatments for women. When a new therapy comes on the market, one of the first things I want to know is how does it work in women compared to men, and all too often that information is simply not available.

For far too long we have simply assumed that if a new drug or medical device works for a man, then it must work for a woman. Thanks to reports such as the National Institute of Medicine's landmark 2001 report "Does Sex Matter?" we know that sex really does make a difference, from womb to tomb. Researchers are learning that sex differences play an increasingly important role in prevention, diagnosis, and treatment. For instance, we have learned from the National Heart, Lung, and Blood Institute–funded WISE study that coronary artery disease may manifest itself differently in women than in men, which suggests that treatment testing regimens that work in men may not work as well in women.

Diagnostic tests, prescription drugs, and medical devices may work differently in women than men. These differences are likely due to a variety of reasons.

***

So in summary, for me as a practicing clinician, it is absolutely important for this Act to be passed so I can take care of women better. Thank you.

Source: Reprinted from Bennett, S. K. 2007. "Hearing Before the Subcommittee on Health of the Committee on Energy and Commerce: House of Representatives One Hundred Tenth Congress, First Session on H.R. 1014." Published May 1. www.gpo.gov/fdsys/pkg/CHRG -110hhrg38951/pdf/CHRG-110hhrg38951.pdf.

CONGRESSIONAL CONFERENCE COMMITTEES

A bill cannot become a law of the land until it has been approved in identical form by both houses of Congress. Once the Senate amends and agrees to a bill that the House already has passed—or the House amends and passes a Senate bill—the two houses may begin to resolve their legislative differences by way of a conference committee or through an exchange of amendments between the houses.

If the Senate does not accept the House's position [or the House does not agree to the Senate's position], one of the chambers may propose creation of a conference committee to negotiate and resolve the matters in disagreement between the two chambers. Typically, the Senate gets to conference with the House by adopting this standard motion: "Mr. President, I move that the Senate insist on its amendment(s) (or "disagree to the House amendment(s)" to the Senate-passed measure), request a conference with the House on the disagreeing votes thereon, and that the Chair be authorized to appoint conferees." This triple motion rolled into one—to insist (or disagree), request, and appoint—is commonly agreed to by unanimous consent. The presiding officer formally appoints the Senate's conferees. (The Speaker names the House conferees.) Conferees are traditionally drawn from the committee of jurisdiction, but conferees representing other Senate interests may also be appointed.

There are no formal rules that outline how conference meetings are to be organized. Routinely, the principals from each chamber or their respective staffs conduct preconference meetings so as to expedite the bargaining process when the conference formally convenes. Informal practice also determines who will be the overall conference chair (each chamber has its own leader in conference). Rotation of the chairmanship between the chambers is usually the practice when matched pairs of panels (the tax or appropriations panels, for example) convene in conference regularly. For standing committees that seldom meet in conference, the choice of who will chair the conference is generally resolved by the conference leaders from each chamber. The decision on when and where to meet and for how long are a few prerogatives of the chair, who consults on these matters with his or her counterpart from the other body.

Once the two chambers go to conference, the respective House and Senate conferees bargain and negotiate to resolve the matters in bicameral disagreement. Resolution is embodied in a conference report signed by a majority of Senate conferees and House conferees. The conference report must be agreed to by both chambers before it is cleared for presidential consideration. In the Senate, conference reports are usually brought up by unanimous consent at a time agreed to by the party leaders and floor managers. Because conference reports are privileged, if any senator objects to the unanimous consent request, a nondebatable motion can be made to take up the conference report. Approval of the conference report itself is subject to extended debate, but conference reports are not open to amendment.

Almost all of the most important measures are sent to conference, but these are only a minority of the bills that the two houses pass each year.

Source: Reprinted from US Senate. 2014. "Legislative Process: How a Senate Bill Becomes a Law." Accessed March 23. www.senate.gov/reference/resources/pdf/legprocessflowchart .pdf.

THE FEDERAL BUDGET PROCESS

This backgrounder describes the laws and procedures under which Congress decides how much money to spend each year, what to spend it on, and how to raise the money to pay for that spending. The Congressional Budget Act of 1974 lays out a formal framework for developing and enforcing a "budget resolution" to guide the process, but in recent years the process has not always worked as envisioned.

We address:

- the President's annual budget request, which is supposed to kick off the budget process;
- the congressional budget resolution—how it is developed, what it contains, and what happens if there is no budget resolution;
- how the terms of the budget resolution are enforced in the House and Senate;
- budget "reconciliation," an optional procedure used in some years to facilitate the passage of legislation amending tax or entitlement law; and
- statutory deficit-control measures—spending caps, pay-as-you-go requirements, and sequestration.

Step One: The President's Budget Request

The process starts when the President submits a detailed budget request for the coming fiscal year, which begins on October 1. (The President's request is supposed to come by the first Monday in February, but sometimes the submission is delayed—particularly when a new Administration takes office or congressional action on the prior year's budget has been delayed.) This budget request—developed through an interactive process between federal agencies and the President's Office of Management and Budget (OMB) that begins the previous spring (or earlier)—plays three important roles.

First, it tells Congress what the President recommends for overall federal fiscal policy, as established by three main components: (1) how much money the federal government should spend on public purposes; (2) how much it should take in as tax revenues; and (3) how much of a deficit (or surplus) the federal government should run, which is simply the difference between (1) and (2). In most years, actual federal spending exceeds tax revenues and the resulting deficit is financed through borrowing.

Second, the President's budget lays out his relative priorities for federal programs—how much he believes should be spent on defense, agriculture, education, health, and so on. The President's budget is very specific, and recommends funding levels for individual federal programs or small groups of programs called "budget accounts." The budget typically sketches out fiscal policy and budget priorities not only for the coming year but also for the next ten years. The budget is accompanied by supporting volumes, including historical tables that set out past budget figures.

The third role of the President's budget is signaling to Congress the President's recommendations for spending and tax policy changes. As discussed later, the budget comprises different types of programs, some that require new funding each year to continue and others that are ongoing and therefore do not require annual action by Congress. While the President must recommend funding levels for annually appropriated programs, he need not propose legislative changes for those parts of the budget that are ongoing.

- **Annually appropriated programs.** These programs fall under the jurisdiction of the House and Senate Appropriations Committees. Funding for these programs must be renewed each year to keep government agencies open and the programs in this category operating. These programs are known as "discretionary" because the laws that establish those programs leave Congress with the discretion to set the funding levels each year. That doesn't mean the programs are optional or unimportant, however. For example, almost all defense spending is discretionary, as are the budgets for a broad set of public services, including environmental protection, education, job training, border security, veterans' health care, scientific research, transportation, economic development, some low-income assistance, law enforcement, and international assistance. Altogether, discretionary programs make up about one-third of all federal spending. The President's budget spells out how much funding he recommends for each discretionary program.

- **Taxes, "mandatory" or "entitlement" programs, and interest.** Nearly all of the federal tax code is set in ongoing law that either remains in place until changed or requires renewal only periodically. Similarly, more than one-half of federal spending is also ongoing. This category is known as "mandatory" spending. It includes the three largest entitlement programs (Medicare, Medicaid, and Social Security) as well as certain other programs (including but not limited to SNAP, formerly food stamps; federal civilian and military retirement benefits; veterans' disability benefits; and unemployment insurance) that are not controlled by annual appropriations. Interest on the national debt is also paid automatically, with no need for new legislation. (There is, however, a separate limit on how much the Treasury can borrow. This "debt ceiling" must be raised through separate legislation when necessary.)

As noted, the President's budget does not need to include recommendations to ensure the continuation of ongoing mandatory programs and revenues, but it will nonetheless typically include proposals to alter some mandatory programs and revenue laws.

- **Recommendations for mandatory programs** typically spell out changes to eligibility criteria and levels of individual benefits but do not specify overall funding levels. Rather, the funding levels effectively are determined by the eligibility and benefits rules set in law.
- **Changes to the tax code will increase or decrease taxes.** Such proposals will be reflected as a change in the amount of federal revenue that the President's budget projects will be collected the next year or in future years, relative to what would otherwise be collected.

Step Two: The Congressional Budget Resolution

Next, Congress generally holds hearings to question Administration officials about their requests and then develops its own budget plan, called a "budget resolution." This work is done by the House and Senate Budget Committees, whose primary function is to draft and enforce the budget resolution. Once the Budget Committees pass their budget resolutions, the bills go to the House and Senate floors, where they can be amended (by a majority vote). A House-Senate conference then resolves any differences, and the budget resolution for the year is adopted when both houses pass the conference report.

The budget resolution is a "concurrent" congressional resolution, not an ordinary bill, and therefore does not go to the President for his signature or veto. It also requires only a majority vote to pass, and its consideration is one of the few actions that cannot be filibustered in the Senate. Because it does not go to the President, a budget resolution cannot enact spending or tax law. Instead, it sets targets for other congressional committees that can propose legislation directly providing or changing spending and taxes.

Congress is supposed to pass the budget resolution by April 15, but it often takes longer. In recent years it has been common for Congress not to pass a budget resolution at all. When that happens, the previous year's resolution, which is a multi-year plan, stays in effect, although the House, the Senate, or both can and typically do adopt special procedures to set spending levels (see box: What if There Is No Budget Resolution?).

- **What is in the budget resolution?** Unlike the President's budget, which is very detailed, the congressional budget resolution is a very simple document. It consists of a set of numbers stating how much Congress is supposed to spend in each of 19 broad spending categories (known as budget "functions") and how much total revenue the government will collect, for each of the next five years or more. (The Congressional Budget Act requires that the resolution cover a minimum of five years, though Congress now generally chooses a longer period, such as ten years.) The difference between the two totals—the spending ceiling and the revenue floor—represents the deficit (or surplus) expected for each year.

- **How spending is defined: budget authority vs. outlays.** The spending totals in the budget resolution are stated in two different

What If There Is No Budget Resolution?

Congress has seldom completed action on the budget resolution by the April 15 target date specified in the Budget Act, and it failed to complete action on a resolution for fiscal years 1999, 2003, 2005, 2007, and each year from 2011 through 2014. In the absence of a budget resolution, the House and Senate typically enact separate budget targets, which they "deem" to be a substitute for the budget resolution. Such deeming resolutions typically provide spending allocations to the Appropriations Committees but may serve a variety of other budgetary purposes. Unless the House or Senate agrees to such a deeming resolution, the multi-year revenue floors and spending allocations for mandatory programs that had been agreed to in the most recent budget resolution remain in effect.

The Bipartisan Budget Act of 2013 described below took a different tack, establishing a "Congressional Budget" for fiscal years 2014 and 2015 in statute as an alternative to the concurrent budget resolution called for in the Congressional Budget Act.

ways: the total amount of "budget authority," and the estimated level of expenditures, or "outlays." Budget authority is how much money Congress allows a federal agency to commit to spend; outlays are how much money actually flows out of the federal Treasury in a given year. For example, a bill that appropriated $50 million for building a bridge would provide $50 million in budget authority for the coming year, but the outlays might not reach $50 million until the following year or even later, when the bridge actually is built.

Budget authority and outlays thus serve different purposes. Budget authority represents a limit on the new financial obligations federal agencies may incur (by signing contracts or making grants, for example), and is generally what Congress focuses on in making most budgetary decisions. Outlays, because they represent actual cash flow, help determine the size of the overall deficit or surplus.

- **How committee spending limits get set: 302(a) allocations.** The report that accompanies the budget resolution includes a table called the "302(a) allocation." This table takes the spending totals that are laid out by budget function in the budget resolution and distributes them by congressional committee instead. The House and Senate tables are different from one another, since committee jurisdictions vary somewhat between the two chambers.

In both the House and Senate, the Appropriations Committee receives a single 302(a) allocation for all of its programs. It then decides on its own how to divide this funding among its 12 subcommittees, creating what are known as 302(b) sub-allocations. Similarly, the various committees with jurisdiction over mandatory programs each get an allocation that represents a total dollar limit on all of the legislation they produce that year.

The spending totals in the budget resolution do not apply to "authorizing" legislation that merely establishes or changes rules for federal programs funded through the annual appropriations process. Unless it changes an entitlement program (such as Social Security or Medicare), authorizing legislation does not actually have a budgetary effect. For example, the education committees could produce legislation that authorizes a certain amount to be spent on the Title I education program for disadvantaged children. However, none of that money can be spent until the annual Labor-Health and Human Services-Education appropriations bill—which includes education spending—sets the actual dollar level for Title I funding for the year, which is frequently less than the authorized limit.

Often the report accompanying the budget resolution contains language describing the assumptions behind it, including how much it envisions certain programs being cut or increased. These assumptions generally serve only as guidance to the other committees and are not binding on them. Sometimes, though, the budget resolution includes more complicated devices intended to ensure that particular programs receive a certain amount of funding.

The budget resolution can also include temporary or permanent changes to the congressional budget process.

Step Three: Enacting Budget Legislation

Following adoption of the budget resolution, Congress considers the annual appropriations bills that are needed to fund discretionary programs in the coming fiscal year and legislation to enact changes to mandatory spending or revenue levels as specified in the budget resolution. Mechanisms exist to enforce the terms of the budget resolution during the consideration of such legislation, and a special mechanism known as "reconciliation" exists to expedite the consideration of mandatory spending and tax legislation.

Enforcing the Terms of the Budget Resolution

The main enforcement mechanism that prevents Congress from passing legislation that violates the terms of the budget resolution is the ability of a single member of the House or the Senate to raise a budget "point of order" on the floor to block such legislation. In some recent years, this point of order has not been particularly important in the House because it can be waived there by a simple majority vote on a resolution developed by the leadership-appointed Rules Committee, which sets the conditions under which each bill will be considered on the floor.

However, the budget point of order is important in the Senate, where any legislation that exceeds a committee's spending allocation—or cuts taxes below the level allowed in the budget resolution—is vulnerable to a budget point of order on the floor that requires 60 votes to waive.

Appropriations bills (or amendments to them) must fit within the 302(a) allocation given to the Appropriations Committee as well as the committee-determined 302(b) sub-allocations for the coming fiscal year. Tax or entitlement bills (or any amendments offered to them) must fit within the budget resolution's spending limit for the relevant committee or within the revenue floor, both in the first year and over the total multi-year period covered by the budget resolution. The cost of a tax or entitlement bill is determined (or "scored") by the Budget Committees, nearly always by relying on the nonpartisan Congressional Budget Office (CBO). CBO measures the cost of tax or entitlement legislation against a budgetary "baseline" that projects mandatory spending and tax receipts under current law.

The Budget "Reconciliation" Process

From time to time, Congress makes use of an optional, special procedure outlined in the Congressional Budget Act known as "reconciliation" to expedite the consideration of mandatory spending and tax legislation. This procedure was originally designed as a deficit-reduction tool, to force committees to produce spending cuts or tax increases called for in the budget resolution. However, it was used to enact tax cuts several times during the George W. Bush Administration, thereby increasing projected deficits. Senate rules now prohibit using reconciliation to consider legislation that would increase the deficit; House rules prohibit using it to increase mandatory spending.

- **What is a reconciliation bill?** A reconciliation bill is a single piece of legislation that typically includes multiple provisions (generally developed by several committees), all of which affect the federal budget—whether on the mandatory spending side, the tax side, or both. A reconciliation bill, like the budget resolution, cannot be filibustered by the Senate, so it only requires a majority vote to pass.

- **How does the reconciliation process work?** If Congress decides to use the reconciliation process, language known as a "reconciliation directive" must be included in the budget resolution. The reconciliation directive instructs committees to produce legislation by a specific date that meets certain spending or tax targets. (If they fail to produce this legislation, the Budget Committee chair generally has the right to offer floor amendments to meet the reconciliation targets for them, a threat which usually produces compliance with the directive.) The Budget Committee then packages all of these bills together into one bill that goes to the floor for an up-or-down vote, with limited opportunity for amendment. After the House and Senate resolve the differences between their competing bills, a final conference report is considered on the floor of each house and then goes to the President for his signature or veto.

- **Constraints on reconciliation: the "Byrd rule."** While reconciliation enables Congress to bundle together several different provisions from different committees affecting a broad range of programs, it faces one major constraint: the "Byrd rule," named after the late Senator Robert Byrd of West Virginia. This Senate rule provides a point of order against any provision of (or amendment to) a reconciliation bill that is deemed "extraneous" to the purpose of amending entitlement or tax law. If a point of order is raised under the Byrd rule, the offending provision is automatically stripped from the bill unless at least 60 senators vote to waive the rule. This makes it difficult, for example, to include any policy changes in a reconciliation bill unless they have direct fiscal implications. Under this rule, changes in the authorization of discretionary appropriations are not allowed, nor, for example, are changes to civil rights or employment law or even the budget process. Changes to Social Security also are not permitted under the Byrd rule, even if they are budgetary.

In addition, the Byrd rule bars any entitlement increases or tax cuts that cost money beyond the five (or more) years covered by the reconciliation directive, unless other provisions in the bill fully offset these "out-year" costs.

What If Appropriations Bills Are Not Passed on Time?

If Congress does not complete action on an appropriations bill before the start of the fiscal year on October 1, it must pass, and the President must sign, a continuing resolution (CR) to provide stopgap funding for affected agencies and discretionary programs. If Congress doesn't pass or the President will not sign a CR because it contains provisions he finds unacceptable, agencies that have not received funding through the ordinary appropriations process must shut down operations.

A dispute over delay or defunding of health reform legislation between President Obama and congressional Republicans led to a 16-day shutdown of ordinary government operations beginning October 1, 2013. A dispute between President Clinton and congressional Republicans in the winter of 1995-96 produced a 21-day shutdown of substantial portions of the federal government.

Statutory Deficit-Control Mechanisms

Separately from the limits established in the annual budget process, Congress operates under statutory deficit-control mechanisms that prevent tax and mandatory spending legislation from increasing the deficit and that constrain discretionary spending.

- **PAYGO.** Under the 2010 Statutory Pay-As-You Go (PAYGO) Act, any legislative changes to taxes or mandatory spending that increase multi-year deficits must be "offset" or paid for by other changes to taxes or mandatory spending that reduce deficits by an equivalent amount. Violation of PAYGO triggers across-the-board cuts ("sequestration") in selected mandatory programs to restore the balance between budget costs and savings.

- **Discretionary funding caps.** The 2011 Budget Control Act (BCA) imposed limits or "caps" on the level of discretionary appropriations for defense and for non-defense programs in each year through 2021. Appropriations in excess of the cap in either category trigger sequestration in that category to reduce funding to the capped level.

- **BCA sequestration.** On top of any sequestration triggered by PAYGO or funding cap violations, the BCA also requires additional sequestration each year through 2021 in discretionary and select mandatory programs, split evenly between defense and non-defense funding. This BCA sequestration was implemented as a result of a BCA-created congressional joint select committee's failure to propose a legislative plan that would reduce deficits by $1.2 trillion over ten years. In the case of discretionary programs, for 2014 and after this special sequestration mechanism operates by reducing the appropriations caps below the level that the BCA originally set.

If budget legislation violates these statutes, the relevant sequestration penalties apply automatically, unless Congress also modifies the requirements. For example, policymakers modified the 2013 BCA sequestration requirement in the American Taxpayer Relief Act of 2012. Similarly, the Bipartisan Budget Act of 2013, worked out by Senate Budget Committee Chair Patty Murray (D-WA) and House Budget Committee Chair Paul Ryan (R-WI), reduced sequestration cuts in 2014 and 2015 while extending BCA sequestration of mandatory programs through 2023.

Conclusion

The annual federal budget process begins with a detailed proposal from the President; Congress next develops a blueprint called a budget resolution that sets limits on how much each committee can spend or reduce revenues over the course of the year; and the terms of the budget resolution are then enforced against individual appropriations, entitlement bills, and tax bills on the House and Senate floors. In addition, Congress sometimes uses a special procedure called "reconciliation" to facilitate the passage of deficit reduction legislation or other major entitlement or tax legislation. Moreover, the budget is subject to statutory deficit-control requirements. Legislation implementing a budget resolution that violates those requirements could trigger across-the-board budget cuts to offset the violations.

Source: Reprinted with permission from the Center on Budget and Policy Priorities. 2014. "Introduction to the Federal Budget Process." Updated September 10. www.cbpp.org/files/3-7-03bud.pdf.

MICHIGAN'S BUDGET PROCESS

Introduction

The Michigan Constitution requires the Governor to propose an Executive Budget for state activities on an annual basis. By law the Executive Budget must be submitted to the Legislature within 30 days after the Legislature convenes in regular session on the second Wednesday in January. However, when a newly elected Governor is inaugurated into office, 60 days are allowed to prepare the proposal. The Executive Budget is more than a statutory requirement. It represents a statement of priorities for the policy activities of state government. Therefore, a detailed budget preparation process is necessary to provide information that will help the Governor and the Legislature allocate state resources most effectively. The budget process can be broken down into the following stages:

- Development of the Governor's Executive Budget
- Enactment by the Legislature
- Budget Revisions

Development of the Governor's Executive Budget

Department Requests

The development of each new fiscal year budget begins in August, approximately 13 to 14 months prior to the beginning of the new fiscal year. The process starts with the State Budget Office issuing program policy guidelines to the departments. The guidelines and directions include assumptions regarding revenue changes, federal funds information, and economic adjustments. The guidelines also include instructions for the preparation of different levels of expenditures for each department. By October, departments submit their budget proposals to the State Budget Office. The State Budget Director makes preliminary budget recommendations to the Governor based on staff evaluations and funding proposals.

First Revenue Estimating Conference

These recommendations are fine-tuned during the next few months. The Revenue Estimating Conference held each January is a major part of the budget process. During the conference, national and state economic indicators are used to formulate an accurate prediction of revenue available for appropriation in the upcoming fiscal year. This conference first convened in 1992, pursuant to Act No. 72 of the Public Acts of 1991. The principal participants in the conference are the State Treasurer and the Directors of the Senate and House Fiscal Agencies or their respective designees. Other participants may include the Governor and senior officials from the Department of Treasury.

Governor's Budget Decisions

Before and after the Revenue Estimating Conference, the State Budget Office, the Executive Office, and the state departments hold briefings and hearings in order to review requests and prepare recommendations. The Governor makes final budget decisions in December prior to the presentation to the Legislature.

Executive Budget Presentation

As indicated above, Act No. 431 of Public Acts of 1984, the Management and Budget Act, requires the budget to be submitted within 30 days after the Legislature convenes in regular session on the second Wednesday in January. When a new governor is elected, 60 days are allowed.

During the budget presentation, the State Budget Director, on behalf of the Governor, presents the budget and accompanying explanations, recommendations, and legislation to the Legislature. This generally takes place in early February during a joint session of the House and Senate Appropriations Committees.

Legislative Action

By custom, all the appropriation bills are introduced in both houses of the Legislature and are divided between the houses for consideration. The bills usually receive more detailed hearings in the house of origin. Generally, all the appropriation bills are introduced by each appropriations committee chair or the ranking member of the Governor's party. Traditionally, only half of the bills are considered in each house initially. Currently, the practice is to alternate the house of origin each year. This practice allows both appropriations committees to work simultaneously on the appropriations bills.

The Appropriations Committees assign the budgets to specific subcommittees. These subcommittees then conduct a series of hearings. State department directors and their staff present an overview of the Governor's proposed budget, followed by briefings from House Fiscal Agency and Senate Fiscal Agency staff. The subcommittees may also hold public hearings in locations across the state. Finally, the subcommittee composes recommendations that are reported to the full Appropriations Committee.

During full House and Senate Committee meetings, state department directors and their staff are expected to provide explanations when their agency's appropriations are considered. A legislative fiscal analyst assigned to that bill is also present. This analyst may prepare a report or series of reports on the bill. The chair of the related subcommittee asks the legislative analyst to summarize the bill. The committee members are then free to ask questions regarding the bill. The appropriations committee may amend the bill or adopt a substitute version. Following approval, the bill is reported to the floor.

Prior to floor consideration, the Democratic and Republican members will discuss the bill during a caucus meeting. In addition to developing a party position, the caucus provides individual legislators with an opportunity to become better informed regarding policy issues incorporated in the budget.

The legislative procedure for consideration of the appropriation bills is basically the same as for other bills except that appropriation measures receive priority on the legislative calendars. In many instances, members who are going to offer amendments will propose the changes to the appropriations committees before floor debate. Floor consideration varies considerably depending on the particular subject matter, issues, and other factors. There may be minimal debate, or it may take a whole day or more for a given bill. Fiscal analysts prepare floor sheets summarizing the appropriation bill, the difference in funding from the prior year, the Governor's recommendation, or between house recommendations, new, expanded, or eliminated programs, and total FTEs (full-time equated positions) authorized.

Second Revenue Estimating Conference

A second Revenue Estimating Conference takes place in May of each year. Its purpose is to provide an updated consensus forecast of anticipated revenues for the Executive Budget. Upon completion of the revised consensus revenue estimate, legislative leadership meets with the Governor and the State Budget Director in an attempt to establish final spending targets for each state department. The process of target setting also involves discussion and attempts for agreement on other overall budget issues including boilerplate language, revenue bills, and other statutory changes to be included in the final budget. Reports of the agreements reached during target setting are then provided to the Legislature.

Conference Committees

Differences between the two houses on each appropriations bill are resolved by a conference committee. The committee consists of six members—three members from the Senate and three members from the House. Traditionally, when differences on any of the appropriation bills necessitate a conference committee, the conferees are usually members of the respective House and Senate appropriations subcommittees. Rule 7 of the Joint Rules of the Senate and the House of Representatives provides:

> The conference committee shall not consider any matters other than matters of difference between the two Houses. When the agreement arrived at by the conferees is such that it affects other parts of the bill, the conferees may recommend amendments to conform with the agreement. The conferees may also recommend corrections to any errors in the bill or title.

Conference committees are expected to ensure that the final levels of appropriations in the conference reports are equal to the appropriations targets established by legislative leadership. This process helps ensure that the enacted appropriations bills do not exceed the consensus estimate of available revenues.

If the conference committee report is approved by both houses, the bill is enrolled and printed (final copy of a bill in the form as passed by both houses) and presented to the Governor. If the conference committee does not reach a compromise and reports that the committee cannot reach an agreement, or if the Legislature does not accept the conference report, a second conference committee may be appointed.

While there is no specific legal time requirement for passage of the budget bills, this task is accomplished prior to the beginning of the new fiscal year. Appropriations bills are usually considered and passed in April by the first house, and in early June by the second house, and usually final action is completed in July.

Governor Signs Bills and/or Vetoes

The same procedures related to gubernatorial approval of other legislation also apply to appropriation bills. However, the Governor has additional authority to veto any distinct item or items appropriating money in any appropriation bill. The parts approved become law. Vetoed items are void unless the Legislature overrules the veto by a two-thirds vote of the members elected to and serving in each house. An appropriation line item vetoed by the Governor and not subsequently overridden by the Legislature is not funded unless another appropriation for that line item is approved.

Budget Revisions

According to the Michigan Constitution, no appropriation is a mandate to spend. The Governor, by Executive Order and with the approval of the appropriations committees, can reduce expenditures whenever it appears that actual revenues for a fiscal period will fall below the revenue estimates on which the appropriations for that period are based. By statute, any recommendation for the reduction of expenditures must be approved or disapproved by both of the appropriations committees within ten days after the recommendation is made. A reduction cannot be made without approval from both committees; not later than 30 days after a proposed order is disapproved, the Governor may submit alternative recommendations for expenditure reductions to the committees for their approval or disapproval.

Since 1970, the Governor has issued 27 Executive Orders to reduce expenditures, but on 11 occasions the Executive Orders did not receive approval of the Appropriations Committees. Subsequently, the Governor issued other Executive Orders that were approved. The Governor may not reduce expenditures for the legislative or judicial branches or expenditures from funds constitutionally dedicated for specific purposes.

Each department prepares the allotment of appropriations and may request revisions, legislative or administrative transfers, or supplemental appropriations. The State Budget Office must approve revisions to allotments. Transfer of funds other than administrative transfers within a department must be submitted by the State Budget Office to the House and Senate Appropriations Committees.

Expenditure increases for a new program or for the expansion of an existing program cannot be made until the availability of money has been determined and the program has been approved and appropriated by the Legislature. The Governor and the Legislature act on supplemental appropriation bills in a manner similar to original appropriations.

Source: Reprinted from Michigan State Budget Office. 2014. "Budget Process." Accessed March 25. www.michigan.gov/budget/0,4538,7-157-11462-34950--,00.html.

OVERSIGHT PLAN OF THE HOUSE COMMITTEE ON ENERGY AND COMMERCE, UNITED STATES HOUSE OF REPRESENTATIVES, 113TH CONGRESS

Rule X, clause 2(d) of the Rules of the House requires each standing Committee to adopt an oversight plan for the two-year period of the Congress and to submit the plan to the Committee on Oversight and Government Reform and to the Committee on House Administration not later than February 15 of the first session of the Congress.

The oversight plan of the Committee on Energy and Commerce for the 113th Congress includes all the areas in which the Committee is expected to conduct oversight during the 113th Congress: HEALTH AND HEALTHCARE ISSUES; ENERGY AND ENVIRONMENT ISSUES; COMMUNICATIONS AND TECHNOLOGY ISSUES; and COMMERCE, MANUFACTURING, AND TRADE ISSUES. The abridged version of the plan presented here covers only the first two areas. The complete oversight plan can be read at https://energycommerce.house.gov/sites/republicans.energycommerce.house.gov /files/20130101Oversight.pdf.

THE HONORABLE FRED UPTON (R, MI), CHAIRMAN

During the 113th Congress, the Committee on Energy and Commerce will hold hearings and conduct rigorous oversight over matters within its jurisdiction. The Committee will conduct thorough oversight, reach conclusions based on an objective review of the facts, and treat witnesses fairly. The Committee will request information in a responsible manner that is calculated to be helpful to the Committee in its oversight responsibilities. The Committee's oversight functions will focus on: 1) cutting government spending through the elimination of waste, fraud, and abuse and 2) ensuring laws are adequate to protect the public interest or are being implemented in a manner that protects the public interest, without stifling economic growth.

Health and Healthcare Issues

Patient Protection and Affordable Care Act

In the 113th Congress, the Committee will continue to examine issues related to the Department of Health and Human Services implementation of Public Law 111-148, The Patient Protection and Affordable Care Act (PPACA) and the related Health Care and Education Reconciliation Act of 2010, Public Law 111-152. This will include the numerous provisions contained within the law that affect the private insurance market in the United States, the creation of health insurance exchanges, and the operation of those exchanges by either the states or the federal government. The Committee will also examine the regulations and requirements imposed on both small and large businesses, and the law's effects on individuals.

The Committee will also evaluate what controls are in place to prevent bias, waste, fraud, and abuse in the management of PPACA and its programs. The Committee will monitor deadlines imposed on HHS by the Patient Protection and Affordable Care Act and examine what procedures HHS has in place for meeting those deadlines and/or complying with missed deadlines. The Committee will examine what programs HHS has in place to improve the availability of reliable, consumer-oriented information on the cost and quality of health care goods, services, and providers. The Committee will also examine the status and future of employer-sponsored health care plans as well as the effects of PPACA's enactment on the states. The Committee will examine the impact of PPACA and its implementing regulations on the economy, consumers, and the health care industry as well as the process by which those regulations are drafted.

Centers for Medicare & Medicaid Services

The Committee will review the management, operations, and activity of the Centers for Medicare & Medicaid Services (CMS) and the programs it administers. The Committee will examine and review Medicare and Medicaid management and activity as it relates to ongoing Committee efforts to prevent bias, waste, fraud, and abuse in federal health care programs, particularly in the implementation of PPACA. The Committee will investigate the process by which CMS implements statutory formulas to set prices for Medicare payment, as well as the effectiveness of those formulas. The Committee will evaluate the competitive bidding process for durable medical equipment and examine ways to use similar programs in Medicare and Medicare Advantage plans. The Committee will examine the effects that the Medicaid expansion included in PPACA will have on state budgets, the budgets of individuals and families, the budgets of providers currently providing uncompensated care, and the impact it may have on access to health insurance and health care. The Committee will investigate the processes by which CMS prevents bias, waste, fraud, and abuse in the award of government contracts.

Food and Drug Administration and Drug Safety

The Committee will review whether the Food and Drug Administration (FDA) is ensuring that regulated drugs are safe, effective, and available to American patients in an expeditious fashion. The Committee will also explore the interplay between these policies and drug innovation, both in the United States and abroad. Further, the Committee will examine FDA's enforcement of current drug safety laws and the issues involved in protecting the nation's supply chains against economically motivated and other forms of adulteration. The Committee will continue its investigation of FDA's handling of the 2012 fungal meningitis outbreak linked to contaminated, compounded drugs.

Public Health

The Committee will examine the roles of various federal agencies involved in insuring and protecting the public health, including the implementation and management of these programs. In particular, the Committee will review federal efforts on mental health and pandemic preparedness, including influenza preparedness.

Tobacco

The Committee will examine the implementation of the 2009 Family Smoking Prevention and Tobacco Control Act, including regulatory actions by the Food and Drug Administration.

Energy and Environment Issues

National Energy Policy

During the 113th Congress, the Committee will examine issues relating to national energy policy, including U.S. policies that relate to production, supply, and consumption of electricity, oil and natural gas, coal, hydroelectric power, nuclear power, hydraulic fracturing, and renewable energy. The Committee will examine the impact of government policies and programs on the exploration, production, and development of domestic energy resources, including issues relating to the nation's current energy infrastructure. The Committee will also continue to examine safety and security issues relating to energy exploration, production and distribution.

Electricity Markets

The Committee will review federal electricity policies of the Department of Energy (DOE) and the Federal Energy Regulatory Commission (FERC) to ensure that those policies promote competitive wholesale power markets, transmission, and generation infrastructure upgrades, and compliance with relevant statutes. It will also examine the activities of the DOE and FERC relating to electric industry restructuring, protection of consumers, and the development of efficient and vigorous wholesale markets for electricity.

Management of the Department of Energy and Its National Laboratories

The Committee will oversee management and operations issues at the Department of Energy (DOE), including oversight, management, and operations of the National Nuclear Security Administration (NNSA) and the national laboratories. The Committee's oversight work will include a review of the implementation of security and safety reforms at NNSA and DOE facilities, ongoing safety and security matters, the Office of Environmental Management's cleanup program, and DOE's implementation of the Nuclear Waste Policy Act.

Yucca Mountain

The Committee will examine the financial and other implications of DOE's decision to abandon licensing for Yucca Mountain as a nuclear waste repository, and the potential impact of this action on the future of nuclear energy in the United States. The Committee will also continue to examine the actions of the Nuclear Regulatory Commission (NRC) in connection with its obligations under the Nuclear Waste Policy Act.

The Nuclear Regulatory Commission

The Committee will review the activities of the Nuclear Regulatory Commission. The Committee will examine NRC's budget requests and conduct oversight of the manner in which the Commission discharges its various responsibilities, including licensing activity, the safety and security of nuclear power facilities, and the agency's post-Fukushima regulatory changes.

Clean Air Act

The Committee will continue to review significant rulemakings under the Clean Air Act and the potential economic and job impacts of those rulemakings on the energy, manufacturing and construction industries and other critical sectors of the U.S. economy, as well as any public health and environmental benefits of the regulations. The Committee's review will include oversight of the Environmental Protection Agency's (EPA) decisions, strategies and actions to meet Clean Air Act standards, and the current role of cost, employment and feasibility considerations in Clean Air Act rulemakings.

Climate Change

The Committee will continue to monitor international negotiations on efforts to control greenhouse gas emissions in connection with concerns about global climate change. In addition, the Committee will examine the EPA's efforts to regulate domestic greenhouse gas emissions under the Clean Air Act based on its endangerment finding. The Committee will consider whether such agreements and regulatory efforts are scientifically well grounded. The Committee will also review the activities undertaken in this area by the Department of Energy (DOE), the Department of Health and Human Services (HHS), and other agencies within the Committee's jurisdiction, including efforts to prepare for and respond to weather events and natural disasters in the future.

EPA Management and Operations

The Committee intends to conduct general oversight of the EPA, including review of the agency's funding decisions, resource allocation, grants, research activities, enforcement actions, relations with State and local governments, public transparency, and respect for economic, procedural, public health, and environmental standards in regulatory actions. The oversight will also include EPA program management and implementation, including efforts to reduce fraud and abuse in the renewable fuels program.

Investment in the Green Energy Sector

The American Recovery and Reinvestment Act (ARRA, or the stimulus) provided $84.6 billion in new spending for the green energy sector, as well as $21.6 billion in tax credits for energy, transport, and climate science. The Committee will continue to review how this money was spent; the development of new technologies, products, and businesses focused on green energy; and how this spending has impacted the domestic suppliers or manufacturers of alternative energy products.

Source: House Committee on Energy and Commerce. 2013. "Oversight Plan for the Committee on Energy and Commerce, U.S. House of Representatives, 113th Congress." Accessed April 1, 2014. https://energycommerce.house.gov/sites/republicans.energy commerce.house.gov/files/20130101Oversight.pdf.

MEDPAC

The Medicare Payment Advisory Commission (MedPAC) is an independent Congressional agency established by the Balanced Budget Act of 1997 (P.L. 10-533) to advise the U.S. Congress on issues affecting the Medicare program. The Commission's statutory mandate is quite broad: In addition to advising the Congress on payments to private health plans participating in Medicare and providers in Medicare's traditional fee-for-service program, MedPAC is also tasked with analyzing access to care, quality of care, and other issues affecting Medicare.

The Commission's 17 members bring diverse expertise in the financing and delivery of health care services. Commissioners are appointed to three-year terms (subject to renewal) by the Comptroller General and serve part time. Appointments are staggered; the terms of five or six Commissioners expire each year. The Commission is supported by an executive director and a staff of analysts, who typically have backgrounds in economics, health policy, public health, or medicine.

MedPAC meets publicly to discuss policy issues and formulate its recommendations to the Congress. In the course of these meetings, Commissioners consider the results of staff research, presentations by policy experts, and comments from interested parties. (Meeting transcripts are available at www.medpac.gov/-public-meetings-). Commission members and staff also seek input on Medicare issues through frequent meetings with individuals interested in the program, including staff from congressional committees and the Centers for Medicare & Medicaid Services (CMS), healthcare researchers, healthcare providers, and beneficiary advocates.

Two reports—issued in March and June each year—are the primary outlet for Commission recommendations. In addition to these reports and others on subjects requested by the Congress, MedPAC advises the Congress through other avenues, including comments on reports and proposed regulations issued by the Secretary of the Department of Health and Human Services, testimony, and briefings for congressional staff.

Source: Reprinted from Medicare Payment Advisory Commission (MedPAC). 2014. "About MedPAC." Accessed April 1. www.medpac.gov/-about-medpac-.

IMPROVING ACCESS TO MENTAL HEALTH SERVICES FOR VETERANS, SERVICE MEMBERS, AND MILITARY FAMILIES

EXECUTIVE ORDER

- - - - - - -

IMPROVING ACCESS TO MENTAL HEALTH SERVICES FOR VETERANS, SERVICE MEMBERS, AND MILITARY FAMILIES

By the authority vested in me as President by the Constitution and the laws of the United States of America, I hereby order as follows:

Section 1. Policy. Since September 11, 2001, more than two million service members have deployed to Iraq or Afghanistan. Long deployments and intense combat conditions require optimal support for the emotional and mental health needs of our service members and their families. The need for mental health services will only increase in the coming years as the Nation deals with the effects of more than a decade of conflict. Reiterating and expanding upon the commitment outlined in my Administration's 2011 report, entitled "Strengthening Our Military Families," we have an obligation to evaluate our progress and continue to build an integrated network of support capable of providing effective mental health services for veterans, service members, and their families. Our public health approach must encompass the practices of disease prevention and the promotion of good health for all military populations throughout their lifespans, both within the health care systems of the Departments of Defense and Veterans Affairs and in local communities. Our efforts also must focus on both outreach to veterans and their families and the provision of high quality mental health treatment to those in need. Coordination between the Departments of Veterans Affairs and Defense during service members' transition to civilian life is essential to achieving these goals.

Ensuring that all veterans, service members (Active, Guard, and Reserve alike), and their families receive the support they deserve is a top priority for my Administration. As part of our ongoing efforts to improve all facets of military mental health, this order directs the Secretaries of Defense, Health and Human Services, Education, Veterans Affairs, and Homeland Security to expand suicide prevention strategies and take steps to meet the current and future demand for mental health and substance abuse treatment services for veterans, service members, and their families.

Sec. 2. Suicide Prevention.

(a) By December 31, 2012, the Department of Veterans Affairs, in continued collaboration with the Department of Health and Human Services, shall expand the capacity of the Veterans Crisis Line by 50 percent to ensure that veterans have timely access, including by telephone, text, or online chat, to qualified, caring responders who can help address immediate crises and direct veterans to appropriate care. Further, the Department of Veterans Affairs shall ensure that any veteran identifying him or herself as being in crisis connects with a mental health professional or trained mental health worker within 24 hours. The Department of Veterans Affairs also shall expand the number of mental health professionals who are available to see veterans beyond traditional business hours.

(b) The Departments of Veterans Affairs and Defense shall jointly develop and implement a national suicide prevention campaign focused on connecting veterans and service members to mental health services. This 12 month campaign, which shall begin on September 1, 2012, will focus on the positive benefits of seeking care and encourage veterans and service members to proactively reach out to support services.

(c) To provide the best mental health and substance abuse prevention, education, and outreach support to our military and their family members, the Department of Defense shall review all of its existing mental health and substance abuse prevention, education, and outreach programs across the military services and the Defense Health Program to identify the key program areas that produce the greatest impact on quality and outcomes, and rank programs within each of these program areas using metrics that assess their effectiveness. By the end of Fiscal Year 2014, existing program resources shall be realigned to ensure that highly ranked programs are implemented across all of the military services and less effective programs are replaced.

Sec. 3. Enhanced Partnerships Between the Department of Veterans Affairs and Community Providers.

(a) Within 180 days of the date of this order, in those service areas where the Department of Veterans Affairs has faced challenges in hiring and placing mental health service providers and continues to have unfilled vacancies or long wait times, the Departments of Veterans Affairs and Health and Human Services shall establish pilot projects whereby the Department of Veterans Affairs contracts or develops formal arrangements with community based providers, such as community mental health clinics, community health centers, substance abuse treatment facilities, and rural health clinics, to test the effectiveness of community partnerships in helping to meet the mental health needs of veterans in a timely way. Pilot sites shall ensure that consumers of community-based services continue to be integrated into the health care systems of the Department of Veterans Affairs. No fewer than 15 pilot projects shall be established.

(b) The Department of Veterans Affairs shall develop guidance for its medical centers and service networks that supports the use of community mental health services, including telehealth services and substance abuse services, where appropriate, to meet demand and facilitate access to care. This guidance shall include recommendations that medical centers and service networks use community-based providers to help meet veterans' mental health needs where objective criteria, which the Department of Veterans Affairs shall define in the form of specific metrics, demonstrate such needs. Such objective criteria should include estimates of wait-times for needed care that exceed established targets.

(c) The Departments of Health and Human Services and Veterans Affairs shall develop a plan for a rural mental health recruitment initiative to promote opportunities for the Department of Veterans Affairs and rural communities to share mental health providers when demand is insufficient for either the Department of Veterans Affairs or the communities to independently support a full time provider.

Sec. 4. Expanded Department of Veterans Affairs Mental Health Services Staffing. The Secretary of Veterans Affairs shall, by December 31, 2013, hire and train 800 peer to peer counselors to empower veterans to support other veterans and help meet mental health care needs. In addition, the Secretary shall continue to use all appropriate tools, including collaborative arrangements with community based providers, pay setting authorities, loan repayment and scholarships, and partnerships with health care workforce training programs to accomplish the Department of Veterans Affairs' goal of recruiting, hiring, and placing 1,600 mental health professionals by June 30, 2013. The Department of Veterans Affairs also shall evaluate the reporting requirements associated with providing mental health services and reduce paperwork requirements where appropriate. In addition, the Department of Veterans Affairs shall update its management performance evaluation system to link performance to meeting mental health service demand.

Sec. 5. Improved Research and Development.

(a) The lack of full understanding of the underlying mechanisms of Post Traumatic Stress Disorder (PTSD), other mental health conditions, and Traumatic Brain Injury (TBI) has hampered progress in prevention, diagnosis, and treatment. In order to improve the coordination of agency research into these conditions and reduce the number of affected men and women through better prevention, diagnosis, and treatment, the Departments of Defense, Veterans Affairs, Health and Human Services, and Education, in coordination with the Office of Science and Technology Policy, shall establish a National Research Action Plan within 8 months of the date of this order.

(b) The National Research Action Plan shall include strategies to establish surrogate and clinically actionable biomarkers for early diagnosis and treatment effectiveness; develop improved diagnostic criteria for TBI; enhance our understanding of the mechanisms responsible for PTSD, related injuries, and neurological disorders following TBI; foster development of new treatments for these conditions based on a better understanding of the underlying mechanisms; improve data sharing between agencies and academic and industry researchers to accelerate progress and reduce redundant efforts without compromising privacy; and make better use of electronic health records to gain insight into the risk and mitigation of PTSD, TBI, and related injuries. In addition, the National Research Action Plan shall include strategies to support collaborative research to address suicide prevention.

(c) The Departments of Defense and Health and Human Services shall engage in a comprehensive longitudinal mental health study with an emphasis on PTSD, TBI, and related injuries to develop better prevention, diagnosis, and treatment options. Agencies shall continue ongoing collaborative research efforts, with an aim to enroll at least 100,000 service members by December 31, 2012, and include a plan for long term follow up with enrollees through a coordinated effort with the Department of Veterans Affairs.

Sec. 6. Military and Veterans Mental Health Interagency Task Force. There is established an Interagency Task Force on Military and Veterans Mental Health (Task Force), to be co-chaired by the Secretaries of Defense, Veterans Affairs, and Health and Human Services, or their designated representatives.

(a) **Membership.** In addition to the Co-Chairs, the Task Force shall consist of representatives from:

    (i)   the Department of Education;

    (ii)   the Office of Management and Budget;

    (iii) the Domestic Policy Council;

    (iv) the National Security Staff;

    (v)   the Office of Science and Technology Policy;

    (vi) the Office of National Drug Control Policy; and

    (vii) such other executive departments, agencies, or offices as the Co-Chairs may designate.

A member agency of the Task Force shall designate a full time officer or employee of the Federal Government to perform the Task Force functions.

(b) **Mission.** Member agencies shall review relevant statutes, policies, and agency training and guidance to identify reforms and take actions that facilitate implementation of the strategies outlined in this order. Member agencies shall work collaboratively on these strategies and also create an inventory of mental health and substance abuse programs and activities to inform this work.

(c) **Functions.**

    (i)   Not later than 180 days after the date of this order, the Task Force shall submit recommendations to the President on strategies to improve mental health and substance abuse treatment services for veterans, service members, and their families. Every year thereafter, the Task Force shall provide to the President a review of agency actions to enhance mental health and substance abuse treatment services for veterans, service members, and their families consistent with this order, as well as provide additional recommendations for action as appropriate. The Task Force shall define specific goals and metrics that will aid in measuring progress in improving mental health strategies. The Task Force will include cost analysis in the development of all recommendations, and will ensure any new requirements are supported within existing resources.

    (ii)   In addition to coordinating and reviewing agency efforts to enhance veteran and military mental health services pursuant to this order, the Task Force shall evaluate:

(1) agency efforts to improve care quality and ensure that the Departments of Defense and Veterans Affairs and community based mental health providers are trained in the most current evidence based methodologies for treating PTSD, TBI, depression, related mental health conditions, and substance abuse;

(2) agency efforts to improve awareness and reduce stigma for those needing to seek care; and

(3) agency research efforts to improve the prevention, diagnosis, and treatment of TBI, PTSD, and related injuries, and explore the need for an external research portfolio review.

(iii) In performing its functions, the Task Force shall consult with relevant nongovernmental experts and organizations as necessary.

Sec. 7. General Provisions.

(a) This order shall be implemented consistent with applicable law and subject to the availability of appropriations.

(b) Nothing in this order shall be construed to impair or otherwise affect:

(i) the authority granted by law to an executive department or agency, or the head thereof; or

(ii) the functions of the Director of the Office of Management and Budget relating to budgetary, administrative, or legislative proposals.

(c) This order is not intended to, and does not, create any right or benefit, substantive or procedural, enforceable at law or in equity by any party against the United States, its departments, agencies, or entities, its officers, employees, or agents, or any other person.

BARACK OBAMA

THE WHITE HOUSE,
August 31, 2012.

Source: Obama, B. 2012. "Executive Order: Improving Access to Mental Health Services for Veterans, Service Members, and Military Families." Accessed April 2, 2014. www.whitehouse .gov/the-press-office/2012/08/31/executive-order-improving-access-mental-health-services -veterans-service.

PERFORMANCE CULTURE IN THE FEDERAL WORKFORCE

The United States Office of Personnel Management (www.opm.gov) conducts the *Federal Employee Viewpoint Survey* to obtain employees' opinions about their supervisors, work experiences, agencies, and senior leaders. Information about performance culture—which evolves out of the policies and practices of an implementing organization, its leadership, and management decisions that shape the work environment—is sought because performance culture is a key component of organizational success. In any work setting, an effective performance culture encourages and motivates employees to put forth effort and helps them achieve satisfaction from their work.

The following table shows the Performance Culture Index obtained in the government-wide surveys in 2012 and 2013. As the director of the Office of Personnel Management observed in her Message from the Director section of the 2013 report,

> Factors such as an unprecedented 3-year pay freeze, automatic reductions from sequester that included furloughs for hundreds of thousands of employees, and reductions in training and other areas are clearly taking their toll on the Federal workforce—and this survey was administered prior to the recent government shutdown. The survey results serve as an important warning about the long-term consequences of the sequestration and budget uncertainty. Without a more predictable and responsible budget situation, we risk losing our most talented employees, as well as hurting our ability to recruit top talent for the future.

Recognition	2012	2013	Difference
In my work unit, differences in performance are recognized in a meaningful way.	34	31	−3
Creativity and innovation are rewarded.	38	35	−3
How satisfied are you with the recognition you receive for doing a good job?	48	45	−3

(continued)

Supervision	2012	2013	Difference
My supervisor supports my need to balance work and other life issues.	77	77	0
Discussions with my supervisor/team leader about my performance are worthwhile.	62	61	−1
Safety	**2012**	**2013**	**Difference**
Physical conditions allow employees to perform their jobs well.	67	66	−1
Work Connection	**2012**	**2013**	**Difference**
The people I work with cooperate to get the job done.	73	73	0
I know how my work relates to the agency's goals and priorities.	84	83	−1
Employees have a feeling of personal empowerment with respect to work process.	45	43	−2
Performance	**2012**	**2013**	**Difference**
My performance appraisal is a fair reflection of my performance.	69	68	−1
In my work unit, steps are taken to deal with a poor performer who cannot or will not improve.	29	28	−1
Promotions in my work unit are based on merit.	34	32	−2
Pay raises depend on how well employees perform their jobs.	22	19	−3

Source: US Office of Personnel Management. 2014. *Federal Employee Viewpoint Survey Results: Employees Influencing Change.* Governmentwide management report. Accessed April 2. www.fedview.opm.gov/2013files/2013_Governmentwide_Management_Report.pdf.

24

STATE EXPERIENCES WITH IMPLEMENTING THE ACA

With support from the Robert Wood Johnson Foundation, the Urban Institute is undertaking a comprehensive monitoring and tracking project to examine the implementation and effects of the Patient Protection and Affordable Care Act of 2010. The project began in May 2011 and will take place over several years. The project will document changes in a sample of states: Alabama, Colorado, Illinois, Maryland, Michigan, Minnesota, New Mexico, New York, Oregon, Rhode Island, and Virginia. The project is intended to help states, researchers, and policymakers learn from the process as it unfolds. This report is one of a series of papers focusing on particular implementation issues in these case-study states. Cross-cutting reports and state-specific reports on case-study states can be found at www.rwjf.org and www.healthpolicycenter.org.

The Patient Protection and Affordable Care Act (ACA) constitutes substantial reform of the US health insurance system. It includes an expansion of Medicaid eligibility to all those with incomes of up to 138 percent of the federal poverty level (FPL), regulatory reforms of private health insurance markets (particularly in the small group and nongroup markets), and financial assistance for the purchase of private insurance plans through newly established Health Insurance Marketplaces (HIMs, or Marketplaces, sometimes also referred to as Exchanges). In addition, the law requires most individuals to enroll in health insurance coverage or pay a penalty (the so-called individual mandate). It also institutes requirements for employers (recently delayed), most notably establishing financial penalties for large employers with workers who obtain subsidized coverage through the HIMs.

While the law established federal minimum standards, the ACA left considerable room for state participation and design flexibility in implementation of its insurance market reforms and the establishment of the Marketplaces. For example, states could establish their own Marketplaces using federal funds (creating State-Based Marketplaces, or SBMs), could leave the entire responsibility for establishing the HIM to the federal government (Federally Facilitated Marketplaces, or FFMs), or could take on particular HIM responsibilities while leaving the lion's share of their establishment to the federal government (FFM-Partnerships [FFM-Ps] or FFM-Marketplace Plan Management arrangements [FFM-MPMs]). States were expected to implement and enforce the new insurance market rules included in the law, but if they could not or would not do so, the rules would be enforced by the federal government. And, while not the original intent of the law as written, a 2012 Supreme Court decision made the ACA's Medicaid expansion an option for states. Many other options were left to states choosing to participate within the rubric of HIM design, insurance reforms, and Medicaid implementation.

As such, the design and effects of the ACA will differ across the states as a function of different policy choices made. Some states demonstrated a strong and consistent commitment to the law's implementation, quickly pursuing options to expand coverage and improve insurance markets as much as possible. Other states—often as a result of powerful political opposition to the law in either the governor's office, the state legislature, or both—chose to play only a limited role in implementation or no role at all. Assessment of the ACA and its potential to reduce the uninsured and to increase access and affordability to adequate insurance coverage will require drawing distinctions between outcomes in states putting maximum effort into the law's implementation and those whose involvement is limited, reluctant, or even obstructionist. The different design and implementation decisions will inevitably result in different outcomes for states, consumers, and other stakeholders

Researchers at the Urban Institute along with colleagues at Georgetown University's Center on Health Insurance Reforms assessed the state of health reform implementation in eight states that exhibit varying levels of support for the law. The findings are contained in a series of papers. These include eight briefs or papers that summarize findings for different kinds of states on a particular topic, including: coverage expansion potential, federal funding flows, information technology (IT) system development, eligibility determination and enrollment outreach, insurance plan participation, competition and premiums, insurance market reforms, Small Business Health Options Program (SHOP) development, and provider capacity. In this paper, we summarize the key findings and discuss the broad implications.

The study states were chosen from among those participating in a multiyear project funded by the Robert Wood Johnson Foundation (RWJF). The project provides in-kind technical support to states to assist them with implementing the reform components each has chosen to pursue; the project also provides funds for qualitative and quantitative research to monitor and track ACA implementation at the state and national levels. The participating states were chosen from among those whose governors expressed interest in participating; governors in all 50 states and the mayor of the District of

Columbia were invited to apply. States did not need to have committed to SBM development to participate, but they had to express interest in exploring potential roles for their state in the implementation of the ACA.

The states ultimately chosen for the larger project from among those expressing interest included Alabama, Colorado, Illinois, Maryland, Michigan, Minnesota, New Mexico, New York, Oregon, Rhode Island, and Virginia. Seven of these states (Colorado, Maryland, Minnesota, New Mexico, New York, Oregon, and Rhode Island) developed their own SBMs. Illinois and Michigan entered into formal partnership arrangements (FFM-Ps, both taking on responsibility for insurance plan management and Illinois also taking responsibility for outreach and enrollment activities) with the federal government, and Virginia developed an FFM-MPM arrangement (taking responsibility for insurance plan management tasks but avoiding the Partnership moniker).

For the current analysis, we chose five states that were actively pro-reform—Colorado, Maryland, Minnesota, New York, and Oregon. These states have demonstrated policy leadership and a strong commitment to effective implementation of the ACA. Each has adopted the Medicaid expansion and developed SBMs. They have engaged with a broad array of stakeholders in designing their state approaches and have pursued significant outreach and enrollment activities in order to increase coverage through their new HIMs and through Medicaid. Each has conducted extensive quantitative analyses of the effects of the law on their states and were quick to engage IT vendors. Each has taken responsibility for implementing insurance market reforms and has moved beyond federal requirements in order to improve stability and sustainability of their insurance markets. Not all of these states have had the same experience—for example, Oregon and Maryland had particularly challenging rollouts of their IT systems and were well behind in enrolling applicants during the initial months of the open enrollment period.

We chose Alabama, Michigan, and Virginia as examples of states taking on a more limited role in the implementation of reform. While all three states explored the possibility of developing their own SBMs early on, none decided to do so. As such, all rely on the federal IT system associated with *healthcare .gov* for eligibility determination and enrollment. But even as problems with the federal website are resolved, these states will face difficulties. None of them participate in consumer outreach and enrollment activities related to their state HIM, and far fewer resources will be devoted to those activities compared with the other five states. Again, the three are not all the same. For example, Michigan and Virginia have taken a responsibility for plan management, but Alabama left that responsibility to the federal government. Michigan chose to expand Medicaid for 2014; Alabama and Virginia may ultimately do so, but at present, they have not. While some factions in each state support the goals of the ACA, in these states there has not been a unified commitment to full participation, and the political leadership has chosen to take a more limited role as a result. These states are not likely to fare as well in expanding coverage and achieving the ACA goals for the foreseeable future.

Findings from this series of papers suggest the following:

- All states will benefit from the establishment of HIMs and income-related subsidies. Employer coverage is not expected to change significantly. States that are expanding Medicaid will ultimately experience larger relative gains in insurance coverage than those states that do not. These states will also see greater reductions in the number of uninsured, in the range of 40 to 50 percent. States not expanding Medicaid have smaller reductions. Because most of the non-expanding states had fewer uninsured to begin with, the ACA will result in increased disparities in coverage, at least in the early years.
- Because of greater increases in Medicaid coverage, expanding states will receive significantly larger relative inflows of federal dollars than those not expanding. The Medicaid expansion, with the very high federal matching rate, will bring in large amounts of federal dollars that will offset the ACA cuts in Medicare provider payment rates and Medicaid and Medicare disproportionate share hospital (DSH) payments. Non-expanding states will still have the ACA cuts with much less in new revenue. New state spending is relatively small, and much of it can be offset by savings in other parts of state budgets.
- SBM states have substantially more federal resources per uninsured person for outreach, education, and enrollment assistance than FFM states have. For public education, our five SBM states are spending, on average, $20.97 per uninsured person versus $5.90 in FFM states. Funding for application assistance per uninsured person is $30.66, on average, in our SBM states versus $8.79 in our FFM states.
- Performance of the IT systems supporting eligibility and enrollment in the five SBM states has been mixed and is reflected in state-specific enrollment numbers. The systems launched by the New York and Colorado Marketplaces are off to a relatively successful start, providing consumer-friendly plan comparison information and a streamlined, automated enrollment experience for a majority of applicants. In Maryland, Oregon, and (to a lesser degree) Minnesota, however, Marketplace IT systems have struggled to overcome technical glitches, defective software, and design flaws. Though these SBMs are committed to improving system functionality, full repairs could take several months (or longer if major software components are replaced) and enrollment numbers are further behind projections. The federal

IT system on which the FFM states rely also stumbled badly in its first two months; but, following a large-scale repair effort, functionality of the *healthcare.gov* site has improved considerably, facilitating a December surge in enrollment that has continued into 2014. The SBM states will continue to benefit from having close coordination between their HIM and Medicaid IT systems, facilitating smooth transitions across programs and greater continuity of coverage for beneficiaries. In contrast, the lack of close coordination between *healthcare.gov* and FFM states' Medicaid IT systems is a disadvantage for these states, relative to the fully participating ones.

- Plan participation and the level of competition is less a function of whether states are SBMs or FFMs and more a function of the pre-ACA insurance market as well as the managed competition framework in the ACA—for example, standardized rules, more information on premiums and benefits, and subsidies that are linked to the second-lowest-cost plan. In both SBM and FFM states, there are a large number of participants in most markets, including large and small commercial insurers and some new entrants, such as Medicaid plans and co-ops. Premiums have been lower-than-expected, reflecting cost-sharing requirements and limited or tiered networks but also intense competition for market share. In essentially monopolistic markets, however, the ACA lacks tools to create competition, and premiums are higher (e.g., some rural markets in Alabama, Michigan, and New York).

- Significant reforms to regulations governing the operation of insurance markets, particularly in the small-employer and nongroup markets, went into effect on January 1, 2014. Although only five of our states— Colorado, Maryland, Minnesota, New York and Oregon—chose to operate their own HIMs, both Michigan and Virginia are playing significant roles in managing the new plans in the HIMs. And, with the exception of Alabama, all the states have been actively involved in developing and implementing processes to review, approve, and monitor insurer compliance with the new rules. However, to date, the SBM states appear to be more proactive in efforts to mitigate potential premium increases during the transition to a reformed market; they have also been more inclined to implement long-term strategies to stabilize health insurance rates and to ensure the sustainability of their HIMs.

- Overall, the SHOP Marketplaces in the SBMs as well as in the FFMs have been slow to make progress, compared with their nongroup Marketplace counterparts. The SBM states with fully functional SHOP websites, however, have committed to providing a choice of plan options in 2014 for workers of participating small employers; employee choice will not be available to the FFM states until 2015. There have been delays in two of the five SBM states studied, Maryland and Oregon, so employer choice will be unavailable until their websites are repaired. SHOP enrollment for the FFM states has been delayed until 2015 due to constraints with *healthcare.gov*. As a result of these delays, SHOP participation for the FFM states is expected to fall below that in many of the SBM states, at least for the first year of operation.

- Likewise, provider supply is a problem in some geographic areas in all states. States that are expected to experience the largest relative increases in insurance coverage—for example, Colorado and Oregon—will see the greatest increase in pressure on this system. States with broad coverage already and those not adopting the Medicaid expansion will see less increase in demand for services. There are several systematic changes taking place to alleviate these demand pressures: increases in Medicaid physician fees, increased funding of community health centers, and increases in hospital ambulatory care capacity.

Source: Extracted from Holahan, J., L. J. Blumberg, T. Coughlin, S. Corlette, B. Courtot, I. Hill, K. Lucia, R. Peters, S. Rifkin, and M. Wilkinson. 2014. *The Launch of the Affordable Care Act in Selected States: State Flexibility Is Leading to Very Different Outcomes.* Reproduced with permission of the Urban Institute. Published March. www.urban.org/UploadedPDF /413035-The-Launch-of-Health-Reform-in-Eight-States-State-Flexibility-Is-Leading-to -Very-Different-Outcomes.pdf.

25

LOWER COSTS, BETTER CARE: REFORMING OUR HEALTH CARE DELIVERY SYSTEM

Fixing America's health care system doesn't stop with guaranteeing that everyone has coverage. To address the rising costs of health care, we must improve the way that health care is delivered, including the coordination and safety of care.

The Affordable Care Act includes tools to improve the quality of health care that can also lower costs for taxpayers and patients. This means avoiding costly mistakes and readmissions, keeping patients healthy, rewarding quality instead of quantity, and building on the health information technology infrastructure that enables new payment and delivery models to work. These reforms and investments will build a health care system that will ensure quality care for generations to come.

Already we have made significant progress:

Health care spending is slowing

According to the annual Report of National Health Expenditures, total U.S. health spending grew 3.7 percent in 2012. This marks the slowest four years on record in overall health expenditures and for the second straight year, overall health costs grew slower than the economy as a whole. Health spending as a share of gross domestic product fell slightly from 17.3 percent in 2011 to 17.2 percent in 2012, the third consecutive year that health spending has held steady or declined as a share of the economy. We have seen low spending growth per enrollee in 2012 for Medicare (0.7 percent), Medicaid (1.3 percent), and private health insurance premiums (2.7 percent). By comparison, over the ten years preceding the recent slowdown (1999 to 2008), those per-enrollee spending growth figures were 7.4 percent for Medicare, 2.8 percent for Medicaid, and 7.4 percent for private health insurance. Slowing private premium cost growth by over 60 percent means real savings for workers, their families, and employers. The Affordable Care Act's 80 / 20 rule (medical loss ratio policy) has led to estimated savings of $5 billion over the past two years. And the strengthened rate review program has resulted in an estimated $1.2 billion in savings in 2012 to consumers of private health insurance.

Health outcomes are improving and adverse events are decreasing

In 2012, we finalized a program that ties Medicare reimbursement for hospitals to their readmission rates, i.e., the percentage of patients who have to return to the hospital within 30 days of being discharged. The 30-day, all-cause readmission rate decreased in 2012 to 18.5 percent, after averaging 19 percent for the past five years. This decline is continuing into 2013 as readmission rates have averaged less than 18 percent over the first eight months of the year. This translates to about 130,000 fewer readmissions for Medicare beneficiaries. Additionally, as part of a new Affordable Care Act initiative, clinicians at some hospitals have reduced their early elective deliveries to close to zero, meaning fewer at-risk newborns and fewer admissions to the NICU.

Providers are engaged

In 2012, Medicare Accountable Care Organizations (ACOs) began participating in the Medicare Shared Savings Program and the Pioneer Accountable Care Organization Model. These programs encourage providers to invest in redesigning care for higher quality and more efficient service delivery, without restricting patients' freedom to go to the Medicare provider of their choice.

Over 360 organizations are participating in the Medicare ACOs, serving approximately 5.3 million Medicare beneficiaries. As existing ACOs choose to add providers and more organizations join the program, participation in ACOs is expected to grow. Medicare ACOs participating in the Shared Savings Program generated $128 million in net savings for the Medicare trust fund to date.

Medicare beneficiaries are shopping for coverage according to quality

The Affordable Care Act tied payment to private Medicare Advantage plans to the quality of coverage they offer. Since those payment changes have been in effect, more seniors are able to choose from a broader range of higher quality Medicare Advantage plans, and more seniors have enrolled in these higher quality plans as well. Over one-third of Medicare Advantage contracts received four or more stars in 2014, which is an increase from 28 percent in 2013. Over half of Medicare Advantage enrollees are enrolled in plans with four or more stars in 2014, a significant increase from 37 percent of enrollees in 2013. Since the health care law passed, enrollment has increased by 32.5 percent and premiums have fallen by 9.8 percent in Medicare Advantage. In 2014, the 14.6 million Medicare beneficiaries currently enrolled in Medicare Advantage have access to 1,625 five- and four-star plans, which is 473 more high-quality plans than were available in the previous year.

Below are specific examples of the reforms and investments that we are making to build a health care delivery system that will better serve all Americans.

PAYING FOR VALUE:

- *Hospitals.* Two important programs that reward hospitals based on the quality of care they provide to patients began in 2012. The Hospital Value-Based Purchasing Program links a portion of hospitals' Medicare payments for impatient acute care to their performance on important quality measures. Examples of measures include whether a patient received an antibiotic before surgery, and how well doctors and nurses communicate with patients. The Hospital Readmissions Reduction Program reduces Medicare payments to hospitals with relatively high rates of potentially preventable readmissions, to financially encourage them to focus on this key indicator of patient safety and care quality.

- *Medicare Advantage Plans.* The Centers for Medicare & Medicaid Services (CMS) strengthened the quality bonus incentives provided by the Affordable Care Act by providing additional payments for plans improving the quality of care.

- *Dialysis Facilities.* The End-Stage Renal Disease (ESRD) Quality Incentive Program ties Medicare payments directly to facility performance on quality measures, resulting in better care at lower cost for over 503,000 Medicare beneficiaries with end-stage renal disease. In addition, a new comprehensive care model announced in January 2013 will test a new payment and service delivery approach to improve care for ESRD beneficiaries, by coordinating primary care with care for their special health needs.

PROMOTING BETTER CARE AND PROTECTING PATIENT SAFETY:

- *Electronic Health Records (EHRs).* Adoption of electronic health records continues to increase among physicians, hospitals, and others serving Medicare and Medicaid beneficiaries helping to evaluate patients' medical status, coordinate care, eliminate redundant procedures, and provide high-quality care. More than 62 percent of health care professionals, and over 86 percent of hospitals, have already qualified for EHR incentive payments for using certified EHR technology to meet the objectives and measures established by the program, known as meaningful use. Electronic health records will help speed the adoption of many other delivery system reforms, by making it easier for hospitals and doctors to better coordinate care and achieve improvements in quality.

- *Partnership for Patients.* The nationwide Partnership for Patients initiative aims to save 60,000 lives by averting millions of hospital-acquired conditions over three years by reducing complications and readmissions, and improving the transition from one care setting to another. At the core of this initiative are 26 Hospital Engagement Networks, which work with 3,700 hospitals, working with health care providers and institutions, to identify best practices and solutions to reducing hospital-acquired conditions and readmissions. National datasets are showing strong progress in 8 of the 10 patient safety priority areas of the Partnership for Patients. The Hospital Engagement Networks have been actively involved in the effort to reduce the rate of early elective deliveries, in conjunction with the Strong Start for Mothers and Newborns Initiative.

- *Healthy infants.* The Strong Start for Mothers and Newborns initiative aims to reduce early elective deliveries as well as test models to decrease preterm births among high-risk pregnant women in Medicaid and the Children's Health Insurance Program (CHIP). The Strong Start initiative builds on the work of the Partnership for Patients, testing ways to support providers in reducing early elective deliveries. It also provides over $11.7 million to 27 awardees to test enhanced prenatal care interventions to lower the risk of preterm birth among pregnant women with Medicaid or CHIP. As part of this initiative, clinicians at some hospitals have reduced their early elective deliveries to close to zero, meaning fewer at-risk newborns and fewer admissions to the NICU. Among 1,321 hospitals reporting common measures, early elective delivery rates have fallen (improved) by 52 percent.

- *Hospital-acquired conditions.* Along with other data available on Hospital Compare, beneficiaries can now find information on the incidence of serious hospital-acquired conditions (HACs) in individual hospitals. In FY 2015, hospitals with high rates of HACs will see their Medicare payments reduced.

- *Community-Based Care.* As part of the Partnership for Patients, the Community-Based Care Transitions Program supports approximately 100 Community-Based Organizations partnering with more than 450 hospitals in 40 states to help patients make more successful transitions from hospital to home or to another post-hospital setting. The Community-Based Care Transitions Program is a five-year program that began in 2011. $300 million in total funding has been appropriated for the program.

ENSURING ALL AMERICANS GET THE RIGHT CARE WHEN THEY NEED IT:

- *Providing states with additional flexibility and resources to enhance care.* The State Innovation Models Initiative aims to help states deliver high-quality health care, lower costs, and improve their health system performance. Nearly $300 million has been awarded to six states (Arkansas, Massachusetts, Maine, Minnesota, Vermont and Oregon) that are ready to implement their health care delivery system reforms and nineteen states to either develop or continue to work on their plans for delivery system reform.

- *Integrating care for individuals enrolled in Medicare and Medicaid.* Many of the ten million Medicare-Medicaid enrollees suffer from multiple or severe chronic conditions. Total annual spending for their care exceeds $300 billion. Nine states (California, Illinois, Massachusetts, Minnesota, New York, Ohio, South Carolina, Virginia, and Washington) have received approval for demonstrations using integrated care teams, health homes, or other interventions to coordinate care for Medicare-Medicaid beneficiaries. The new demonstrations are designed to provide participants with a person-centered, integrated care program that provides a more easily navigable and seamless path to all covered Medicare and Medicaid services.

- *Greater independence for Americans with disabilities and long-term care needs.* The Affordable Care Act includes a number of policies to promote non-institutional long-term care programs that will help keep people at home and out of institutions:

  - Fourteen additional states have joined the Money Follows the Person Program to help rebalance their long-term care systems to transition Medicaid beneficiaries from institutions to the community. Forty-four states and the District of Columbia are now participating in Money Follows the Person. Over 31,000 people with chronic conditions and disabilities have transitioned from institutions back into the community through Money Follows the Person programs as of December 2012.

  - Seventeen states are participating in the Balancing Incentive Program, which gives states incentives to increase access to non-institutional long-term services and supports and provides new ways to serve more Medicaid beneficiaries in home- and community-based settings.

- Fourteen states have approved Health Home State Plan Amendments to integrate and coordinate primary, acute, behavioral health, and long-term services and supports for Medicaid beneficiaries.

- *Promoting care at home.* A new Affordable Care Act demonstration, Independence at Home, tests whether providing chronically ill beneficiaries with primary care in the home will help them stay healthy and out of the hospital. Fifteen physician practices and three consortia of physician practices are participating in the Independence at Home Demonstration.

CONTINUOUS QUALITY IMPROVEMENT:

- *Center for Medicare and Medicaid Innovation.* The Innovation Center is charged with testing innovative payment and service delivery models to reduce expenditures in Medicare, Medicaid, and CHIP, and at the same time, preserving or enhancing quality of care. Already the Innovation Center is engaged in projects with more than 50,000 health care providers to improve care.

- *Pioneer Accountable Care Organization (ACO) Model.* 23 ACOs are participating in the Pioneer ACO Model that is designed for health care organizations and providers that are already experienced in coordinating care for patients across care settings. Preliminary initial results from the independent evaluation of the Pioneer ACO Model show that Pioneer ACOs have generated gross savings of $147 million in their first year while continuing to deliver high-quality care.

- *Bundled Payments for Care Improvement initiative.* 232 organizations are testing how bundling payments for episodes of care can result in more coordinated care for Medicare beneficiaries and lower costs for Medicare. Bundling payment for services that patients receive across a single episode of care, such as heart bypass surgery or a hip replacement, is one way to encourage doctors, hospitals and other health care providers to work together to better coordinate care for patients, both when they are in the hospital and after they are discharged.

- *Health Care Innovation Awards.* The Health Care Innovation Awards are funding up to $1 billion in awards to 107 organizations that are implementing the most compelling new ideas to deliver better health, improved care and lower costs to people enrolled in Medicare, Medicaid and the Children's Health Insurance Program (CHIP). The

Health Care Innovation Awards Round Two will fund up to $1 billion in awards to applicants across the country that test new payment and service delivery models.

REDUCING HEALTH COSTS:

- *Lower cost health care equipment and supplies.* In 100 metropolitan areas, a strong Medicare Durable Medical Equipment, Prosthetics, Orthotics, and Supplies (DMEPOS) competitive bidding program set new, lower payment rates for medical equipment and supplies. This program has already saved more than $400 million for Medicare and its beneficiaries, and CMS estimates even larger savings as a result of the Round 2 expansion and the National Mail Order program for diabetic testing supplies, which both went into effect in July 2013. Overall, the initiative is expected to save the Medicare program an estimated $25.8 billion, and beneficiaries an estimated $17.2 billion, over the next 10 years.

- *Fighting fraud.* The Affordable Care Act's landmark steps to improve and enhance the Administration's ongoing efforts to prevent and detect fraud and crack down on individuals who attempt to defraud Medicare, Medicaid, and CHIP has resulted in a record level of recoveries—$4.2 billion in fiscal year 2012—and a record return on investment—$7.90 for every dollar invested. Total recoveries over the past four years were $14.9 billion compared to $6.7 billion over the prior four years. Efforts include tough new rules and sentences for criminals; enhanced screening and enrollment requirements; increased coordination of fraud-fighting efforts; sharing data across federal agencies to fight fraud; and new tools to target high-risk providers and suppliers. We have also prioritized engaging beneficiaries in fighting fraud through providing more claims data to beneficiaries in an easy-to-read format and proposing to increase the rewards available for fraud referrals.

Source: Reprinted from Centers for Medicare & Medicaid Services. 2014. "Lower Costs, Better Care: Reforming Our Health Care Delivery System." Fact sheet. Published January 30. www.cms.gov/Newsroom/MediaReleaseDatabase/Fact-Sheets/2014-Fact-sheets -items/2014-01-30-03.html.

OBSERVATIONS ON THE DEPARTMENT OF HOMELAND SECURITY'S (DHS'S) EFFORTS TO IDENTIFY, PRIORITIZE, ASSESS, AND INSPECT CHEMICAL FACILITIES

Facilities that produce, store, or use hazardous chemicals could be of interest to terrorists intent on using toxic chemicals to inflict mass casualties in the United States. DHS has established the Chemical Facility Anti-Terrorism Standards (CFATS) program through which it issued regulations establishing standards for the security of these facilities. DHS established the CFATS program to assess risk at facilities covered by the regulations and inspect them to ensure compliance. . . .

This statement provides observations on DHS efforts related to the CFATS program. It is based on the results of previous GAO reports in July 2012 and April 2013, with selected updates conducted in February 2014. In conducting the earlier work, GAO reviewed DHS reports and plans on the program and interviewed DHS officials. In addition, GAO interviewed DHS officials to update information. . . .

In a July 2012 report, GAO recommended that DHS measure its performance implementing actions to improve its management of CFATS. In an April 2013 report, GAO recommended that DHS enhance its risk assessment approach to incorporate all elements of risk, conduct a peer review, and gather feedback on its outreach to facilities. DHS concurred with these recommendations and has taken actions or has actions underway to address them.

GAO provided a draft of the updated information to DHS for review, and DHS confirmed its accuracy.

What GAO Found in the Updated Report of February 2014

In managing its Chemical Facility Anti-Terrorism Standards (CFATS) program, the Department of Homeland Security (DHS) has a number of efforts underway to identify facilities that are covered by the program, assess risk and prioritize facilities, review and approve facility security plans, and inspect facilities to ensure compliance with security regulations.

- **Identifying facilities.** DHS has begun to work with other agencies to identify facilities that should have reported their chemical holdings to CFATS, but may not have done so. DHS initially identified about 40,000 facilities by publishing a CFATS rule requiring that facilities with certain types of chemicals report the types and quantities of these chemicals. However, a chemical explosion in West, Texas last year demonstrated the risk posed by chemicals covered by CFATS. Subsequent to this incident, the President issued Executive Order 13650 which was intended to improve chemical facility safety and security in coordination with owners and operators. Under the executive order, a federal working group is sharing information to identify additional facilities that are to be regulated under CFATS, among other things.

- **Assessing risk and prioritizing facilities.** DHS has begun to enhance its ability to assess risks and prioritize facilities. DHS assessed the risks of facilities that reported their chemical holdings in order to determine which ones would be required to participate in the program and subsequently develop site security plans. GAO's April 2013 report found weaknesses in multiple aspects of the risk assessment and prioritization approach and made recommendations to review and improve this process. In February 2014, DHS officials told us they had begun to take action to revise the process for assessing risk and prioritizing facilities.

- **Reviewing security plans.** DHS has also begun to take action to speed up its reviews of facility security plans. Per the CFATS regulation, DHS was to review security plans and visit the facilities to make sure their security measures met the risk-based performance standards. GAO's April 2013 report found a 7- to 9-year backlog for these reviews and visits, and DHS has begun to take action to expedite these activities. As a separate matter, one of the performance standards—personnel surety, under which facilities are to perform background checks and ensure appropriate credentials for personnel and visitors as appropriate— is being developed. As of February 2014, DHS has reviewed and conditionally approved facility plans pending final development of the personal surety performance standard.

- **Inspecting to verify compliance.** In February 2014, DHS reported it had begun to perform inspections at facilities to ensure compliance with their site security plans. According to DHS, these inspections are to occur about 1 year after facility site security plan approval. Given the backlog in plan approvals, this process has started recently and GAO has not yet reviewed this aspect of the program.

Source: Reprinted from Caldwell, S. L. 2014. "Observations on DHS Efforts to Identify, Prioritize, Assess, and Inspect Chemical Facilities." Highlights of GAO-14-365T, a testimony before the Subcommittee on Cybersecurity, Infrastructure Protection, and Security Technologies, Committee on Homeland Security, House of Representatives. Published February. http://gao.gov/assets/670/661181.pdf.

OPTIONS FOR REDUCING THE DEFICIT: INCREASE ALL TAXES ON ALCOHOLIC BEVERAGES TO $16 PER PROOF GALLON

In 2012, the federal government collected $9.7 billion in revenue from excise taxes on distilled spirits, beer, and wine. The different alcoholic beverages are taxed at different rates. Specifically, the alcohol content of beer and wine is taxed at a much lower rate than the alcohol content of distilled spirits because the taxes are determined on the basis of different liquid measures. Distilled spirits are measured in proof gallons (a standard unit for measuring the alcohol content of a liquid). The current excise tax levied on those spirits, $13.50 per proof gallon, translates to about 21 cents per ounce of alcohol. Beer, by contrast, is measured by the barrel, and the current tax rate of $18 per barrel translates to about 10 cents per ounce of alcohol (under the assumption that the average alcohol content of beer is 4.5 percent). The current levy on wine is $1.07 per gallon, or about 8 cents per ounce of alcohol (assuming an average alcohol content of 11 percent). Last raised in 1991, current excise tax rates on alcohol are far lower than historical levels when adjusted for inflation.

This option would standardize the base on which the federal excise tax is levied by using the proof gallon as the measure for all alcoholic beverages. The tax would be raised to $16 per proof gallon, thus increasing revenues by $64 billion over the 2014–2023 period as shown in the following table. (Because excise taxes reduce producers' and consumers' income, higher excise taxes would lead to reductions in revenues from income and payroll taxes. The estimates shown here reflect those reductions.)

											Total	
(Billions of dollars)	2014	2015	2016	2017	2018	2019	2020	2021	2022	2023	2014–2018	2014–2023
Change in Revenues	4.7	6.3	6.4	6.4	6.5	6.6	6.6	6.7	6.8	6.9	30.3	63.8

A tax of $16 per proof gallon would equal about 25 cents per ounce of alcohol. Under this option, the federal excise tax on a 750-milliliter bottle (commonly referred to as a fifth) of distilled spirits would rise from about $2.14 to $2.54. The tax on a six-pack of beer would jump from about 33 cents to 81 cents, and the tax on a 750-milliliter bottle of wine would increase by a similar amount, from about 21 cents to 70 cents.

Experts agree that the consumption of alcohol creates costs for society that are not reflected in the pretax price of alcoholic beverages. Examples of those "external costs" include spending on health care that is related to alcohol consumption and covered by the public, losses in productivity stemming from alcohol consumption that are borne by others besides the consumer, and the loss of lives and property that results from alcohol-related accidents and crime. Calculating such costs is difficult. However, one study found that the external economic costs of alcohol abuse exceeded $130 billion in 2006—an amount far greater than the revenues currently derived from taxes on alcoholic beverages.

One argument in favor of raising excise taxes on alcoholic beverages is that they would reduce alcohol use—and thus the external costs of that use—and make consumers of alcoholic beverages pay a larger share of such costs. Research has consistently shown that higher prices lead to less alcohol consumption, even among heavy drinkers.

Moreover, raising excise taxes to reduce consumption might be desirable, regardless of the effect on external costs, if lawmakers believed that consumers under-estimated the harm they do to themselves by drinking. Heavy drinking is known to cause organ damage and cognitive impairment; and the links between highway accidents and drinking, which are especially strong among the young, are well-documented. Substantial evidence also indicates that the use of alcohol from an early age can lead to heavy consumption later in life. When deciding how much to drink, people—particularly young people—may not adequately consider such long-term risks to their health.

An increase in taxes on alcoholic beverages would have disadvantages as well. It would make a tax that is already regressive—one that takes up a greater percentage of income for low-income families than for middle- and upper-income families—even more so. In addition, it would affect not only problem drinkers but also drinkers who imposed no costs on society and who thus would be unduly penalized. Furthermore, higher taxes would reduce consumption by some moderate drinkers whose intake of alcohol is believed to have health benefits. (Moderate alcohol consumption, particularly of wine, has been linked to lower incidence of heart disease, obesity, and stroke and to increases in life expectancy in middle age.) With regard to the argument that some drinkers underestimate the personal costs of alcohol consumption, some opponents of raising taxes on alcohol argue that the government should not try to modify consumers' private behavior. Finally, as to effects on the federal budget, in the longer term, overall savings to the federal government from this tax would be at least partially offset by additional spending, as healthier people lived longer and relied more on federal health care, disability, and retirement programs. Those longevity-related offsets would grow over time.

Source: Reprinted from Congressional Budget Office. 2013. *Options for Reducing the Deficit: 2014 to 2023.* Published November. www.cbo.gov/sites/default/files/cbofiles /attachments/44715-OptionsForReducingDeficit-3.pdf.

28

OPENING STATEMENT: HEARING ON "WHERE HAVE ALL THE PATIENTS GONE? EXAMINING THE PSYCHIATRIC BED SHORTAGE"

The Honorable Tim Murphy
Chairman, Subcommittee on Oversight and Investigations of the Energy &
Commerce Committee of the US House of Representatives
March 26, 2014

Right after the December 14, 2012 elementary school shootings in New-
town, Connecticut, the Subcommittee on Oversight and Investigations
began a review of federal programs and resources devoted to mental health
and serious mental illness.

Recent events have shown the continuing importance of this inquiry,
including the September 2013 Navy Yard shooting just a couple of miles
from where we sit this morning, in Washington, D.C.

Other tragic cases, like Seung-Hui Cho, James Holmes, Jared Lough-
ner, and Adam Lanza, all exhibited a record of untreated severe mental illness
prior to their crimes. It is a reflection of the total dysfunction of our current
mental health system that despite clear warning signs, these individuals failed
to receive inpatient or outpatient treatment for their illnesses that might have
averted these tragedies.

They all leave us wondering what would have happened if . . .

What would have happened if Aaron Alexis was not just given sleep-
ing pills at the VA? Or if there was an available hospital bed or outpatient
treatment available for others who later became violent, involved in a crime,
unable to pay bills, or tossed out on the street?

Part of the problem is that our laws on involuntary commitment are
in dire need of modernization—it is simply unreasonable, if not a danger to
public safety, that our current system often waits until an individual is on
the brink of harming himself or others, or has already done so, before any
action can be taken. The scarcity of effective inpatient or outpatient treatment options in the community, as illustrated by the premature release of

Gus Deeds, son of Virginia senator Creigh Deeds, from emergency custody because of the lack of psychiatric beds, is also to blame. A sad ending that in our heart we cannot begin to imagine a parent's grief when told there is no place for your son to get help.

Nationwide, we face an alarming shortage in inpatient psychiatric beds that, if not addressed, will result in more tragic outcomes. This is part of the long-term legacy of deinstitutionalization, the emptying out of state psychiatric hospitals resulting from the financial burden for community-based care being shifted from the state to the federal government. With deinstitutionalization, the number of available inpatient psychiatric beds has fallen considerably. On the whole, the number of beds has decreased from 559,000 in the 1950s to just 43,000 today. We needed to close those old hospitals that had become asylums, lock-ups, and dumping grounds.

But where did all the patients go? They were supposed to be in community treatment—on the road to recovery—but for many that did not happen.

The result is that individuals with serious mental illness who are unable to obtain treatment through ordinary means are now homeless or entangled in the criminal justice system, including being locked up in jails and prisons.

Right now, the country's three largest jail systems—in Cook County, Illinois; Los Angeles County; and New York City—have more than 11,000 prisoners receiving treatment on any given day and are, in fact, the largest mental health treatment facilities in the country. These jails are many times larger than the largest state psychiatric hospitals.

Not surprisingly, neither living on the streets nor being confined to a high-security cellblock are known to improve the chances that an individual's serious mental illness will stabilize, let alone prepare them, where possible, for eventual reentry into the community, to find housing, jobs, and confidence for their future.

It is an unplanned, albeit entirely unacceptable consequence of deinstitutionalization that the state psychiatric asylums, dismantled out of concern for the humane treatment and care of individuals with serious mental illness, have now effectively been replaced by confinement in prisons and homeless shelters.

What can we do earlier in people's lives to get them evidence-based treatment, community support, and on the road to recovery not recidivism?

Where is the humanity in saying there are no beds to treat a person suffering from schizophrenia, delusions, and aggression so we will sedate you and restrain you to an ER bed for days?

This morning, to provide some perspective on the far-reaching implications of the current psychiatric bed shortage and to hear some creative approaches to address it, we'll be receiving testimony from individuals with a wealth of experience across the full range of public services consumed by the seriously mentally ill. These include:

- Lisa Ashley, the mother of a son with serious mental illness who has been boarded multiple times at the emergency department;
- Dr. Jeffrey Geller, a psychiatrist and co-author of a report on the trends and consequences of closing public psychiatric hospitals;
- Dr. Jon Mark Hirshon, an ER physician and Task Force Chair on a recent study of emergency care compiled by the American College of Emergency Physicians;
- Chief Mike Biasotti, Immediate Past President of the New York State Association of Chiefs of Police and parent of a daughter with serious mental illness;
- Sheriff Tom Dart, of the Cook County, IL Sheriff's Office, who oversees one of the largest single site county pre-detention facilities in the U.S.;
- The Honorable Steve Leifman, Associate Administrative Judge, Miami-Dade County Court, 11th Judicial Circuit of Florida;
- Gunther Stern, Executive Director of Georgetown Ministry Center, a shelter and clubhouse caring for Washington D.C.'s homeless;
- Hakeem Rahim, a mental health educator and advocate;
- LaMarr Edgerson, a clinical mental health counselor and Director at Large of the American Mental Health Counselors Association; and
- Dr. Arthur Evans, Jr., Commissioner of Philadelphia's Department of Behavioral Health and Intellectual Disability Services.

I thank them all for joining us this morning.

Source: Reprinted from Murphy, T. 2014. "Opening Statement of the Honorable Tim Murphy, Subcommittee on Oversight and Investigations, Hearing on 'Where Have All the Patients Gone? Examining the Psychiatric Bed Shortage.'" Published March 26. http://energycommerce.house.gov/sites/republicans.energycommerce.house.gov/files/Hearings/OI/20140326/HHRG-113-IF02-MState-M001151-20140326.pdf.

A PROPOSED RULE ON REVISION OF NUTRITION LABELS

DEPARTMENT OF HEALTH AND HUMAN SERVICES

Food and Drug Administration

21 CFR Part 101

[Docket No. FDA–2012–N–1210]

RIN 0910–AF22

Food Labeling: Revision of the Nutrition and
Supplement Facts Labels

AGENCY: Food and Drug Administration, HHS.

ACTION: Proposed rule.

SUMMARY: The Food and Drug Administration (FDA, the Agency, or we) is proposing to amend its labeling regulations for conventional foods and dietary supplements to provide updated nutrition information on the label to assist consumers in maintaining healthy dietary practices. The updated information is consistent with current data on the associations between nutrients and chronic diseases or health-related conditions, reflects current public health conditions in the United States, and corresponds to new information on consumer behavior and consumption patterns. We are proposing to update the list of nutrients that are required or permitted to be declared; provide updated Daily Reference Values and Reference Daily Intake values that are based on current dietary recommendations from consensus reports; amend requirements for foods represented or purported to be specifically for children under the age of 4 years and pregnant and lactating women and establish nutrient reference values specifically for these population subgroups; and revise the format and appearance of the Nutrition Facts label.

CURRENT LABEL

Nutrition Facts

Serving Size 2/3 cup (55g)
Servings Per Container About 8

Amount Per Serving

Calories 230   Calories from Fat 40

	% Daily Value*
Total Fat 8g	**12%**
Saturated Fat 1g	**5%**
Trans Fat 0g	
Cholesterol 0mg	**0%**
Sodium 160mg	**7%**
Total Carbohydrate 37g	**12%**
Dietary Fiber 4g	**16%**
Sugars 1g	
Protein 3g	

Vitamin A	10%
Vitamin C	8%
Calcium	20%
Iron	45%

* Percent Daily Values are based on a 2,000 calorie diet. Your daily value may be higher or lower depending on your calorie needs.

	Calories:	2,000	2,500
Total Fat	Less than	65g	80g
Sat Fat	Less than	20g	25g
Cholesterol	Less than	300mg	300mg
Sodium	Less than	2,400mg	2,400mg
Total Carbohydrate		300g	375g
Dietary Fiber		25g	30g

PROPOSED LABEL

Nutrition Facts

8 servings per container

Serving size   2/3 cup (55g)

Amount per 2/3 cup

Calories   **230**

% DV*

12%	**Total Fat** 8g
5%	Saturated Fat 1g
	Trans Fat 0g
0%	**Cholesterol** 0mg
7%	**Sodium** 160mg
12%	**Total Carbs** 37g
14%	Dietary Fiber 4g
	Sugars 1g
	Added Sugars 0g
	Protein 3g

10%	**Vitamin D** 2mcg
20%	**Calcium** 260mg
45%	**Iron** 8mg
5%	**Potassium** 235mg

* Footnote on Daily Values (DV) and calories reference to be inserted here.

Source: Reprinted from *Federal Register.* 2014. "Food Labeling: Revision of the Nutrition and Supplement Facts Labels." 21 C.F.R. 101 (March 3, 2014), 11880-11987. Accessed January 23, 2015. www.gpo.gov/fdsys/pkg/FR-2014-03-03/pdf/2014-04387.pdf.

SUMMARY OF THE FDA'S OPHTHALMIC DEVICES PANEL MEETING

Department of Health & Human Services

Public Health Service

Food and Drug Administration

Silver Spring, MD 20993-0002

Introduction:
The Ophthalmic Devices Panel of the Medical Devices Advisory Committee to the Food and Drug Administration met on March 14, 2014 to discuss, make recommendations, and vote on information related to the premarket approval (PMA) application, P030016/S001 for the Visian Toric Implantable Collamer® Lens (TICL) sponsored by STAAR Surgical Company.

The applicant has proposed the following Indication for Use:
The Visian TICL is indicated for use in adults 21–45 years of age:

1. for the correction of myopic astigmatism in adults with spherical equivalent ranging from −3.0D to ≤−15.0D with cylinder of 1.0D to 4.0D
2. for the reduction of myopic astigmatism in adults with spherical equivalent ranging from greater than −15.0D to −20.0D with cylinder 1.0D to 4.0D
3. with an anterior chamber depth (ACD) of 3.0 mm or greater, when measured from the corneal endothelium to the anterior surface of the crystalline lens and a stable refractive history (within 0.5 Diopter for 1 year prior to implantation).
4. The Visian TICL is intended for placement in the posterior chamber (ciliary sulcus) of the phakic eye.

Panel Deliberations/FDA Questions:
The Panel evaluated the data generated from the TICL study (including but not limited to 3,646 data points affected by the protocol deviations; significant amount of missing data; within-window accountability of 70.5% at 12 months; and 68% (143/210) of eyes implanted with lenses not according

to protocol), and concluded that the data generated from the TICL study are not sufficient to represent valid scientific evidence for assessment of the device safety and effectiveness.

The Panel stated that since the directions for use for the TICL are the same as that of the approved Implantable Collamer® Lens for Myopia (MICL) and have not changed, the directions for use concerning sizing provides adequate guidance to reasonably ensure predictable and safe postoperative vaulting. The Panel also stated that the labeling does provide adequate instruction for the evaluation of postoperative lens vault, since it has not changed from the MICL labeling.

Given the available treatment alternatives for lower myopes and the safety profile of the TICL, the Panel expressed concern regarding use of the device in lower myopes and discussed limiting the range of spherical equivalent powers compared to the proposed range (−3D to −16D).

Regarding rotational stability, the Panel was not able to determine, based on the quality of the data from the TICL study, whether rotational and axial stability for the TICL was established.

Regarding the fixation angle in the proposed labeling, the Panel expressed concerns with the validity of the data in order to adequately assess the proposed maximum fixation angle.

Regarding the proposed post-approval study (PAS), the Panel generally believed that, should the TICL be approved, a PAS would be necessary. The Panel believed that the PAS should include an active control arm and be powered to detect significant differences in the proportion of eyes with large changes in endothelial cell density (ECD) loss. The Panel recommended that additional endpoints be evaluated, including transillumination defects, imaging to confirm the footplate location, pigment dispersion in the angle, and a validated questionnaire to address issues related to visual distortion.

Panel Vote:

Voting Question 1, the Panel voted 5-1-3 (yes, no, abstain) that the data shows there is reasonable assurance that the Visian Toric Implantable Collamer® Lens is safe for use in patients who meet the criteria specified in the proposed indication.

Voting Question 2, the Panel voted 7-1-1 (yes, no, abstain) that there is reasonable assurance that the Visian Toric Implantable Collamer® Lens is effective for use in patients who meet the criteria specified in the proposed indication.

Voting Question 3, the Panel voted 6-0-3 (yes, no, abstain) that the benefits of the Visian Toric Implantable Collamer® Lens do outweigh the risks for use in patients who meet the criteria specified in the proposed indication.

Source: Reprinted from US Food and Drug Administration. 2014. "Summary of the Ophthalmic Devices Panel Meeting." Published March 14. www.fda.gov/downloads/Advisory Committees/CommitteesMeetingMaterials/MedicalDevices/MedicalDevicesAdvisory Committee/OphthalmicDevicesPanel/UCM389566.pdf.

INDEX

Note: Italicized page locators refer to figures or tables in exhibits.

Eunice Kennedy Shriver National Institute of Child Health and Human Development, 437
Evaluating: defined, 245
Evaluating activity: focus and, 310; implementation phase of policymaking and, 93–94, 221, 245–54; within matrix of opportunities to influence policymaking, *311*; modification through, 285–87
Evaluations: timing of, 247–48; types of, 246–47
ex-ante policy evaluation, 247
Excise taxes, distilled spirits, *541, 541–43*
Executive branch, 472–73; bills drafted in, 174; of federal government, 50, *51,* 52; health policies and, 71; policy ideas and, 173; policy implementation role, *86,* 97, 109, 240; policy modification and, *86,* 273–75; of state government, 55, 56
Executive communications: legislative proposals and, 172–73
Executive officeholders: budget role, 185–86, 491–93, 501–2; policy evaluation and analysis and, 248; policy modification and, 270; policy roles, 70–71; role in agenda setting, 158–59; role in policy implementation, 197, 198; as suppliers of health policies, 70–71
Executive orders, 236, 244, 273–75
Expert power, 77, 308–9
Ex-post policy evaluation, 248
External environmental factors, 138; dynamic, policymaking in context of, *86,* 95–96; health-related organizations, interest groups, and, 322, *323*; of policy, *303,* 304; redesign within implementing organizations and, 222

Factions, Madison's definition of, 65
Families USA, 148
Family Planning Services and Population Research Act, 391
Family Smoking Prevention and Tobacco Control Act, 29, 131, 426, 509

FBI. *See* Federal Bureau of Investigation
FCLAA. *See* Federal Cigarette Labeling and Advertising Act
FDA. *See* Food and Drug Administration
FDA Amendments Act of 2007, 29
FDA Export Reform and Enhancement Act of 1996, 29
FDA Food Safety Modernization Act of 2011, 29, 433
FDAMA. *See* Food and Drug Administration Modernization and Accountability Act
FDA v. Brown & Williamson Tobacco Corporation, 118
FDCA. *See* Food, Drug, and Cosmetic Act
FEC. *See* Federal Election Commission
Federal agencies: rulemaking process, 224, *225*
Federal Anti-Tampering Act of 1983, 29
Federal budget process, 173; audit and review of expenditures, 188; important roles of, 186; legislation development for, 184–88; steps in, *185*
Federal Bureau of Investigation, 362, 472
Federal Cigarette Labeling and Advertising Act, 12, 387
Federal Coal Mine Health and Safety Act, 390, 393
Federal Coal Mine Health and Safety Amendments, 393
Federal coercion: "cooperative federalism" and, 120–22
Federal Council on Aging, 394
Federal courts: jurisdiction of, 108; policy modification and, 275; system structure, 54–55
Federal Election Campaign Act, 152
Federal Election Commission, 152, 484
Federal Employees Health Benefits Act, 385
Federal Employee Viewpoint Survey, 521
Federal Energy Regulatory Commission, 510

ABOUT THE AUTHOR

Beaufort B. Longest, Jr., PhD, FACHE, is professor of health policy and management in the Graduate School of Public Health at the University of Pittsburgh (Pitt). He is the founding director of Pitt's Health Policy Institute, which he led from 1980 to 2011.

He received his undergraduate education at Davidson College and his MHA and PhD from Georgia State University. He is a Fellow of the American College of Healthcare Executives and holds memberships in the Academy of Management, AcademyHealth, and the American Public Health Association. He has the unusual distinction of being an elected member of both Beta Gamma Sigma, the international honor society in business, and Delta Omega, the honor society in public health.

His research on modeling managerial competence, issues of governance in healthcare organizations, and health policymaking has generated substantial grant support and has appeared in numerous peer-reviewed journals. In addition, he has authored or coauthored 11 books and 32 chapters in other books. His book *Managing Health Services Organizations and Systems*, coauthored with Kurt Darr, is now in its sixth edition.

He has consulted with healthcare organizations and systems, universities, associations, and government agencies on health policy and management issues, and he has served on several editorial and organization boards.

ABOUT THE CONTRIBUTOR

Mary Crossley, JD, is professor of law and former dean at the University of Pittsburgh School of Law. She received her BA in history from the University of Virginia and her JD from Vanderbilt University School of Law. She is an expert in health law and policy and teaches courses in health law, legislation and regulation, family law, and torts. Her research has focused on the law's response to instances of inequality in healthcare financing and delivery.